W9-AUX-926

Analysis of
Human Genetic Linkage

Analysis of
Human Genetic Linkage
Revised Edition

JURG OTT
Professor, Department of Genetics and Development and
Department of Psychiatry, Columbia University

The Johns Hopkins University Press
Baltimore and London

The Johns Hopkins University Press
2715 North Charles Street
Baltimore, Maryland 21218-4319
The Johns Hopkins Press Ltd., London

In Table 9.2 the data for family 29 are taken from G. Romeo, M. Devoto, G. Costa, L. Roncuzzi, L. Catizone, P. Zuchelli, G. G. Germino, T. Keith, D. J. Weatherall, and S. T. Reeders, A second genetic locus for autosomal dominant polycystic kidney disease, *Lancet* 2, no. 8601: 8–11. © 1988 The Lancet Ltd.

Library of Congress Cataloging-in-Publication Data

Ott, Jurg.
    Analysis of human genetic linkage / Jurg Ott. — Rev. ed.
      p.   cm. — (The Johns Hopkins series in contemporary medicine and public health)
    Includes bibliographical references and index.
    ISBN 0-8018-4257-3 (hard : alk. paper).
    1. Linkage (Genetics) 2. Human genetics. I. Title. II. Series. [DNLM: 1. Linkage (Genetics)   QH 445.2 089a]
QH445.2.O88   1991
573.2′13—dc20
DNLM/DLC
for Library of Congress   91-7048

A catalog record for this book is available from the British Library.

To my wife, Salome

Contents

List of Illustrations

List of Tables

Preface

The warm and vivid response to the first edition of this book has been gratifying. Personal discussions with colleagues, particularly with Dr. Robert Elston, pointed out areas in the first edition which needed enhancement. I would also like to acknowledge helpful discussions with Drs. Lodewijk Sandkuijl, Daniel Weeks, and Neil Risch, and I am grateful to Joseph Terwilliger for critical reading of the manuscript and for making numerous constructive comments.

I have tried to present the material in a generally simpler and more intuitive manner. The book sections are of varying mathematical difficulty; theoretical aspects are generally concentrated towards the end of each section. Each chapter ends with a collection of problems whose solutions are given at the end of the book. Some of these problems cover particular theoretical aspects that seemed too specialized to be taken up in the general text.

For one to follow the theoretical aspects of linkage analysis presented, some facility with equations and simple algebra will be beneficial. As in the first edition, no introduction to probability calculus is given. The reader without knowledge of probability laws will have to accept some statements at face value but should still be able to follow much of this book. However, an outline of some statistical methods, particularly significance testing, is provided.

The topics and problems of linkage analysis have changed dramatically since the first edition of this book was written. Also, a considerable shift in the available techniques has occurred. Naturally, multipoint linkage analysis now takes up much more room than previously, and a few very specialized sections (e.g., on mating types) were shortened or deleted. Also, computer simulation methods—not covered before—are emerging as powerful tools and are given broad coverage.

No background is furnished on population genetics, since excellent

xvii

treatments of this important topic exist (e.g., Cavalli-Sforza and Bodmer 1971; Hartl 1988; Maynard Smith 1989). Hartl (1988) also provided an introduction to molecular genetic aspects of population genetics, and Maynard Smith (1989) covered modern genetic concepts from an evolutionary standpoint. A mathematical treatment of a wide range of topics in classical and population genetics, including statistical methods for DNA sequence data, was given by Weir (1990). For more general aspects of human genetics, the reader is referred to one of the human genetics texts, particularly the one by Vogel and Motulsky (1986). A general short overview of the principles of linkage analysis was presented by Conneally and Rivas (1980). Theory and sampling in pedigree analysis may be found in Thompson (1986). Various facets of gene mapping and sequencing, as well as an easy-to-read introduction to the various mapping techniques, is covered in the book issued by the U.S. Congress, Office of Technology Assessment (1988).

In a field such as linkage analysis, in which experts from several diverse disciplines collaborate, using technical terms in accordance with their definition is important but evidently very difficult. There is quite a confusion of technical terms, and it must often be difficult for researchers not intimately familiar with a particular subspecialty to know the current meaning of terms. Technical terms in a specialized field of research often take on a new meaning when they are used by individuals who are not very familiar with that field. As a few examples, *linkage* and *gene map* were used earlier in a purely genetic sense: *linkage* referred to genetic linkage (linkage groups), and *gene map* was a theoretical construct representing the linear arrangement of genes. Thus, for example, *physical mapping methods* is a contradiction when mapping is used in the original sense of the word. Many of these terms and their new meanings are so well established now in human genetics that it would not be meaningful to be too puristic.

My guide in defining and using technical terms has been to minimize confusion. For example, *mutation* used to refer to the process by which one allele turns into another one; now, however, it is often used as a synonym for *mutated allele* or just *disease allele*. In some instances, avoiding confusion means to reject some of the newer meanings. For example, *assortative mating* originally referred to the phenotypes of two mates, but it is now sometimes used to designate similarity between the phenotypes of the relatives (ancestors) of two mates, irrespective of the mates' phenotypes. The latter usage of the term should be discouraged. Also, unfortunately, *support intervals* are often called *confidence intervals*. Occasionally, it is truly difficult to grasp in which sense a term is used. The best example seems to be *linkage disequilibrium*, which originally was a purely descriptive expression for the fact that alleles do not occur independently of each other in haplotypes. Now, it is often used to refer to a particular cause of that phenomenon, namely tight linkage.

Linkage analysis is sometimes perceived as a matter of simply using the proper computer program, so that anyone with sufficient computer expertise could "do the linkage analysis" after family data and marker typing have been obtained. Such claims are not usually made in other fields of research and should not be made here either. It is dangerous to have linkage analyses carried out by individuals without the necessary theoretical background. The table of contents lists the book's sections, for those readers who are interested in only a cursory reading of this material.

List of Symbols

α Significance level (type I error) in a statistical test (lowercase Greek alpha); or
Proportion of a particular family type in a mixture of families

β Type II error in a statistical test $(1 - \beta = \text{power})$ (lowercase Greek beta)

δ Indicator variable, $\delta = 0$ or $\delta = 1$ (lowercase Greek delta), identifying the intervals of a map, which constitute a given region A of the map; or
Difference operator

Δ Difference operator

ε Indicator variable, $\varepsilon = 0$ or $\varepsilon = 1$ (lowercase Greek epsilon), identifying the intervals of a map in which a crossover occurs

θ Recombination fraction as a variable in log likelihoods or lod scores (lowercase Greek theta); occasionally also the true value (r) of the recombination fraction when there is no danger of confusing it with the variable

θ_0, θ_1 Specific assumed values of θ. In the first edition of this book, θ_0 denoted the true value of the recombination fraction (now r).

$\hat{\theta}$ Maximum likelihood estimate of the recombination fraction

$\bar{\theta}$ Asymptotic estimate of the recombination fraction, that is, the value of θ at which the expected log likelihood (expected lod score) attains its maximum

λ	Exponent in power transformation of θ (lowercase Greek lambda)
Λ	Average of likelihood ratio (capital Greek lambda)
μ	Mean (lowercase Greek mu)
ρ	Correlation coefficient (lowercase Greek rho)
σ	Standard deviation/standard error (lowercase Greek sigma)
Σ	Summation operator (capital Greek sigma)
ϕ	Power, probability of significant result (lowercase Greek phi)
E	Expectation operator, $E(x)$, average of quantity x, where x may be a function
$E[Z(\theta)]$	Expected lod score, evaluated at θ
ELOD	Expected lod score evaluated at its maximum value
f	Penetrance; or Density of a random variable
F	Distribution function of a random variable
G	Joint or n-fold recombination fraction (as a function of ε, section 6.1)
i	Expected Fisher information (average per observation)
I	Total Fisher information for all observations
$\hat{\imath}$	Observed average Fisher information
$\hat{I}$	Observed total Fisher information
L	Likelihood
L^*	Rescaled likelihood, or likelihood ratio
p	Empirical significance level, p-value
r	True value of the recombination fraction (when used together with a formal θ parameter in the same context; otherwise, θ sometimes denotes the true recombination fraction)
R	Ratio, often likelihood ratio, or (relative) risk, or linkage value (as a function of δ, section 6.1)
s	Reduction from full penetrance ($1 - s =$ penetrance), or misclassification probability, or conditional rate of false positives (sporadic cases) (s is typically a small value)
Z	Lod score, log likelihood ratio with respect to recombination fraction, $\log_{10}(R)$, $R = L(\theta)/L(\frac{1}{2})$

Analysis of
Human Genetic Linkage

1.

Basic Genetics and Cytogenetics

1.1. Mendelian Inheritance

Genes and genetic linkage are often introduced with reference to chromosomes. Conceptually, however, genetic and cytologic phenomena are very different. In this and the next section, *genes* and *genetic linkage* will be defined in purely genetic terms, but later it will be convenient to use genetic, cytogenetic, and molecular genetic terms interchangeably.

In crossing experiments with peas, Gregor Mendel hypothesized what are now called Mendel's laws in 1865 (Mendel 1866; Bateson 1913). After the rediscovery of these laws in 1900 by Correns, Tschermak, and de Vries, Sutton and Boveri formulated the chromosomal theory of inheritance in 1902–4. A proper understanding of chromosomes gave Mendel's laws the plausibility that they had been lacking. Below is a brief and simplistic description of autosomal mendelian inheritance in the current terminology. More detailed introductions to basic genetics and cytogenetics may be found in many textbooks. An interesting historical and sociologic perspective of mendelism was given by Bowler (1989).

Heritable characters are determined by *genes*, where different genes are responsible for the expression of different characteristics. In modern terminology, a gene is a specific coding sequence of DNA (Elandt-Johnson 1971, 3; Hartl 1988), the unit of transmission, recombination, and function (Vogel and Motulsky 1986). Estimates of the total number of genes are 50,000 in the human and 5,000 in the fruitfly, *Drosophila melanogaster* (see references in McKusick and Ruddle 1977). A number of 1,000 essential genes in *Drosophila* has also been quoted (Maynard Smith 1989, 59). Each individual carries two copies of each gene, of which one was received from the mother and the other from the father. A gene may occur in different forms or states called *alleles*, each potentially having a different physical expression. For example, three major alleles of the *ABO*

1

gene interact to determine the various ABO blood types. It is often difficult to distinguish whether different characteristics are caused by different genes or by different alleles of the same gene, and the solution to this question will be deferred to the next section.

The relative frequencies in the population of the different alleles of a gene are called *gene frequencies*, where each individual contributes two alleles (for an autosomal gene) to the population gene pool. For example, the three alleles, *A*, *B*, and *O*, of the *ABO* gene occur with approximate gene frequencies in Caucasians of $p_A = 0.28$, $p_B = 0.06$, and $p_O = 0.66$. A gene is called *polymorphic* when its most common allele has a population frequency of less than 95 percent (a less stringent criterion of 99 percent is sometimes used).

The pair of alleles in an individual constitutes that individual's *genotype*. With *n* alleles, $n(n + 1)/2$ genotypes can be formed. For example, for the *ABO* blood group gene ($n = 3$), the six genotypes are *A/A*, *A/B*, *A/O*, *B/B*, *B/O*, and *O/O*. The two alleles in an individual are either the same (*A/A*, *B/B*, and *O/O*), in which case a genotype is called *homozygous* and the individual with such a genotype is said to be a *homozygote*, or they are different (*A/B*, *A/O*, and *B/O*), in which case the genotype is *heterozygous* and the individual with such a genotype is called a *heterozygote*. In X linkage, the same terms are used in females, but in males the genotype at X-linked genes is called *hemizygous* (e.g., *A/y,* where *y* stands for the *Y* chromosome). Finally, when the two alleles in a homozygous genotype are known to be copies of the same ancestral allele (identical by descent), that genotype is termed *autozygous*.

The expression of a particular genotype is called a *phenotype*. At the *ABO* gene, the six genotypes determine four phenotypes (blood groups)—type A, type B, type AB, and type O. The relation between genotypes and (qualitative) phenotypes for a particular gene is conveniently represented in the form of a table, in which the rows correspond to genotypes and the columns correspond to phenotypes. Each cell in the table then contains a *penetrance*, that is, a conditional probability of observing the corresponding phenotype given the specified genotype. In simple cases, penetrances are either 0 or 1; for many diseases, however, intermediate values of penetrances occur. An example is given in table 1.1, which shows the penetrances for the *ABO* gene. The two genotypes *A/A* and *A/O* have the same phenotype (A blood type) or, as geneticists say, *A* is *dominant* over *O* ($A > O$), since the *A* allele is expressed irrespective of the presence of an *O* allele. Conversely, *O* is said to be *recessive* with respect to *A* since it has no effect on the phenotype in the presence of *A*; it is only "seen" in the genotype *O/O*, which leads to the O

Table 1.1. Relation between Genotypes and Phenotypes (Penetrances) at the *ABO* locus

	Phenotype			
Genotype	Type A	Type B	Type AB	Type O
A/A	1	0	0	0
A/B	0	0	1	0
A/O	1	0	0	0
B/B	0	1	0	0
B/O	0	1	0	0
O/O	0	0	0	1

blood type. Also, *B* is dominant over *O*, while *A* and *B* are *codominant* because *A* and *B* are both expressed when present in the same genotype, *A/B*.

Through the formation of gametes, each parent passes to each of his or her children one of the two alleles with probability ½. The allele received from the mother and that from the father constitute a child's genotype. For example, if two parents have the respective blood types AB and O (genotypes *A/B* and *O/O*), then half of their children are expected to have the genotype *A/O*, and the other half, the genotype *B/O*. If the assumed mode of inheritance is correct, deviations from this 1:1 ratio will be due to chance fluctuations. When a new gene has been discovered and a particular mendelian mode of inheritance is hypothesized for it, it is common practice to predict for given parental matings the proportion of children with different phenotypes and to test whether observed and expected proportions agree. For example, Juneja et al. (1988) studied four alleles of the plasma α_1B-glycoprotein gene. They grouped fifty-seven families by their mating types (parental genotypes) and verified that the offspring genotypes were observed as predicted by mendelian inheritance. Two or more genotypes are termed genetically *inconsistent* or incompatible when they are not in agreement with the mendelian laws. For example, a mother's genotype *A/B* is inconsistent with an offspring's genotype *O/O*.

Under conditions of random mating and the absence of disturbing forces such as migration, mutation, and selection at the gene in question, a population is said to be in *Hardy-Weinberg equilibrium* (HWE), meaning that the genotype frequencies in the population depend only on the gene frequencies (Hartl 1988). For example, $P(A/A) = p_A^2$, $P(A/B) = 2p_A p_B$. Notice that the genotype *B/A* is the same as *A/B*. A salient feature of the Hardy-Weinberg principle is that for autosomal genes, whatever the genotype distribution in the parental generation was, HWE will be obtained after one generation of random mating. In other words, the genotype frequencies in the children's generation depend only on the allele frequencies and not on the genotype frequencies in the parental generation. In a finite population, however, the genotype frequencies are not constant. By random fluctuation, allele frequencies in generation 2 may deviate somewhat from those in generation 1, and it is then the new allele frequencies in generation 2 that determine the expected genotype frequencies in generation 3. This random force of divergence is called *genetic drift* (Maynard Smith 1989).

The existence of HWE is often taken to imply that mating is random. Although random mating implies HWE, however, the reverse is not necessarily true. Certain patterns of deviations from random mating (termed *pseudo-random mating*) have been shown to lead also to HWE in the offspring generation (Li 1988).

Instead of a single gene, consider now two genes simultaneously, gene 1 with two alleles, A and a, and gene 2 also with two alleles, B and b. For example, figure 1.1 shows an artificial family in which the two grandparents are both doubly homozygous: the grandmother is homozygous for the alleles A (at gene 1) and B (at gene 2), and the grandfather is homozygous for the alleles a and b. In experimental organisms, such homozygosity can be achieved through successive inbreeding and selection of the desired genotypes. The father (son of the two grandparents) must have received alleles A and B from the grandmother and alleles a

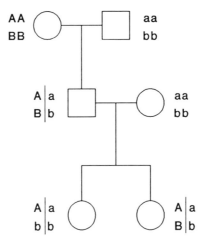

Figure 1.1. Artificial family with assumed genotypes at two loci showing one recombinant and one nonrecombinant offspring.

and *b* from the grandfather. The alleles (at different genes) received by an individual from one parent are called a *haplotype*. The father thus received the haplotype *AB* from his mother and the haplotype *ab* from his father.

In principle, a doubly heterozygous individual (*A/a*, *B/b*) received his or her *A* allele in coupling with either the *B* or the *b* allele from one parent. These two possibilities are distinguished as the two *phases* of a double heterozygote (more than two phases exist in individuals heterozygous for more than two genes). Depending on the alleles of interest, one of the two phases is called the *coupling*, or *cis* phase, and the other is called the *repulsion*, or *trans* phase. Often, the phase of a double heterozygote is unknown, that is, it is unclear which two alleles were received as a haplotype from one parent. For the father in figure 1.1 (middle generation) the phase is known, which is indicated by the vertical bar in his genotype separating maternal (left side of bar) from paternal alleles. For genotypes in which at most one gene is heterozygous, the phase is always known because it is clear which alleles must have come as a haplotype from one of the parents, although one may be unable to indicate which haplotype came from which parent.

In analogy to the notion of gene frequency at a single gene, a population haplotype frequency can be defined. If n_i is the number of alleles for the *i*th gene, $i = 1 \ldots N$, the total number, H, of possible haplotypes for all N genes is given by the product of the n_i, $H = \Pi n_i$. The total number of different genotypes is then calculated as $H(H + 1)/2$, where multiple heterozygotes differing in their phase but not in the genotype for single genes are counted as different multigenic genotypes. For example, when three genes have 4, 2, and 3 alleles respectively, there are 24 possible haplotypes and 300 possible genotypes. When alleles of different genes occur independently in haplotypes, the population frequency of a haplotype is given by the product of the gene frequencies of its constituent alleles. Deviations from random occurrence of alleles in haplotypes are referred to as *allelic association* or *linkage disequilibrium* and will be covered in detail later (section 11.4).

1.2. Recombination and Genetic Linkage

In figure 1.1, it is assumed that the (doubly heterozygous) father is married to a doubly homozygous individual, *ab/ab*, who has the same genotype as one of the parents in the previous generation (one of the grandparents). Such a mating is called a *backcross*, a phase-known double backcross in this case. Also, a cross between two doubly heterozygous (*A/a*, *B/b*) individuals is called an *intercross*. If the two genes assumed in figure 1.1 are inherited independently of each other, the father is expected to pass the four haplotypes, *AB*, *ab*, *Ab*, and *aB*, to his offspring in the ratio of $1:1:1:1$. The haplotypes *AB* and *ab* look the same as the ones he received from his parents (from the grandparents). Children receiving these are called parental types in classical genetics (for example, the child on the right side of figure 1.1). The other two haplotypes, *Ab* and *aB*, are unlike any haplotypes received by the father from the grandparents and contain one allele from each grandparent (a "re-combination" of grandparental alleles must have occurred in the father). In classical genetics, offspring carrying such haplotypes are designated as nonparental types. In human genetics, the nonparental types, *Ab* and *aB*, are called *recombinants*, and the other two haplotypes (*AB* and *ab*) are called *nonrecombinants*. A *recombination* between two genes denotes the event that two different grandparents contribute one allele at each of the two genes to a haplotype in an individual, whereas a *nonrecombination* is said to have occurred when a haplotype in an individual contains two alleles (one at each gene) which originate from the same grandparent of that individual. Also, an offspring is termed recombinant or nonrecombinant depending on whether or not the offspring indicates that a recombination has occurred in one of the parents. Thus, in figure 1.1, daughter 1 is a recombinant and daughter 2 is a nonrecombinant.

When two genes are inherited independently of each other, recombinants and nonrecombinants are expected in equal proportions among the offspring. For some pairs of genes, one observes a consistent deviation from the $1:1$ ratio of recombinant to nonrecombinant offspring in the sense that the alleles in the haplotype passed from a grandparent to a parent tend to be passed again as the same haplotype from the parent to the offspring. In other words, alleles of different genes appear to be genetically coupled, and this phenomenon is called *genetic linkage*. Two genes are completely linked when a doubly heterozygous parent can produce only nonrecombinant gametes, and linkage is absent (recombination is free) when a parent produces both recombinant and nonrecombinant haplotypes in equal proportions.

The extent of genetic linkage is measured by the *recombination fraction*, which is the probability that a gamete produced by a parent is a recombinant. Traditionally, in human genetics, the recombination fraction is denoted by the Greek letter θ (theta). Thus, genes segregating independently are unlinked and are characterized by a recombination fraction of $\theta = \frac{1}{2}$ between them, whereas linked genes are characterized by $\theta < \frac{1}{2}$. Some pairs of genes are very tightly linked so that θ approaches 0, that is, only very rarely does a recombination occur between them. The estimation of θ and tests of the hypothesis of free recombination ($\theta = \frac{1}{2}$) versus linkage ($\theta < \frac{1}{2}$) are the objects of linkage analysis.

Genetic linkage between two or more genes is characterized by the following features:

1. Since recombination events can only be recognized on the basis of haplotypes passed from parents to children, linkage analysis cannot be carried out with unrelated individuals but requires observations on relatives. Therefore, for a linkage analysis, researchers collect phenotypic information on members of family pedigrees.

2. Recombinant and nonrecombinant haplotypes produced by a parent cannot always be distinguished. Consider, for instance, the *Ab* haplotype produced by a parent with genotype *Ab/ab*. Because of homozygosity for the second gene, *Ab* could be a recombinant or a nonrecombinant haplotype. For these to be distinguishable, the parent must thus be doubly heterozygous. Only then is he or she potentially *informative for linkage*, as geneticists say. A mating is potentially informative for linkage between two specific genes when at least one of the parents is a double heterozygote.

3. For many pairs of genes, linkage analyses show that the recombination fraction differs depending on the sex of the parent producing gametes. Therefore, one distinguishes a male recombination fraction, θ_m, from a female recombination fraction, θ_f. The distinction between the two refers to the gender of the parent in which recombination takes place and not to the gender of the children who may be counted as recombinant or nonrecombinant offspring. Sex dependency of the recombination fraction will be covered in greater detail later (section 9.1).

The evolutionary significance of recombination is discussed in chapter 12 of Maynard Smith (1989). Its major aspect seems to be that recombination increases variability and thus accelerates evolution by natural selection.

1.3. Linkage Groups and Synteny

If gene 1 is genetically linked to gene 2 and gene 2 is linked to gene 3, gene 1 may or may not appear to be linked to gene 3. A *linkage group* is defined as a set of genes in which each gene is linked with at least one other gene in the same set. Experience shows that partitioning genes into linkage groups is unique in the sense that two genes belonging to different linkage groups are unlinked. For the early geneticists, the interpretation of the genetic phenomenon of a linkage group became clear with the observation that, in each (diploid) species investigated, the number of linkage groups coincided with the number of chromosome pairs. The linkage groups can now be interpreted as being the genetic equivalents of the chromosomes on which the genes are arranged linearly. That genes occur in pairs is explained by the fact that chromosomes also exist in pairs, the so-called two *homologs*. Linked genes are localized on the same chromosome. Finally, as a consequence of the process of meiosis, gametes contain only a haploid set of chromosomes, which explains why parents pass only a single allele of each gene to their offspring.

Genes located on the same chromosome are said to be *syntenic*. Synteny of a pair of genes has always been shown to imply that the two genes belong to the same linkage group, although they are not necessarily genetically linked. The converse, that nonsyntenic genes show linkagelike associations, has occasionally been observed and called *quasilinkage* or affinity (Bailey 1961). An example in the mouse and a discussion of various possible mechanisms can be found in Stockert et al. (1976).

The fact that two alleles of different genes occur in the same haplotype does not imply synteny of these genes. The vertical bar in the genotype of the father in figure 1.1 simply indicates that phase is known, but this says nothing about the linkage or synteny relationship of the two genes involved. This situation is a source of confusion for many students of linkage analysis, and it is very important that these relationships are clearly understood before one proceeds.

In humans, as is well known, in addition to the twenty-two pairs of chromosomes called *autosomes*, there exist two chromosomes, X and Y, called *sex chromosomes*, of which women carry two X and men carry one X and one Y. Everything said thus far about genes and chromosomes implicitly referred to autosomal genes. The X and Y chromosomes also carry genes that show a characteristic *sex-linked* mode of inheritance, since boys (X/Y) receive their X from the mother and the Y from the father and girls (X/X) receive one X each from mother and father. For an X-linked gene, each female contributes two alleles and each male contributes one allele to the total number of alleles in the population. Therefore, assuming equal numbers of females and males in a population, the gene frequency of a particular allele of an X-linked gene is given by $(2p_f + p_m)/3$, where p_f is the gene frequency among females and p_m that among males. Under equilibrium conditions, $p_f = p_m$. (For X-linked genes, HWE is not reached after one generation of random mating but after a gradual stabilization.) Well-known examples of X-linked genes are color blindness and hemophilia. For many autosomal genes, X-linked inheritance is mimicked in that the same genotype is expressed differently in males and females. This phenomenon, *sex-limited inheritance*, must not be confused with sex-linked inheritance.

Progress in molecular genetics has been extremely rapid in recent years, and much has been learned about the structure and function of genes. These are known to correspond to sequences of nucleotides along a DNA molecule. They contain active sequences of DNA, the so-called *exons*, which are interspersed with stretches of nonactive DNA, the so-called *introns* or intervening sequences. Some genes are very long; for example, the gene that when defective leads to Duchenne's muscular dystrophy (DMD) consists of at least sixty-five exons spread over approximately 2,000 kb (Koenig et al. 1987). Furthermore, there are DNA sequences, called *transposons*, which can change their location within the genome and which can be acquired by infection (Shapiro 1983, Maynard Smith 1989). A brief presentation of population genetic and molecular aspects of genes and their expression may be found in Hartl (1988). The precise nature of the biochemical process of recombination is only partly understood. Studies in phages and plants suggest that recombination occurs at discrete, predefined sites in the genome (White and Lalouel 1987). Cellular enzymes have been implicated in this process in that they actively induce recombination during meiosis by making occasional breaks along a pair of chromosomes (Watson et al. 1987a). Consequently, recombination frequency may not be a good indicator of physical distance between linked genes.

In addition to the nuclear genes that reside on the chromosomes within the cell nucleus, the mitochondria also contain DNA (mtDNA) ("The other human genome", *Science* 249:1104–5, 1990). The phenotypes under the control of mitochondrial genes follow a *maternal mode of inheritance* (Wallace 1989). The mitochondrial genome has been completely sequenced (Anderson et al. 1981). A well-known example of a maternally inherited disease, Leber's disease, was shown to be due to a single nucleotide change in the mitochondrial DNA (Wallace et al. 1988), but in some families the disease seems to be caused by different mitochondrial genes (Vilkki, Savontaus, and Nikoskelainen 1989). Owing to a high mutation rate and the absence of recombination, mtDNA is well suited for studies of genetic diversity (e.g., Excoffier 1990). It has been suggested that the mitochondrial DNA of all present-day human beings stems exclusively from one woman who lived about 200,000 years ago in Africa (Cann et al. 1987), but alternative interpretations of the mitochondrial evolutionary clock have also been given (Krüger and Vogel 1989; Excoffier and Langaney 1989). Most modern Africans are closer to the ancestral mitochondrial DNA sequence than are modern Caucasians (Watson et al. 1987b). Investigations of Y-chromosomal DNA analogous to those of mitochondrial DNA are conceivable but are proving difficult (Maynard Smith 1990).

As an aside, it may be mentioned that the chloroplasts of plants also contain genes. Mitochondria and chloroplasts are about the same size as bacteria and, like bacteria, have circular DNA genomes (Watson et al. 1987b), which suggests that they are derived from free-living bacteria.

Gene expression not only depends on allelic status but is also determined by modifications of the DNA, higher order chromosome structure, and interaction among genes (epistasis). Many of these effects are due to methylation of DNA, and some are clearly heritable (*epigenetic inheritance*) (Monk 1990). A particular form of such effects is genomic imprinting; that is, genes are expressed differently depending on whether they were received from the mother or the father. Imprinting has been observed for many human disorders (Reik 1989; Hall 1990).

1.4. Crossing Over and Map Distance

In meiosis (the cell division leading to the formation of gametes, i.e., egg or sperm cells), homologous chromosomes pair up. At that stage, each homologous chromosome consists of two strands (chromatids), so that a chromosome pair consists of four strands. In the course of meiosis, the two homologous chromosomes separate from each other at most places but maintain one or more zones of contact known as *chiasmata* (Ayala and Kiger 1984). Each chiasma involves one chromatid from each of the two homologous chromosomes. Chiasmata reflect the occurrence of crossing over between chromatids, which is the genetic process leading to recombinant haplotypes.

In a simplified manner, the chromosomal interpretation of recombination is depicted in figure 1.2, which shows three genes and two points of crossover. An exchange of single strands between the parental chromosomes leads to the formation of a cross-bridged structure, the Holliday structure (see fig. 14.1 in Ayala and Kiger 1984). According to the current model for recombination, the Holliday structure may be resolved by cutting of single strands, where the cuts can occur in two different directions, both leading to linear molecules (strands). One type of cut (shown in fig. 1.2) results in strands that are recombinant for parental genetic markers on either side of the cut. The other type of cut results in nonrecombinant strands (not shown in fig. 1.2) (Ayala and Kiger 1984). Meiosis results in the production of four sperm cells, or one egg cell and three polar bodies,

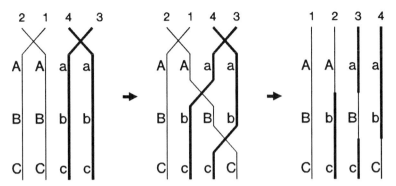

Figure 1.2. Schematic representation of two crossovers between two homologous chromosomes carrying three genes.

each of which receives one chromatid of each chromosome. The exact relation between chiasmata and recombinant haplotypes is unclear; conventionally, it is assumed that one chiasma corresponds to two recombinant and two nonrecombinant haplotypes (see section 1.5).

In figure 1.2, two crossovers are assumed to occur between the genes with alleles *A, a* and *C, c*. After meiosis, a chromatid having experienced a single crossover between the two genes will correspond genetically to a recombinant haplotype. When two crossovers occur between two genes, however, the result is the same as without a crossover. Generally, an odd number of crossovers between two genes results in a recombination, whereas an even number leads to a nonrecombination.

I will only briefly mention here that, in male meioses, the X and Y chromosomes also pair up. Recombination then takes place in the small region of homology between X and Y (Rouyer et al. 1986), the pseudoautosomal region (Ellis and Goodfellow 1989). Linkage analysis involving pseudoautosomal genes is covered in section 8.4.

A phenomenon often related to recombination is that of *gene conversion*: when two alleles pair up at meiosis, one is "converted" to resemble the other (Maynard Smith 1989). On the surface, this phenomenon resembles mutation, but its characteristics are quite distinct from those of mutation. Details and genetic models of gene conversion may be found in Ayala and Kiger (1984). In some organisms, gene conversion is relatively frequent. In humans, improved molecular techniques have only recently made it possible to show the occurrence of gene conversion (Nakashima et al. 1990; Urabe et al. 1990).

When many genes along a chromosome are studied, one observes that recombinations and, thus, crossovers occur randomly along the chromosome in the sense that there is no observable constancy of time and location in their occurrence. This is not to say that their distribution along the chromosome is uniform. On the contrary, recombination intensity varies with the region of the chromosome investigated and is, for example, almost totally suppressed in regions of chromosomal inversion. Also, as discussed in more detail in section 6.4, occurrence of a new crossover seems to be suppressed in the immediate vicinity of an existing crossover (chiasma interference). Occurrence of crossovers is "semirandom" (Watson et al. 1987a), which is the basis for our ability to construct genetic maps (see below). Genes located in close proximity to each other have only a small chance of experiencing a recombination between them. With increasing distance between two genes, an increasing number of crossovers is expected to occur between them. Since each crossover affects only two of the four chromatids, for genes far apart on the same chromosome the recombination fraction between such genes approaches 50 percent. Also, as seen above, genes on different chromosomes most often segregate independently so that they recombine with a frequency of 50 percent. For this reason, the recombination fraction is usually restricted to the range between 0 for tightly linked genes and 50 percent for distant genes.

Which of the two homologous strands of a chromosome are involved in a crossover appears to be random and independent from one crossover to the next (absence of so-called chromatid interference). In the absence of chromatid interference, it has been shown that θ cannot exceed 50 percent (Mather 1938), and the theoretical possibility that it might slightly exceed 50 percent in the presence of chromatid interference is not generally considered to be important in human genetics.

For completeness, it should be mentioned here that aberrant patterns of nonrandom assortment have been found leading to recombination fractions of much more than 50 percent between genes on the same chromosome. One species exhibiting such so-called *pseudolinkage* is cutthroat trout (*Salmo clarki*), in which recombination fractions of 80 percent and more are regularly observed (Wright et al. 1983).

The above considerations suggest that the rate of crossovers or the recombination rate between two genes could serve as a stochastic measure of distance between them. The genetic *map distance* (in units of Morgans) between two genes is defined as the expected number of crossovers occurring on a single chromosome strand (chromatid) between the genes. However, crossovers are not directly observable, but recombinations are. In small intervals, when the probability of multiple crossovers is negligible, recombinations may be counted as crossovers. Then the probability of a recombination (the recombination fraction) is the same as the expected number of crossovers on one strand, which is also expressed in formula (1.1). The relation between crossovers, recombinations, and chiasmata may be seen in the assumed example pictured in figure 1.2. For the two flanking genes, after meiosis, one chromatid shows two crossovers, two chromatids show one crossover each, and one chromatid shows no crossover. On average, in this example, there is one crossover per chromatid (strand). On the other hand, the two crossovers are visible under the microscope as two chiasmata. One may, thus, also define map distance as one half of the expected number of chiasmata. Observing chiasmata shows that (1) there appears to be always at least one chiasma per chromosome per meiosis, and (2), in male meioses an average number of about fifty-three chiasmata occur over all of the autosomes. The total male autosomal map length is thus estimated as approximately 26.5 Morgans (Renwick 1969), or 2,650 centimorgans (cM). Based on higher recombination rates in female than in male meioses, the female map length is approximately 1.5 times that of the male map (i.e., the female map length measures approximately 39 Morgans), and a sex-averaged autosomal map length of 33 Morgans may thus be quoted (Renwick 1969). The "average" human chromosome is then 1.5 Morgans long; that is, it experiences an average of 1.5 crossovers.

In classical genetics, a set of linearly arranged genes with map distances determined between them is termed a *genetic map* and the position of a gene on the map is called its *locus* (plural: loci). In modern terminology, a *locus* (also called a system) comprises not only genes but also genetic units without a known function, for example, DNA polymorphisms (section 2.5). For example, several polymorphic sites—loci—are known in the gene for DMD mentioned above. Alleles are now alternative forms of a locus, not only of a gene, and a *polymorphism* is a polymorphic locus, not just a polymorphic gene. Also, *gene map* is no longer strictly a genetic term. Instead, it generally refers to everything that is known about the physical and genetic location of genetic loci on the chromosomes. Also, mapping a gene generally means to locate its position on the chromosomes by any available technique, not just through linkage to known loci.

For larger distances, the recombination fraction is not an additive distance measure. For example, consider three loci numbered 1, 2, and 3. If the recombination fraction between loci 1 and 2 and that between loci 2 and 3 is each assumed to be equal to $\theta = 0.30$, then the recombination fraction between loci 1 and 3 cannot be 2θ, since that value would exceed 50 percent. One therefore needs to transform the recombination fraction,

θ, into additive map distance, x. Such transformations are called mapping functions or *map functions* and are covered in the subsequent section.

The concept of map distance has been covered here in a relatively simple manner, the emphasis being on application rather than on theory. Mathematically inclined readers may be interested in a more thorough treatment of this subject, which may be found, for example, in Mather 1938, Barratt et al. 1954, Bailey 1961, Karlin 1984, and Liberman and Karlin 1984.

1.5. Map Functions

This section presents an overview of various map functions with little mathematical complexity. Theoretical aspects of map functions will be covered in section 6.4 on interference.

As discussed above, when the occurrence of multiple crossovers between two loci can be excluded (complete interference), the appropriate map function is simply

$$x = \theta, \tag{1.1}$$

since the probability, θ, of a recombination is equal to the expected number of crossovers between the two loci when at most one crossover occurs. This assumption is usually warranted for closely linked genes, say, when $\theta < 0.10$. For example, when the recombination fraction between two loci is equal to $\theta = 0.06$, the map distance between them is approximately equal to 0.06 Morgan, i.e., a recombination fraction of 6 percent corresponds to ≈ 6 cM. When many closely linked genes are available on a chromosome and their order is known, then the simplest method of determining map distances among these genes is to estimate the recombination fractions in each interval of adjacent loci. The map distance between two more distant loci is then obtained as the sum of the map distances in the intervals between these loci (Sturtevant 1913). Equation (1.1) is also known as Morgan's map function (Morgan 1928).

The major reason for the nonadditivity of θ as a distance measure is the occurrence of multiple crossovers between two loci. Under the assumptions that crossovers in different intervals occur according to the Poisson probability law, Haldane (1919) expressed map distance as

$$x = \begin{cases} -\tfrac{1}{2}\ln(1 - 2\theta) & \text{if } 0 \le \theta < \tfrac{1}{2}, \\ \infty & \text{otherwise,} \end{cases} \tag{1.2}$$

whose inverse is

$$\theta = \tfrac{1}{2}[1 - \exp(-2|x|)],$$

where exp denotes the exponential function (inverse of natural logarithm) and $|x|$ stands for the absolute value of x. For example, to convert a recombination fraction of 22 percent into a map distance according to the Haldane map function, $\theta = 0.22$ is entered in equation (1.2) so that it yields $x = 0.29$ Morgan, that is, 29 cM. As a distance measure, x may in principle be taken to be positive or negative, which is why absolute signs are used above. Throughout the remainder of this section, however, map distance will be assumed to be positive.

Depending on the assumed mechanism by which interference operates, many other map functions have been derived. Here, only a few more shall be mentioned. For simplicity, it will be assumed that θ is less than 0.5 so that the case $\theta = \tfrac{1}{2}$ will not have to be considered separately. By making particular assumptions on marginal interference to be covered later, Kosambi (1944) derived the map function

$$x = \tfrac{1}{2} \tanh^{-1}(2\theta) = \tfrac{1}{4} \ln \frac{1 + 2\theta}{1 - 2\theta}, \tag{1.3}$$

with inverse

$$\theta = \tfrac{1}{2} \tanh(2x) = 1/2 \frac{\exp(4x) - 1}{\exp(4x) + 1}.$$

This map function has been widely used in genetics. Using the same example as above, $\theta = 0.22$ in equation (1.3) yields a map distance of 23.6 cM.

For the relatively strong interference in the mouse, Carter and Falconer (1951) made other assumptions on marginal interference and found the following map function to fit observed data rather well:

$$x = \tfrac{1}{4}[\tan^{-1}(2\theta) + \tanh^{-1}(2\theta)]. \tag{1.4}$$

Its inverse cannot be obtained in closed form, but the following equation allows an iterative computation of θ from x when the value of θ on the right side is initially set equal to x:

$$\theta = \tfrac{1}{2} \tanh[4x - \tan^{-1}(2\theta)].$$

The map functions considered thus far incorporate fixed assumptions on how interference operates. Interference is strongest in (1.1), where no more than a single crossover is allowed, and is absent in (1.2). To provide for an adjustable level of interference, Haldane (1919) proposed the compound map function,

$$x = (1 - p)\theta - \tfrac{1}{2}p \ln(1 - 2\theta), \quad 0 \le p \le 1. \tag{1.5}$$

It is a weighted average of the map functions (1.1) and (1.2) with weights $1 - p$ and p, where Haldane chose $p = 0.7$. For $p = 0$, (1.5) reduces to (1.1). For $p = 1$, (1.5) is identical with the regular Haldane map function (1.2). Thus, the compound map function (1.5) allows any level of positive interference, but it is not generally used in human genetics.

Rao et al. (1979) extended this concept by defining a mapping parameter, p, such that x reduces to x_1, x_2, x_3, and x_4, given by (1.2), (1.3), (1.4), and (1.1), respectively, when p assumes the respective values 1, $\tfrac{1}{2}$, $\tfrac{1}{4}$, and 0. This map function is a weighted average, $x = \Sigma_{i=1}^4 w_i x_i$, where $w_1 = p(1 - 2p)(1 - 4p)/3$, $w_2 = -4(1 - p)(1 - 4p)p$, $w_3 = 32(1 - p)(1 - 2p)p/3$, $w_4 = (1 - p)(1 - 2p)(1 - 4p)$, and $\Sigma w_i = 1$. The inverse of Rao's map function as well as that of (1.5) are unavailable in closed form but may be calculated by standard numerical methods.

Another map function with a variable level of interference was given by Felsenstein (1979) as

$$x = \frac{1}{2(2 - k)} \ln \left[1 + \frac{2\theta(2 - k)}{1 - 2\theta} \right], \quad 0 \le k < 2, \tag{1.6}$$

with inverse

$$\theta = 1/2 \, \frac{\exp[2x(2 - k)] - 1}{\exp[2x(2 - k)] + 1 - k}.$$

With $k = 1$, (1.6) is identical with the Haldane map function (1.2), and with $k = 0$ it is identical with the Kosambi map function (1.3). The strongest level of interference allowed by this map function is the one incorporated in Kosambi's function (1.3).

Postulating an obligatory crossover and assuming that additional crossovers are distributed at random, Sturt (1976) developed the map function

$$\theta = \begin{cases} \tfrac{1}{2}[1 - (1 - x/L)\exp(-2x + x/L)] & \text{if } x < L \\ \tfrac{1}{2} & \text{otherwise,} \end{cases} \tag{1.7}$$

where $L \ge \tfrac{1}{2}$ is the chromosome length in Morgans. For example, when two loci are 29 cM apart and are located on a chromosome of length 150 cM ($L = 1.5$), formula (1.7) predicts a recombination fraction of 23 percent between the two loci. The inverse of (1.7) may be obtained by standard numerical procedures and furnishes, for example, a map distance of $x = 0.25$ for $\theta = 0.20$ and $L = 1.5$. For $L = \frac{1}{2}$, the graph of (1.7) is a straight line, corresponding to (1.1). For large L, however, (1.7) becomes identical to the inverse of Haldane's map function (1.2). The parameter L in (1.7) may also be interpreted as the map distance between two unlinked loci ($\theta = \frac{1}{2}$).

All of the above map functions except equation (1.1) postulate a theoretically unlimited number of crossovers. If one assumes at most N crossovers, independently distributed in an interval of length x according to the binomial law (Karlin 1984), one obtains the binomial map function,

$$\theta = \begin{cases} \frac{1}{2}[1 - (1 - 2x/N)^N] & \text{if } x < N/2 \\ \frac{1}{2} & \text{otherwise,} \end{cases} \tag{1.8}$$

with inverse

$$x = \frac{1}{2}N[1 - (1 - 2\theta)^{1/N}]. \tag{1.9}$$

It follows from equation (1.9) that the map distance between unlinked loci is equal to $N/2$. Graphs of several map functions discussed above are shown in figure 1.3.

Map functions incorporate different levels of interference, which may depend on map distance. Consequently, for three loci, 1, 2, and 3, they yield different predictions of the recombination fraction, θ_{13}, between the

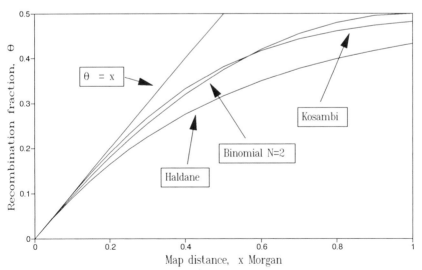

Figure 1.3. Graphs of several mapping functions.

flanking loci based on the recombination fractions θ_{12} and θ_{23} in the two intervals. For the Haldane map function, such an addition formula is obtained as follows: To find θ_{13}, one must convert θ_{12} and θ_{23} into the respective map distances, x_{12} and x_{23}, which can then be summed to yield x_{13}. This, in turn, is then transformed back into a recombination fraction, θ_{13}. Equation (1.2) furnishes x_{12} and x_{23} so that one obtains $x_{13} = -\frac{1}{2} \ln[(1 - 2\theta_{12})(1 - 2\theta_{23})]$. Substituting x_{13} for x in the right side of the inverse of (1.2) gives the desired solution, $\theta_{13} = \theta_{12} + \theta_{23} - 2\theta_{12}\theta_{23}$. An interpretation of this formula is given in section 6.4 on interference.

The MAPFUN computer program (section 8.5) interactively calculates map distances from recombination fractions and vice versa for the map functions mentioned above. It allows, for example, numerical calculation of the predicted recombination fraction between the flanking loci based on the recombination fractions in the two adjacent intervals. In many multipoint computer programs, absence of interference is assumed for the calculation of haplotype probabilities. Researchers then often use the Haldane map function (absence of interference) to convert the estimated recombination fractions to map distances, but other map functions are employed as well. In fact, it seems preferable to use a map function with interference such as Kosambi's as it appears to produce more realistic map distance values than does Haldane's formula.

If one wants to convert a map distance into a recombination fraction, one needs to know by what metric the map distance was obtained. It has, therefore, been recommended (Keats, Ott, and Conneally 1989) that map distances be identified through an appropriately modified symbol such as x_H, x_K, x_R, x_C, or x_F for the Haldane, Kosambi, Rao ($p = 0.35$), Carter-Falconer, or Felsenstein map function, respectively, or by labeling the measurement units as cM(H), cM(K), cM(R), cM(C), or cM(F). To compare results in which map distances are based on different metrics, one needs to convert map distances from one to another metric. Consider, for example, figure 1 in Keats, Ott, and Conneally (1989), which gives an artificial example of four loci on a map, where locus 1 has map location 0 and the map locations for the other loci are known to have been obtained through the Haldane map function. The object is to convert Morgans, M(H), based on Haldane into Morgans, M(K), based on Kosambi. One might see two possible ways of doing this, but simply converting the map *locations* into recombination fractions between locus 1 and each of the other loci and converting these recombination fractions into M(K) units will generally furnish wrong results. Presumably, the map locations in M(H) units were originally obtained from transformations of the recombination fractions in the various map intervals. The different addition formulas of the different map functions then render the procedure just discussed inappropriate. The correct way of converting map locations from M(H) units into M(K) units is first to calculate the map *distance* in each interval. Then, transform these map distances into recombination fractions which, in turn, are transformed into map distances in M(K) units.

For a recombination fraction of $\theta = 0.10$, the Kosambi map function yields a map distance that is approximately 1 percent longer than $x = \theta$, and for map functions with stronger interference the length difference is even smaller. Therefore, for recombination fractions up to about $\theta = 0.10$, one may use θ directly as a map distance. On the other hand, for $\theta = 0.10$, the Haldane map function yields a map distance 12 percent longer than $x = \theta$.

1.6. The Human Chromosomes

Physical distance between two points on a chromosome may be determined by measuring the length of that section under the microscope. Ultimately, however, one would like to be able to measure physical distances in numbers of base pairs (bp) or units of 1,000 base pairs (kb) of DNA. Length measurements are often given in percentage of total chromosome length (Lichter et al. 1990). Refined methods of in situ hybridization allow the visualization of loci (Lichter and Ward 1990; Lawrence, Singer, and McNeil 1990). A rough estimate of the ratio of physical to genetic distance may be obtained for the interval between the loci HRAS and PTH on the distal portion of the short arm of chromosome 11. The physical distance between these loci corresponds to 8 percent of the chromosome length (Lichter et al. 1990) or, since chromosome 11 comprises approximately 4.6 percent of the human autosomal genome (table 1.2), to a fraction of 0.00368 of the total autosomal length. On the other hand, the male recombination fraction estimate between HRAS and PTH is 0.14 (Keats, Ott, and Conneally 1989; their tables are based on the Rao map function), which translates into a map distance of 14.12 cM when the Rao map function with parameter $p = 0.35$ is used. This map distance corresponds to a proportion of $14.12/2577 = 0.00548$ of the male genetic map length. Thus, in that portion of the genome, map length is roughly 1½ times the physical length.

Assuming a total genetic map length of 3,000 cM and a number of 3×10^9 bp in the haploid genome, a genetic distance of 1 cM approximately corresponds to 1,000 kb or 1 million base pairs (1 megabase) (Donis-Keller et al. 1987). Such indirect estimates of the kb/cM ratio have been shown to vary considerably between species and between chromo-

Table 1.2. Male Map Lengths and Physical Volume (Proportional to Physical Length) of the Human Chromosomes

No.	Map Length[a] cM	%	Volume[b] %	I	No.	Map Length[a] cM	%	Volume[b] %	I
1	195	7.57	8.82	47	14	88	3.41	3.64	11
2	173	6.71	8.38	38	15	96	3.73	3.46	14
3	150	5.82	6.90	46	16	108	4.19	3.10	39
4	138	5.36	6.78	28	17	109	4.23	2.96	31
5	137	5.32	6.12	28	18	98	3.80	2.84	24
6	131	5.08	6.00	36	19	97	3.76	2.36	45
7	136	5.28	5.34	37	20	99	3.84	2.12	45
8	131	5.08	5.34	32	21	54	2.10	1.62	17
9	115	4.46	4.88	36	22	60	2.33	1.72	26
10	127	4.93	4.72	31					
11	110	4.27	4.60	39	Total	2,577	100.00	100.00	—
12	137	5.32	4.62	28	X	—	—	5.10	42
13	88	3.41	3.66	9	Y	—	—	2.30	18

[a] Data from an analysis of chiasma counts (Morton et al. 1982).
[b] Data from a cytologic reconstruction (Heslop-Harrison et al. 1989); I = centromere index.

somal regions within a species; direct measurements of actual physical distance (bp) as well as determinations of genetic distance (cM) have been made for only a few pairs of loci in eukaryotic systems (Meagher, McLean, and Arnold 1988).

Map distance is a genetic distance, which need not correlate well with physical distance. The only assumption is that at a given point on the gene map, genetic distance and physical distance are monotonic, that is, an increase in map distance from a given locus translates into a larger physical distance to it. However, the same map distance in different regions of the map may refer to different physical distances. An important characteristic of map distance is that it can be translated into a recombination fraction, and this rather than physical distance is what is relevant in genetic counseling.

If recombination intensity and interference were constant throughout the genome, map distances obtained by the appropriate map function from recombination fractions would show constant proportionality to physical distances. This is not, however, what one observes. For example, the region of the Duchenne's muscular dystrophy (DMD) gene has been described as a hot spot for recombination (Grimm et al. 1989). Also, the pseudoautosomal region appears to be a hot spot of recombination in males, presumably because of the requirement of one obligate crossover between the X and Y chromosomes occurring over a relatively short region (Rouyer et al. 1986). The physical length of the pseudoautosomal region extends over at most 5,000 kb so that the recombination rate for two pseudoautosomal loci is expected to be at most 5 percent. In male meiosis, however, the two pseudoautosomal loci *DXYS14* and *DXYS17* recombine at the rate of 36 percent. In female meioses, the recombination rate of 4 percent between these two loci approximately corresponds to expectation (Rouyer et al. 1986). With the Haldane map function, this difference in recombination rates translates into a ratio of female to male map distances of approximately $0.066 \approx 1/15$.

As pointed out above, the normal karyotype in men comprises twenty-two pairs of autosomes and two sex chromosomes, X and Y. The morphology of the chromosomes is described by a nomenclature that was defined in a series of conferences (*Paris Conference [1971]* 1972; *Paris Conference [1971], Supplement* 1975). Each chromosome comprises two arms separated by a primary restriction, the centromere. The short arm is denoted by p (*petit* in French $=$ small); the long arm by q. A secondary restriction (the centromere being the primary chromosomal restriction) is denoted by h. For example, 9qh designates the secondary restriction on the long arm of chromosome 9. The relative position of the centromere on a chromosome is indicated by the centromere index, $c = 100 \, p/(p + q)$, where p and q refer to the arm lengths of the chromosome. Recently, the cubic volumes of chromosomes were measured by cytologic reconstruction and shown to correlate well with measurements of DNA content and chromosome length (Heslop-Harrison et al. 1989). These volumes are listed in table 1.2. For comparison, genetic lengths based on male chiasma counts (Morton et al. 1982) are also given. The total haploid male autosomal map length is obtained as 2,427 cM or 24.3 Morgans, which is less than Renwick's (1969) figure of 26.5 Morgans and probably represents a lower bound to the actual map length of the male genome. As table 1.2 shows, a rough proportionality exists between chromosome volume (representing DNA content or physical length) and genetic length.

Various staining methods show many different chromosome bands that allow unequivocal identification of each chromosome and of portions of chromosomes. The chromosome band nomenclature (*Paris Conference [1971]* 1972) defines a *landmark* as a consistent and distinct morphologic feature, such as the ends of chromosome arms, the centromere, and certain bands. A *region* is defined as any area of a chromosome lying between two adjacent landmarks. Regions and bands are numbered consecutively from the centromere outward along each chromosome arm. For a detailed analysis, some bands are divided into subbands, whose numbers are separated from the band number by a decimal point. For example, the ABO blood group locus is at 9q34, that is, in band 34 on the long arm of chromosome 9 (McAlpine et al. 1989). The positions of some loci can only be assigned to a larger chromosome area. For example, the Huntington's disease gene (HD) lies in the area 4pter-p16.3 (McAlpine et al. 1989), which extends from the end (terminus) of the short arm of chromosome 4 to band 16.3 of that arm.

Problems

Problem 1.1. Consider three gene loci numbered 1, 2, and 3, and assume that the recombination fractions in the two intervals are θ_{12} and θ_{23}. What is the recombination fraction, θ_{13}, between loci 1 and 3 in terms of θ_{12} and θ_{23} as predicted by the Kosambi formula?

Problem 1.2. Using the same assumptions as in problem 1.1, derive the expression for θ_{13} in terms of θ_{12}, θ_{23}, and k, where k is the parameter in Felsenstein's map function (1.6). Then solve the resulting equation for k, thus finding an estimator for the level of interference. Verify your results by setting $k = 1$, which should yield the results obtained for the Haldane map function.

Problem 1.3. Assume that for four loci, based on estimates of the recombination fractions in the three intervals, map positions are given as 0, 14, 18, and 37 cM (Haldane). Convert these map positions to units of Kosambi-centimorgans.

Problem 1.4. Explain why under complete interference the map length between two points can be no longer than ½ Morgan.

2.

Genes and
Genetic Polymorphisms

As we saw in the previous chapter, linkage analysis investigates genetic distance between loci, particularly the relationships between disease genes and *genetic markers*, i.e., genetic entities known to follow a mendelian mode of inheritance (a narrower definition of genetic marker also requires that its map location be known). This chapter gives an overview of the number and types of human loci. The first section covers questions of nomenclature and gene classification. In the sections below, the major categories of marker polymorphisms used in human linkage analysis are discussed. These presentations involve few technical details and are intended only as a brief reference for linkage analysts.

2.1. Nomenclature and Characterization of Genes

Classically, the presence of genes has been recognized by the variability of their effects, that is, only polymorphic genes were readily detectable. Modern molecular genetics methods allow the recognition and location of genes based on the proteins they produce; the genes themselves may or may not be polymorphic. The estimated proportion of genes that are polymorphic varies from roughly 15 percent in fishes to close to 50 percent in *Drosophila* (Hartl 1988). In humans, the proportion of genes that are polymorphic has been estimated as 32 percent (Harris, Hopkinson, and Edwards 1977). Newer data confirm this; of the reported 945 cloned genes (Kidd et al. 1989), 41 percent are polymorphic. Of all 4,362 mapped DNA clones known in 1989 (genes and anonymous sequences), 43 percent were polymorphic (Kidd et al. 1989). Thus, of the estimated total number of 50,000 genes in humans, one would expect about 20,000 to be polymorphic.

Probably the largest database of genes identified in humans is Mc-

Kusick's (1990) *Mendelian Inheritance in Man* (*MIM*). That book was first published in 1966 and has been regularly updated. There is also an on-line version (OMIM[TM]), so its contents may be accessed electronically via a computer terminal and the telephone line. *MIM* describes disease genes as well as marker genes, each provided with a unique number (referred to as the MIM number). Its latest edition has a total of 4,937 entries.

Many of the known human genes have been mapped. A standing committee has set up and maintains rules for their nomenclature (McAlpine et al. 1989). The official locus symbols are regularly published in the proceedings of the international Human Gene Mapping Workshops (Ruddle and Kidd 1989) and are also used in this book. The tenth human gene-mapping workshop (HGM10) was held in 1989 in New Haven, and HGM11 will be held in August 1991 in London. For DNA polymorphisms, special rules apply (see section 2.5).

The *1989 catalog of mapped genes* (McAlpine et al. 1989) contains three general types of markers: functional genes, DNA segments of unknown function, and inherited chromosomal variants such as fragile sites. Each of these types is presented in the subsequent sections. The total number of loci (excluding fragile sites and DNA segments) in that catalog is 1,631. In addition, there are 113 fragile sites, over 3,300 DNA segments, and some 54 mitochondrial loci (McAlpine et al. 1989). In addition to the official gene symbols, the catalog lists the MIM number when known, the marker name, the map location, and a few other useful indications.

Genetic markers that follow a dominant or codominant mode of inheritance are referred to as *factor-union systems* (Cotterman 1969). Their phenotypes are often reactions to certain tests, and these reactions (called factors) are either positive (present) or negative (absent). Characterization of such phenotypes is particularly simple in factor-union notation—that is, by a sequence of binary digits in which each element is either a one or a zero, where the one stands for presence and the zero for absence of a particular factor. Examples will be found, for example, in the discussion of the ABO blood groups, below. Factor-union notation is also used in some computer programs to describe the phenotypes of codominant and dominant allele systems.

Although it is not necessary for a linkage analyst to understand the molecular genetics of a marker, he or she must know exactly the relation between genotypes and phenotypes of each marker used in the linkage analysis. Representative examples will be given below, but for more complete information the reader is referred to the literature.

2.2. The Degree of Polymorphism

The term *polymorphism* denotes the fact that a locus is polymorphic, but it is also used as a synonym for polymorphic locus. A general discussion of human polymorphisms may be found in section 6.1.2 of Vogel and Motulsky (1986).

It was established in chapter 1 that, for a mating to be (potentially) informative for linkage between two gene loci, at least one of the two parents must be doubly heterozygous. Therefore, a marker's usefulness for linkage analysis depends on the number of its alleles and their gene frequencies (i.e., its degree of polymorphism), in the sense that an increased polymorphism leads to an increased probability of heterozygosity. Marker "usefulness" is discussed here purely in terms of degree of polymorphism, but other characteristics of gene markers determine their usefulness in a more general sense. For example, a DNA polymorphism may have a large number of alleles which are recognized as bands on a Southern blot, but the bands may be so little separated from each other that unique identification of the different alleles is difficult, leading to phenotypic misclassification.

Two measures of the degree of polymorphism are in general use. One is the so-called *heterozygosity*,

$$H = 1 - \sum p_i^2, \tag{2.1}$$

where p_i is the population frequency of the ith allele, and H is simply the probability that a random individual is heterozygous for any two alleles at a gene locus with allele frequencies, p_i. For example, the three alleles with frequencies of 0.28, 0.06, and 0.66 at the *ABO* locus yield a heterozygosity of 0.48 so that almost half of all individuals are expected to be heterozygous at the *ABO* locus.

Strictly speaking, the proportion of heterozygotes is determined by the gene frequencies (and thus by H) only under random mating. Assortative mating (matings occur preferentially between individuals with similar phenotypes) and inbreeding (mating between relatives) tend to reduce heterozygosity but do not change gene frequencies (Hartl 1988). In human populations, however, these effects are not strong enough to reduce heterozygosity noticeably. Under inbreeding, the expected proportion of heterozygotes is $(1 - F)H$ (Hartl 1988), where F is the inbreeding coefficient. Vogel and Motulsky (1986) gave a lucid discussion of inbreeding and provided an extensive table of estimates of F for various human populations. The largest values found are around $F = 0.005$, but the values are in most cases much smaller than that. Therefore, predictions of the proportion of heterozygotes based on H are not much biased by inbreeding.

For a gene with n alleles, heterozygosity is largest when the alleles are equally frequent, $p_i = p_j = 1/n$. Then, the heterozygosity takes the simple form,

$$H = 1 - 1/n. \tag{2.2}$$

For example, a locus with three alleles has a maximum heterozygosity of $\frac{2}{3} = 0.67$. Solving $H = 1 - 1/n$ for n leads to $n = 1/(1 - H)$, which allows one to calculate the number of equally frequent alleles (or the minimum number of alleles with any frequencies) needed to attain a specified heterozygosity, H. For example, for a heterozygosity of 0.90, a gene must have at least ten alleles, but its heterozygosity will be 0.90 only when each allele has a population frequency of 10 percent; otherwise, heterozygosity will be less than 0.90.

In human genetics, another measure of the degree of polymorphism often used is the PIC (polymorphism information content) value (Botstein et al. 1980). It was derived for the situation of a (rare) dominant disease in a nuclear family and a codominant marker. One of the parents is assumed to be affected (heterozygous for the disease allele). The PIC value is defined as the probability that the marker genotype of a given offspring will allow deduction of which of the two marker alleles of the affected parent it had received. PIC is calculated as

$$\begin{aligned} \text{PIC} &= 1 - \sum_{i=1}^{n} p_i^2 - \sum_{i=1}^{n-1} \sum_{j=i+1}^{n} 2p_i^2 p_j^2 \\ &= 2 \sum_{i=1}^{n-1} \sum_{j=i+1}^{n} p_i p_j (1 - p_i p_j), \end{aligned} \tag{2.3}$$

where p_i is the population frequency of the ith allele. For the ABO example used above, PIC is equal to 0.41.

As one can see from comparing (2.3) with (2.1), the PIC value is always smaller than the heterozygosity. For alleles with equal population frequencies, $p_i = p_j = 1/n$, equation (2.3) reduces to

$$\text{PIC} = (n - 1)^2 (n + 1)/n^3. \tag{2.4}$$

A comparison of equations (2.2) and (2.4) shows that, for large numbers n of alleles, heterozygosity and PIC tend to become very close. This can also be seen in figure 2.1, which shows pairs of points (PIC, H). The figure was obtained by evaluating, for loci of two through five alleles, all possible combinations of gene frequencies in steps of 0.05. Each set of gene frequencies furnished a pair of values, PIC and H (there are 2,826

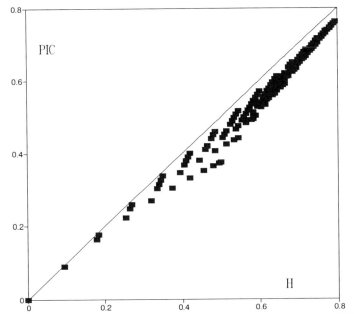

Figure 2.1. Correspondence between polymorphism information content, PIC, and heterozygosity, *H*, for loci between two and five alleles.

such pairs, but in fig. 2.1 many of them overlap). The two values are generally very close, with the greatest divergence occurring around a heterozygosity of 50 percent.

In chapter 1, a gene was defined to be polymorphic when its most common allele has a population frequency of at most 95 percent. Equations (2.1) and (2.3) then imply $H \geq 0.10$ and PIC ≥ 0.10, respectively. Thus, a polymorphic gene may be defined as one with a heterozygosity (or a PIC value) of at least 10 percent.

Both of these measures of polymorphism are functions of the marker gene frequencies and do not take into account whether a marker is codominant or dominant. There exists a measure of the degree of polymorphism which takes dominance relations among the marker alleles into account (Chakraborty, Fuerst, and Ferrell 1979), but it has not found much practical use.

2.3. Blood Cell Antigens

When the body is challenged by a foreign substance, it reacts by producing an immune response, manufacturing *antibodies* (Vogel and Motulsky 1986). These are protein molecules that have the ability to bind specifically to the foreign substance, or *antigen*, that triggered their production (antibody-antigen reaction). Many substances on the surface of the blood cells of an individual act as antigens when they are brought into the body of another individual. The observation that blood from a given individual may evoke an immune response in one individual but not in another led to the discovery of the first blood groups and to the recognition that these are genetic polymorphisms. In practice, the blood cell antigens produced by different genotypes at a gene locus are distinguished most often by *serologic* techniques, that is, an antigen is tested against a battery of antisera containing specific antibodies. Molecular genetic aspects of red cell surface antigens, which determine the blood groups, were recently reviewed by Anstee (1990). For an account of the terminology of blood groups and their alleles, see Lewis et al. 1990.

The *ABO blood group* locus produces two major antigens, *A* and *B*, located on the surface of the red blood cells. These antigens can be probed with two antisera containing the respective antibodies, anti-A and anti-B. Cells with the A antigen will show a reaction (agglutination) to anti-A, and cells with the B antigen will react to the anti-B antiserum but not to the anti-A. It is convenient to code the presence or absence of an antibody-antigen reaction by the respective symbols 1 and 0 (factor-union notation). The reaction of the red blood cells of some individual to anti-A and anti-B is then coded as two digits. For example, 01 represents reaction to anti-B but not to anti-A; cells with this reaction carry the B antigen but not the A antigen on their surfaces. A total of four different reactions can be observed: 10, 01, 00, and 11, corresponding to the blood groups A, B, O, and AB, respectively. It is a peculiarity of the ABO system that individuals always have in their blood serum the antibodies against those antigens not present on their red blood cells. For example, individuals showing reaction 10 (blood group A) have the A antigens on their red blood cells and the anti-B antibodies in their serum.

The genetic interpretation of the four phenotypes (blood groups) is that they are under the control of three alleles. Two alleles, *a* and *b*, produce the respective antigens A and B (codominant inheritance), whereas a third allele, *o*, does not produce any antigens, so that $o < a$ and $o < b$, that is, *o* is recessive to *a* and *b*. These three alleles combine in pairs to form a total of six possible genotypes, and the relations between genotypes and phenotypes are shown in table 1.1. On the molecular level, the *a*, *b*, and *o* alleles were recently shown to differ in a few single-base substitutions (Yamamoto et al. 1990).

Table 2.1. Penetrances and Expected Phenotype and Genotype Frequencies at the *ABO* Locus with Four *ABO* Alleles

Genotypes	Phenotypes						Genotype Frequency
	A_1	A_2	A_1B	A_2B	B	O	
a_1/a_1	1	0	0	0	0	0	0.0441
a_1/a_2	1	0	0	0	0	0	0.0294
a_1/b	0	0	1	0	0	0	0.0252
a_1/o	1	0	0	0	0	0	0.2772
a_2/a_2	0	1	0	0	0	0	0.0049
a_2/b	0	0	0	1	0	0	0.0084
a_2/o	0	1	0	0	0	0	0.0924
b/b	0	0	0	0	1	0	0.0036
b/o	0	0	0	0	1	0	0.0792
o/o	0	0	0	0	0	1	0.4356
Phenotype frequency	0.3507	0.0973	0.0252	0.0084	0.0828	0.4356	1

Blood type A may be subdivided into at least two subgroups called A_1 and A_2. Usually, the blood cells are first tested for a general A antigen. Those that respond negatively contain neither A_1 nor A_2. Those that respond positively are then tested for the A_1 antigen. A positive reaction indicates blood type A_1; a negative reaction, blood type A_2. Table 2.1 shows the relation between genotypes and phenotypes, assuming four different alleles at the *ABO* locus, a_1, a_2, b, and o. In Caucasian populations, their respective gene frequencies are approximately equal to 0.21, 0.07, 0.06, and 0.66, which amounts to a heterozygosity of 0.51 and a PIC of 0.47. From these frequencies, under the assumptions of Hardy-Weinberg equilibrium, the expected frequencies of the genotypes and phenotypes can be calculated (table 2.1). The *ABO* gene is located on the long arm of chromosome 9, in the 9q34.1-q34.2 region (McAlpine et al. 1989). Associations between ABO blood groups and diseases are well known, and the world distribution of ABO gene frequencies suggests influences of natural selection (Vogel and Motulsky 1986).

Another group of antibodies on the red blood cells belongs to the *Rhesus (RH) blood group* system (Vogel and Motulsky 1986). It is generally assumed that the RH phenotypes are determined by three closely linked loci, with recombination occurring very rarely between them. The description below is an adaptation of this topic as presented by Cavalli-Sforza and Bodmer (1977).

The RH polymorphism can generally be explained by assuming two alleles at each of the three tightly linked loci. At the first of these loci, the two alleles produce the antigens c and C, which can be detected by the respective antibodies anti-c and anti-C. The second locus produces antigens *d* and *D*; *D* can be detected by anti-D (originally called Rh +), while no anti-d is known. Similarly, the antigens e and E, produced by the third locus, are detectable with anti-e and anti-E. With two alleles at each of three loci, one has eight different haplotypes. Among Caucasians, the most frequent haplotype is *CDe*, with a population frequency of about 40 percent.

Typing results are often reported as 1 or 0 depending on whether or not an antibody has led to a serologic reaction (factor-union notation). Here, reactions of the antigens are assumed in the order DCEce so that the phenotype consists of a sequence of five 0s or 1s. For example, an individual with genotype *cde/cDe* will show an antigenic reaction pattern of 10011. Owing to allelism, at least one of the two antibodies anti-e and anti-E must always show a reaction. Occasionally, it happens that neither anti-c nor anti-C provokes a reaction. In that case, a third allele, C^w, is segregating, and the individual in question is homozygous, C^w/C^w. With three alleles, *C, c*, and C^w, at the first locus, twelve different haplotypes exist. They are listed along with their population frequencies in Caucasians in table 2.2. The corresponding heterozygosity is equal to 0.66, and PIC is 0.60.

In a linkage analysis, one may treat the RH system as a set of three loci with zero recombination fraction between them; the order assumed for these loci is then irrelevant. Should a recombination occur between

Table 2.2. RH Haplotypes and Their Frequencies in Caucasians

Number	Symbol	Frequency
1	*CDe*	0.4036
2	*cDE*	0.1670
3	*cde*	0.3820
4	*cDe*	0.0186
5	C^wDe	0.0198
6	*Cde*	0.0049
7	*cdE*	0.0029
8	*CDE*	0.0008
9	C^wde	0.0003
10	*CdE* ⎫	
11	C^wDE ⎬	0.0001
12	C^wdE ⎭	

Source: Cavalli-Sforza and Bodmer 1971.

Table 2.3. Relation between Genotypes and Some Phenotypes (Penetrances) at the RH Locus

Genotype	Phenotype							
	00011	00111 01011	01111 10011	10110	10111	11001	11011	11111
1/1	0	0	0	0	0	1	0	0
1/2	0	0	0	0	0	0	0	1
1/3	0	0	0	0	0	0	1	0
1/4	0	0	0	0	0	1	1	1
2/2	0	0	0	1	0	0	0	0
2/3	0	0	0	0	1	0	0	0
2/4	0	0	0	1	1	0	0	1
3/3	1	0	0	0	0	0	0	0
3/4	0[a]	1	1	0	0[a]	0	0	1
4/4	0	0	1	0[a]	1	0[a]	1	1

Note: Alleles *1* through *3* correspond to haplotypes *1* through 3 in table 2.2, whereas haplotypes *4* through *12* in table 2.2 are lumped together to form allele *4*. Phenotypes reflect typing results for the antigens DCEce.

[a] If allele C^w is to be allowed for, 0 should be replaced by 1.

one of the component loci, a small recombination fraction (e.g., $\theta = 0.001$) has to be specified. Alternatively, assuming absence of recombination within the component loci, the eight or twelve haplotypes may be used as alleles of a single compound locus. Since several of these haplotypes have very small population frequencies, it is most unlikely that more than one of them will occur simultaneously in the same pedigree. Therefore, one may generally lump them into a single haplotype with only minimal loss of informativeness, but if the presence of several rare alleles is detected in a pedigree they should, of course, be distinguished from each other. If in table 2.2, haplotypes 4 through 12 are combined into a single allele with frequency 0.0474, heterozygosity is still equal to 0.66 to two decimal places. Table 2.3 shows the relations between genotypes and phenotypes when haplotypes 4 through 12 are treated as a single fourth allele. The RH gene complex is located on the short arm of chromosome 1, in the region 1p36.2-p34 (McAlpine et al. 1989).

A particular role in human genetics is played by the *HLA gene complex* (Bodmer 1981; Ryder, Svejgaard, and Dausset 1981; Vøgel and Motulsky 1986). Its antigens are located on the white blood cells and are concerned with histocompatibility. At least four closely linked loci—designated *HLA-A*, *B*, *C*, and *D/DR*—determine these antigens and are located on the short arm of chromosome 6. The gene order is D-B-C-A (from proximal to distal) with the respective male map distances between

Table 2.4. Relation between *LU* Genotypes and Phenotypes (Penetrances)

	Phenotype				
	Using Anti-A and Anti-B			Using Anti-A Only	
Genotype	A + B −	A + B +	A − B +	A +	A −
A/A	1	0	0	1	0
A/B	0	1	0	1	0
B/B	0	0	1	0	1

them of 1.0, 0.1, and 0.7 cM (Lamm and Olaisen 1985). The HLA system is highly complex and extremely polymorphic (Spence, Spurr, and Field 1989). Some of its haplotypes show a peculiar association to diseases.

There are several other polymorphisms of cell surface antigens. Only one more shall be mentioned here briefly. At the *Lutheran (LU) blood group* locus, two major alleles exist, *A* and *B*, with the respective approximate allele frequencies 0.04 and 0.96 (among Asians only *B* occurs; see table 11.7 in Cavalli-Sforza and Bodmer 1971). The antigens can be detected by antibodies anti-A and anti-B, so that heterozygous *A/B* individuals can be distinguished from both types of homozygotes (codominant inheritance). Sometimes only anti-A is used in laboratories. In that case, *A* is "dominant" since *A/A* homozygotes cannot be distinguished from *A/B* heterozygotes. The relation between LU genotypes and phenotypes is given in table 2.4. The map location of the LU locus is 19q12-q13, which was found only in the early 1980s. LU was long known to be linked with the Secretor blood group (FUT2, earlier Se); in fact, this was the first autosomal linkage detected in humans (Mohr 1954).

2.4. Blood Proteins

Many proteins (among them many enzymes) in the blood, either in the serum or in the blood cells, can be shown to be polymorphic. Most have been detected by *electrophoretic techniques*, that is, by separation of the protein molecules according to differences in electric charge and molecular weight. Only one example will be given here. A simple technical description of protein electrophoresis may be found in Hartl (1988).

The locus for phosphoglucomutase-1 (PGM1), an enzyme in the red blood cells, is on chromosome 1, in the region 1p22.1 (McAlpine et al. 1989). For many years, the alleles, *1* and *2*, with the respective gene frequencies 0.74 and 0.26 (heterozygosity = 0.38), were known to exist at this locus. The three genotypes can be distinguished by their electrophoretic pattern. By isoelectric focusing methods, two additional alleles were detected (Sutton and Burgess 1978), leading to the four alleles $1+$, $1-$, $2+$, and $2-$, with the respective gene frequencies 0.62, 0.12, 0.14, and 0.12 (heterozygosity $= 0.57$).

2.5. DNA Polymorphisms and the Genome Project

The rapid progress in molecular genetics has been a boon to human linkage analysis. In a seminal paper, Botstein et al. (1980) proposed to treat differences in the DNA sequence like allelic variants of a gene and use them as genetic markers for gene mapping. Based on a technique described by Southern (1975), such differences can be made visible by the use of restriction enzymes, which cut DNA at specific sequences (the recognition sites), resulting in DNA fragments of various lengths. If the DNA sequence at a cutting site is different in a homologous chromosome, DNA will not be cut there so that fragments of different sizes occur. The size differences will then lead to differential migration in electrophoresis and can be made visible as different banding patterns. Details of this technique can be found in many textbooks. Polymorphisms obtained in this manner are appropriately called restriction fragment length polymorphisms (RFLPs). As they presumably have no physiologic function, they can be expected not to interfere with the phenotypic expressions at other loci and to be free of the influences of selection. RFLPs thus are well suited as genetic markers. Researchers developing new polymorphisms or investigating polymorphisms in a new population generally compare the observed distribution of the genotypes with that expected under Hardy-Weinberg equilibrium (section 1.1). For example, Väisänen et al. (1988) investigated four RFLPs in the type II collagen gene in the Finnish population and found satisfactory agreement between observed and predicted genotype distributions.

In simple cases, the interpretation of the banding pattern poses no problems. However, in more complex situations, it may not be easy to identify alleles uniquely, and different genotypes may correspond to the same phenotype (Lange and Boehnke 1983). Although it generally is the responsibility of the molecular geneticist to interpret his or her blots, it is useful for a linkage analyst to be aware of potential problems.

RFLPs are generally based on single nucleotide changes, but another type of polymorphism results from a variable number of tandem repeats of a relatively short oligonucleotide sequence. Such polymorphisms, called VNTRs (Nakamura et al. 1987), are much more polymorphic than

RFLPs. However, with a high degree of polymorphism, the different bands are sometimes not well separated on the gel, which introduces the danger of misclassifying alleles. Also, the probes used often recognize DNA at various locations on the genome, which produces additional bands and thus an additional possibility of uncertainty in interpreting the banding pattern. Although these difficulties may give the impression that homozygotes are more frequent than expected under Hardy-Weinberg equilibrium (HWE), statistical analyses do not show deviations from HWE (Devlin, Risch, and Roeder 1990), particularly when single alleles are recognizable (Chakraborty and Boerwinkle 1990). VNTRs are sometimes said to show considerable mutation rates; in light of their being in HWE, however, mutation rates cannot be extremely high.

Multiple occurrences of very short sequences, so-called minisatellites, often differ in the number of these repeats and thereby can serve as extremely useful polymorphic marker loci (for example, CA repeats; Weber and May 1989). These short stretches of DNA can be amplified directly with the polymerase chain reaction (PCR) technique so that a large number of copies of these DNA segments are synthesized; these can then be put on a gel and subjected to electrophoresis.

Probes recognizing repetitive sequences at not one but several loci are extremely polymorphic (Jeffreys, Wilson, and Thein 1985). However, the resulting banding patterns are difficult to interpret and alleles cannot generally be recognized. Such probes furnish a genetic "fingerprint" that is practically unique for each individual and is, among other things, often used in linkage analyses to establish paternity. However, an occasional crossover or DNA slippage during replication might lead to unexpected differences between parents and offspring, and this may occur at a rate of one in several hundred (section 6.1.2 in Vogel and Motulsky 1986).

Names for DNA polymorphisms are assigned according to strict rules. They all begin with the letter D (and are thus called D numbers) followed by the number of the chromosome on which they are located. After that, a letter indicating the complexity of the DNA sequence and a unique sequential number are assigned. For details, the reader is referred to the literature (Kidd et al. 1989).

The already large number of loci is expected to become enormous quickly, although plans to establish a 1-cM map are somewhat behind schedule ("Whatever happened to the genetic map?" *Science* 247: 281–82, 1989). A general outline of the genome project and its technical and financial aspects may be found in *Mapping Our Genes* (U.S. Congress OTA 1988; see also Watson 1990). To facilitate the ordering of loci on the chromosomes and the integration of information from different sources, at least two types of 'anchor genes' are defined. On the gene mapping and cytogenetics level, well characterized (recognized by a specific clone) and mapped polymorphic loci are designated as assigned reference points (ARPs) (previously called arbitrary reference points), and the map position of other loci may then be given relative to their nearest ARPs (Kidd et al. 1988). For example, HLA on chromosome 6 is an ARP (Spence, Spurr, and Field 1989). On the molecular genetics level, it has been proposed (Olson et al. 1989) to define a large number of so-called sequence-tagged sites (STSs), which will serve as the basic landmarks on the physical map. A number of 33,000 STSs has been recommended so that on average STSs will be spaced 100 kb apart. Each STS is to consist of a short, unique DNA sequence that can be recognized by a PCR assay. STSs will not necessarily be polymorphic, but the map position of well-defined polymorphic loci may be indicated with reference to an STS nearby. Loci for which order on a linkage map is well supported are termed *framework loci* (Keats et al. 1991; see section 6.1).

Many laboratories are working on mapping whole chromosomes or particular portions of a chromosome. A predominant concerted effort at constructing a human genetic map is based on a set of 40 reference families, the so-called CEPH families (Dausset et al. 1990). These families consist of one pair of parents, many offspring, and four or fewer grandparents. Their mean sibship size is 8.3.

2.6. Variants in Chromosome Morphology

Chromosomes exhibit a fair degree of morphologic variability. Not infrequently, such variants were observed in parents and offspring as well, so that inheritance had to be assumed. For example, Cooper and Hernits (1963) described an elongated chromosome 1 in a mother and a daughter. They were unable to decide whether the elongation was due to the presence of an extra segment in the long arm, near the centromere, or whether it was the consequence of an alteration in the coiling structure at that place. They nonetheless regarded the unusual spot on chromosome 1 as a chromosome marker and carried out linkage studies between it and nine genetic markers. All genetic markers were uninformative, but the Duffy blood group was consistent with linkage, although the smallness of the family did not permit any conclusions. In contrast to other researchers, these authors tended to believe that the occurrence of the chromosome variant and the phenotypic abnormality in the proband was fortuitous, since chromosome studies were carried out preferentially on phenotypically abnormal individuals.

Donahue et al. (1968) and Ying and Ives (1968) independently reported families segregating apparently the same chromosome variant, and both found good evidence for linkage to the Duffy blood group. This established the first assignment of a human gene to an autosome. The particular chromosome variant (a secondary restriction) occurs in about 0.5 percent of the population and is dominantly inherited (Vogel and Motulsky 1986).

On many chromosomes, *fragile sites* have been observed (McAlpine et al. 1989). These are chromosome sites showing an increased risk of breakage, particularly under special cell culture conditions. Most of them do not seem to be associated with any phenotypic abnormalities. A well-known exception is the fragile site at Xq27.3 (gene symbol *FRAXA*), which is associated with a characteristic form of mental retardation, the mar(X) or Martin-Bell or fragile X syndrome (Vogel and Motulsky 1986). It is inherited as an X-linked dominant condition with incomplete penetrance (Sherman et al. 1985).

2.7. Marker Coverage of the Human Genome

In the "pre-RFLP" era, the number of markers was severely limited and, even with excellent family data, linkage analyses had little prospect of success. Mohr (1964) investigated the a priori probability of success assuming a varying number, m, of markers, even though at the time only sixteen useful autosomal marker systems were available. He posed the question: Given a map length of L Morgans, what is the probability of an arbitrary locus being not more than $d = 20$ cM from the nearest known marker system? (This probability is 1 when all markers are spaced 40 cM apart.) Using computer simulation, assuming a map length of $L = 28.57$ Morgans, he found, for example, a probability of 32 percent for thirty markers and 54 percent for sixty markers.

This question was treated analytically (i.e., using algebraic methods) by Elston and Lange (1975). They assumed a total autosomal map length of $L = 33$ Morgans and considered, among other things, that, for a linkage to be detectable at all, the recombination fraction between a locus and the nearest marker must not exceed $\theta = 0.40$ (corresponding to a map distance of $d = 44$ cM, Carter-Falconer map function, equation [1.4]). With this, they found a prior probability of linkage ($\theta \leq 0.40$) of 2 percent for 1 marker, of 50 percent for 30 markers, and of 89 percent for 100 markers. (This prior probability would be 1 if all markers were spaced $2d = 88$ cM apart.)

Lange and Boehnke (1982) turned these questions around and asked:

Given a prescribed probability, P, of success (prior probability of linkage), what is the number, m, of markers required for a random new locus to fall within a distance, d, of the nearest marker? Although this question could have been answered by the methods mentioned above, Lange and Boehnke (1982) sought a statistically different solution. Treating m as a random variable and requiring that, in the search for RFLPs, no gap between adjacent markers be larger than $2d = 20$ cM, they found a mean number of markers required of 797 to 1,749 (95 percent confidence interval).

A few years earlier, Botstein at al. (1980) also calculated the number of markers it takes to span the assumed length of 33 Morgans of the human genome, but they assumed that markers should be equally spaced $2d = 20$ cM apart so that any gene to be mapped will be within $d = 10$ cM of the nearest markers. Under these assumptions, $3,300/20 = 165$ markers would be required.

For a relatively dense map of markers, if one assumes that RFLPs are found at random along the genome, the number of markers required to map a gene may be calculated to a good approximation as follows: The probability, P, that a gene is within a distance, d, of a random marker, disregarding the possibility that the marker may be located at the end of a chromosome, is approximately equal to $2d/L$, where L is the total map length, usually assumed as 33 Morgans. For m markers, the probability that a gene is *not* within a distance d of any of them, assuming independence, is equal to $(1 - 2d/L)^m$, so that the gene is within a distance d of at least one of the m markers with probability

$$P = 1 - (1 - 2d/L)^m.$$

This equation may be solved for the number of markers,

$$m = \ln(1 - P)/\ln(1 - 2d/L) \approx -[L/(2d)] \ln(1 - P). \qquad (2.5)$$

For example, if one demands a probability $P = 90$ percent that a gene be located within $d = 1$ cM of a marker, approximately $m = 3,800$ randomly placed markers are required (a fixed 2-cM map would ensure that a gene is never more than 1 cM from the next marker), and, if a higher certainty of 99 percent is postulated, about 7,600 markers are required. Equation (2.5) shows that, approximately, the number of markers required increases linearly with the total map length and with the inverse of the postulated marker distance.

These calculations indicate the potentially large number of markers needed for dense coverage of the genome. Today, of course, markers are no longer detected at random on the genome but can be searched for in the vicinity of an existing marker. The number of 7,600 markers required for the equivalent of a 2-cM map may thus be somewhat too high. On the other hand, technical difficulties and varying ratios of physical to genetic distance will probably require many more than the minimum of 1,650 equally spaced markers.

Problems

Problem 2.1. For a marker locus with n equally frequent alleles, what is the difference between heterozygosity, H, and polymorphism information content, PIC? What is the minimum number of alleles such that this difference is no greater than 0.01?

Problem 2.2.   A chromosome of length 100 cM should be covered with n marker loci such that, with probability $P = 95$ percent, a gene with unknown location on this chromosome will be at most 5 cM away from the nearest marker. Approximately what number n of markers are required?

3.

Aspects of
Statistical Inference

This chapter provides a selection of technical statistical tools for readers with little background in statistics. Their knowledge is not absolutely necessary for a fruitful study of the remainder of this book, although a deeper understanding of linkage analysis, especially of the methods to be presented in chapter 4, requires familiarity with basic principles of statistical inference. Of course, researchers who want to carry out independent and original work in linkage analysis methods need to know much more than what is presented here.

The discussion of statistical methods given below is not intended as a rigorous outline of statistical methods nor as a historical overview. The modest goal of this chapter is to define some statistical terms and to explain rationale and technique of a selection of statistical methods. As will be seen in the next chapter, elements from more than one "school" of thought are in current use in linkage analysis. I see nothing wrong with that. Some statistical approaches are better than others at solving a particular problem, and the situation may be reversed for another problem. What is missing to a large extent in this chapter is a discussion of bayesian inference methods—a reflection of my personal bias. Of course, where prior information is available, it should not be disregarded, and using the Bayes theorem does not make one a bayesian. However, translating ignorance on a parameter into a uniform distribution for it and the arbitrariness inherent in rules of assigning prior distributions (section 5b.3 in Rao 1973) do not appeal to me.

A brief discussion of the concepts of prior and posterior probability of linkage is given in chapter 4. Readers interested in a broader outline of statistical methods than that presented here are referred to the literature (e.g., Smith 1959; A. W. F. Edwards 1984; A. W. F. Edwards 1989). Interesting aspects of statistical methodology were also discussed by Cohen (1990). Lod scores are briefly introduced in this chapter; a more detailed and elementary discussion follows in chapter 4.

As pointed out in the preface, no introduction to probability calculus is provided in this book. A brief outline is given in the appendix of Thompson 1986. For its practical importance in probability calculations, the Bayes theorem (an application of conditional probability calculus) is briefly discussed in the last section of this chapter.

3.1. Likelihood

To "explain" a particular phenomenon in nature, scientists build a *model* (also called a *hypothesis*) of the phenomenon, that is, a description that accounts for most or all of the phenomenon's known properties. Models may be of a biochemical, physical, statistical, etc., nature. Good models are those that explain and accurately predict a large number of properties. For example, the mendelian laws are a model for the inheritance of genetic markers and many diseases. Consider a gene locus with two alleles, A and a, where A is dominant over a. The three genotypes, A/A, A/a, and a/a, then give rise to two phenotypes, $A+$ under A/A and A/a and $A-$ under a/a. Assume that two parents each have phenotypes $A+$ and that their genotypes are known to be A/a each (see problem 3.1). A child of such an $A/a \times A/a$ mating is predicted to have phenotype $A+$ with probability ¾ and phenotype $A-$ with probability ¼. Once the first child is born, the same probabilities hold for each subsequent child because, according to Mendel's laws of inheritance, one child's phenotype does not influence that of another. In other words, with given parental genotypes, the phenotypes of the offspring are mutually independent. Among a large number of children, one expects a proportion of roughly 75 percent to be of phenotype $A+$. On the basis of these assumptions, using probability calculus, one may make further predictions. For example, the probability that among two children at least one has the $A+$ phenotype (which is the same as saying that not both children are $A-$) is given by $1 - (¼)^2 = 0.9375$, or the probability that both children are either $A+$ or $A-$ is equal to $(¾)^2 + (¼)^2 = 0.625$.

Hypotheses are verified on the basis of observations. The better the data conform with a hypothesis, the more readily we tend to accept it as being "true." But how are we to measure the degree by which certain observations agree with a hypothesis, or whether they agree better with hypothesis H_1 or H_2? The statistical quantity that seems most suitable to serve as a measure for our belief in a particular hypothesis is the likelihood (Fisher 1970; Edwards 1984). The *likelihood* for a hypothesis H given a set of observations F is defined as the probability, $L(H) = P(F; H)$, with which the observations have occurred, the probability being calculated under the targeted hypothesis. For example, using the hypothesis of the previous paragraph, if the parents have three children, the first two with A+ phenotypes and the third with an A− phenotype, the likelihood is calculated as ($\frac{3}{4}$) × ($\frac{3}{4}$) × ($\frac{1}{4}$) = $\frac{9}{64}$ (see problem 3.3).

As will be seen in the next paragraph, it is often different values of an unknown parameter (rather than different hypotheses) whose likelihoods are of interest. The likelihood, although defined as a probability, is used as a function of the unknown parameter values, whereas probability is a function of an event. The two quantities, likelihood and probability, thus have very different properties and follow different laws (Fisher 1970).

When comparing hypotheses (or values of an unknown parameter), the absolute values of their likelihoods are not generally meaningful so that they are often scaled by suitable constants. The *odds* in favor of hypothesis H_1 versus H_2 are expressed by the likelihood ratio, $R = L(H_1)/L(H_2)$, often written as $R{:}1$. For example, in gene mapping of several linked markers, the hypotheses of interest may be the different locus orders (e.g., O'Connell et al. 1987). The natural logarithm of the likelihood, $S(H) = \ln[L(H)]$, is referred to as the *support* for hypothesis H (or for a particular value, H, of an unknown parameter).

In linkage analysis between two loci, the two basic hypotheses are free recombination (H_0) and linkage (H_1). They are defined through the value of the recombination fraction, free recombination corresponding to $\theta = \frac{1}{2}$ and linkage corresponding to $\theta < \frac{1}{2}$. Conventionally (see section 4.1), the common (decimal) logarithm of the likelihood ratio, the so-called lod score

$$Z(\theta) = \log_{10}[L(\theta)/L(\frac{1}{2})], \tag{3.1}$$

is used as the measure of support for linkage versus absence of linkage. For example, if observations consist of k recombinants and $n - k$ nonrecombinants, the corresponding lod score is given by

$$Z(\theta) = \begin{cases} n \log(2) + k \log(\theta) + (n - k) \log(1 - \theta) & \text{if } \theta > 0 \\ n \log(2) & \text{if } \theta = 0, \end{cases} \tag{3.2}$$

where the domain is usually $0 \leq \theta \leq \frac{1}{2}$.

3.2. Maximum Likelihood Estimation

Many models or hypotheses contain variables, called *parameters*, whose values are unknown and have to be estimated on the basis of observations. In the example used above, the population gene frequency p of allele A is such a parameter. In statistical terminology, observations are random variables. Any function of random variables which does not depend on unknown parameters is termed a *statistic*. In particular, *estimates* or *estimators* are functions of the observations which are constructed to estimate unknown parameter values. For instance, consider a sample of individuals of size n, k of whom are of phenotype A + (genotypes A/A or A/a), the remaining $n - k$ being of phenotype A − (genotypes a/a). Under Hardy-Weinberg equilibrium, the proportion of A − individuals in the population is expected to be equal to $q = (1 - p)^2$. The commonly used estimate of that proportion is simply the observed proportion of A − individuals in the sample, $(n - k)/n = 1 - (k/n)$. Since $p = 1 - \sqrt{q}$, the estimate of p is taken to be $1 - [1 - (k/n)]^{1/2}$.

Various statistical methods of parameter estimation exist. A very general one is the method of maximum likelihood (Fisher 1921). It is based on the likelihood function of a parameter, which is, as defined above, the probability of the observations used as a function of the unknown parameter or parameters. For example, take the sample of n observations considered in the previous paragraph, k of whom are A + (occurring with probability $1 - q$) and $n - k$ of whom are A − (occurring with probability q). The log likelihood is then proportional to $S(q) = \ln L(q) = (n - k) \ln(q) + k \ln(1 - q)$. The *maximum likelihood estimate* (MLE) $\hat{q}$ of q is defined as that value of q which maximizes $S(q)$. An MLE of a parameter is usually symbolized by the parameter symbol with a hat on top. Maximization of S may be carried out analytically by taking the first derivative, dS/dq, of S and setting it equal to zero. When $dS/dq = 0$ (the so-called likelihood equation) is solved for q, it results in the MLE, provided that the solution represents a maximum rather than a minimum. For the present example, this procedure leads to the estimate, $\hat{q} = 1 - (k/n)$, which shows that the estimate obtained above is an MLE.

In linkage analysis, as will be seen later, the likelihood cannot generally be maximized analytically. Instead, MLEs must be found numerically by varying the values of the parameters of interest and recomputing the likelihood for many trial values of the parameter until an approximate maximum is found. An outline of numerical methods will be covered in chapter 5.

3.3. Statistical Properties of Maximum Likelihood Estimates

Maximum likelihood estimates have certain well-known properties, some of which are briefly discussed here. For a more detailed treatment of this subject, see Elandt-Johnson (1971).

1. It is often easier to find the *MLE of a function of a parameter* rather than of the parameter itself. In the example of the previous section, the MLE of the proportion q of A− individuals was simply given by $1 - (k/n)$, the observed proportion of A− individuals in the sample. It is a function of the parameter of interest, the gene frequency p: $q = (1 - p)^2$. For any monotonic function (one-to-one transformation), $p = f(q)$, if $\hat{q}$ is the MLE of q, then $\hat{p} = f(\hat{q})$ is the MLE of p. This rule provides the justification for the derivation of the estimate of p in the previous section, since $q = (1 - p)^2$ is monotonic in the domain of p. As another example, assume that in a genetic counseling situation one needs to know the probability, θ^2, that a recombination has occurred in both of two parents. An MLE, $\hat{\theta} = k/n$ (the proportion of recombinants out of n phase-known meioses), is available for θ. The MLE estimate of θ^2 is then given by $(k/n)^2$ because θ^2 is monotonic for $\theta \geq 0$.

2. Maximum likelihood estimates are often *biased*. In repeated samples of the same data type, the MLE can occur in a variety of values. For example, consider the estimate of the recombination fraction, $\hat{\theta} = k/n$, where k is the number of recombinants and $n - k$ is the number of nonrecombinants. This estimate can assume $n + 1$ values ($0/n$, $1/n$, etc.), and the probability of each outcome is given by the binomial formula, $\binom{n}{k}\theta^k(1 - \theta)^{n-k}$. In general, if $\hat{\theta}_i$ denotes the ith outcome of a particular MLE of θ, and p_i is the probability with which it occurs, then the weighted average,

$$E(\hat{\theta}) = \sum p_i \hat{\theta}_i, \qquad (3.3)$$

is the expected value or *expectation* of the estimator $\hat{\theta}$ (an example is calculated below). If it is equal to the (true) parameter value θ, then $\hat{\theta}$ is said to be unbiased. The quantity,

$$b(\hat{\theta}) = E(\hat{\theta}) - \theta, \qquad (3.4)$$

is called the bias of $\hat{\theta}$. For binomial and multinomial proportions, the observed class frequencies are unbiased estimators of the class proportions (probabilities), but estimates of nonlinear functions of the class probabilities are generally biased. In the example given above, the frequency $(n - k)/n$ is an unbiased estimate of the proportion q of A− individuals, but the estimate of the gene frequency $p = 1 - \sqrt{q}$ must be biased. Bias reduction techniques for this case were proposed by Huether and Murphy (1980). A general method for bias reduction is the jackknife procedure (see discussion in Weir 1990).

Bolling and Murphy (1979) demonstrated strong biases in the estimate of the recombination fraction from certain family types. These biases are

Table 3.1. Calculation of Expected Value $E(\hat{\theta}) = 0.095$ for $n = 3$ Recombination Events and Known Recombination Fraction 0.1 (k = Number of Recombinants; $P(k)$ = binomial probabilities)

	k	$P(k)$	$\hat{\theta}$	$\hat{\theta} \times P(k)$
	0	0.729	0	0
	1	0.243	1/3	0.0810
	2	0.027	1/2	0.0135
	3	0.001	1/2	0.0005
Sum		1		0.0950

at least partially due to truncation: if θ is estimated from k recombinants and $n - k$ nonrecombinants, then $\hat{\theta} = \frac{1}{2}$ if $k > n/2$. For example, with $n = 3$ and an assumed known recombination fraction of 0.1, table 3.1 demonstrates the calculation of $E(\hat{\theta})$ and shows that it is different from θ. As will be seen later, in linkage analysis the statistical bias due to truncation is not a matter of concern; the really serious biases are those arising from selected sampling when only a portion of the data is analyzed.

Generally, if T is the value of θ in the interval $(0, 1)$ at which the log likelihood is maximized, the recombination fraction estimate is defined as

$$\hat{\theta} = \begin{cases} T \text{ if } T < \frac{1}{2} \\ \frac{1}{2} \text{ otherwise.} \end{cases}$$

If T is unbiased, $\hat{\theta}$ is clearly biased because $T > \frac{1}{2}$ is truncated to $\frac{1}{2}$. However, since $\theta \leq \frac{1}{2}$, the *mean square error* of $\hat{\theta}$ is smaller than that of T: $E[(\hat{\theta} - \theta)^2] < E[(T - \theta)^2]$ (Rao 1973).

In linkage analysis, the recombination fraction θ is generally a complicated function of multinomial proportions and is thus usually biased (for examples, see end of section 6.3 and end of section 7.3). This statistical bias has not received much attention, probably because it tends to vanish with increasing sample size (see paragraph 3).

3. In general, MLEs are *asymptotically unbiased*, that is, their bias tends to vanish when the number of observations becomes large, where *observations* refers to either the number of families or the number of individuals within a family (Bailey 1961).

4. MLEs generally are *consistent*, that is, they are asymptotically unbiased, and their variance becomes zero in the limit for a large number of observations. In other words, the accuracy of MLEs increases with increasing sample size; they "close in" on the true parameter value, so to

speak. In the presence of ascertainment biases, as will be seen in chapter 10, MLEs are often inconsistent, which is a most unfortunate situation because with the accumulation of more and more data, one will find an increasingly precise estimate of a quantity that is different from the one to be estimated.

If an MLE is consistent, the maximum of the expected support function occurs at the true parameter value, under which the expectation is calculated (see inequalities 5f.2.1 on p. 364 in Rao 1973 and section 7.2 in Edwards 1984). This property provides a simple method to prove or disprove consistency (see chapter 10). A simple numerical example may be found in section 5.2.

MLEs are also asymptotically normally distributed, which allows the calculation of approximate confidence intervals from asymptotic variances (see section 5.3).

3.4. Significance Tests

The object of estimating an unknown parameter is often to prove a hypothesis that a researcher suspects is correct. For example, in linkage analysis, a researcher is convinced that two loci are genetically linked. The investigation of five recombination events in one family showed that one was a recombination, whereas four were nonrecombinations. The estimated recombination fraction is thus 20 percent. Is this convincing evidence for linkage? Statistical tests discussed below are designed to answer such questions. Two hypotheses may be distinguished, the null hypothesis, H_0, and the alternative hypothesis, H_1, where H_1 is the one a researcher would like to prove. The principle of significance testing is to assume that H_0 is true until one has good evidence to the contrary. A researcher thus must make an effort to *dis*prove H_0.

On the basis of an experiment and some predefined decision rules discussed below, either a significance test will reject H_0 (the investigator accepts H_1), in which case the experiment is said to have furnished a significant result, or the test will fail to reject H_0, in which case the result is said to be nonsignificant. Depending on the state of nature (i.e., whether H_0 or H_1 is true), the test result is associated with one of two types of errors whose conditional probabilities of occurrence are displayed in table 3.2. A *type I error* (false-positive result) occurs with probability $\alpha = P$(test is significant$|H_0$) when the test rejects H_0 although it is true. A *type II error* (false-negative result) occurs with probability $\beta = P$(test is not significant$|H_1$) when the test fails to reject H_0 although it is false. The power $1 - \beta$ of the test is the probability that it rejects H_0 when it is false.

Table 3.2. Conditional Probabilities of Test Results Given State of Nature

State of Nature	Test Rejects H_0		Sum
	No	Yes	
H_0	$1 - \alpha$	α	1
H_1	β	$1 - \beta$	1

The probability of a type I error is also known as the *significance level* of the test. Significance tests are carried out assuming H_0 is true. Hence, if a test is nonsignificant one cannot say that it accepts H_0. It may be nonsignificant because H_0 is in fact true or because of low power.

Hypotheses are often defined by the values of an unknown parameter. A hypothesis specified by a single parameter value (e.g., $\theta = \frac{1}{2}$) is called a simple hypothesis, whereas a hypothesis admitting a whole range of parameter values (e.g., $\theta < \frac{1}{2}$) is a composite hypothesis.

Consider two simple hypotheses, the null hypothesis $H_0: \theta = \frac{1}{2}$ of free recombination and the alternative hypothesis $H_1: \theta = \theta_1$, where $\theta_1 < \frac{1}{2}$ is some fixed value of the recombination fraction such as 0.1. To test H_0 on the basis of observations, one may use the likelihood ratio, $T(\theta_1) = L(\theta_1)/L(\frac{1}{2})$, as a test statistic. If H_0 is true, one expects small values of T, but if H_1 is true, a tendency towards larger T values is expected. The statistical test consists of the decision rule to reject H_0 if T exceeds a critical point, T_c, and not to reject H_0 if T falls below T_c. Any test such as this, based on the likelihood ratio, is called a *likelihood ratio (LR) test*.

To determine the error probabilities associated with this test, one must work out the distribution of the test statistic, T, where $\alpha = P(T \geq T_c | H_0)$ and $\beta = P(T < T_c | H_1)$. If the assumed distribution for T deviates from its true distribution, the assumed or nominal significance level, α_N, may be different from the actual significance level, α. A test is called *conservative* if $\alpha < \alpha_N$ and nonconservative or anti-conservative if $\alpha > \alpha_N$. In the latter case, under H_0, the test will be significant more often than one anticipates on the basis of the assumed wrong distribution of T.

Not knowing the distribution of the test statistic, one can give an upper bound to α (Haldane and Smith 1947; Smith 1953). With $T(\theta_1) \geq 0$, probability calculus leads to the Chebyshev-type inequality (Johnson and Kotz 1970):

$$\alpha = P[T(\theta_1) \geq T_c | H_0] \leq \frac{E[T(\theta_1)]}{T_c}, \qquad T_c > E[T(\theta_1)]. \tag{3.5}$$

Furthermore, under H_0 the average value of the likelihood ratio is easily shown to be equal to 1 (Haldane and Smith 1947), so that

$$\alpha \leq 1/T_c, \qquad T_c > 1. \tag{3.6}$$

For example, assume a critical limit of $T_c = 10$. The type I error associated with this limit is at most 0.10 (with $T_c = 100$, $\alpha \leq 0.01$). Consider now our previous hypothetical example of one recombinant and four nonrecombinants. For these data, the likelihood ratio is calculated as $T_{obs} = 0.1 \times (0.9)^4/(0.5)^5 = 2.1$. The test of H_0 is thus not significant relative to the critical limit of 10.

In significance tests, one often does not set a rigorous critical boundary for the test statistic. Instead, with an observed value of the test statistic, one calculates the smallest value of α for which T_{obs} is still significant and calls it the *p*-value or *empirical significance level*, $p = P(T > T_{obs}|H_0)$. Notice that p is not the probability that H_1 is true; rather, it represents the probability, given that H_0 is true, that T turns out as large or larger than T_{obs}. With our data, the *p*-value is at most as large as $1/2.1 = 0.48$. Equations (3.5) and (3.6) are discussed further in section 4.6.

The upper bound (3.6) on the significance level is useful when H_0 is tested against a simple alternative hypothesis. In practice, of course, one wants to consider not just a single alternative but the whole range of values, $0 \leq \theta < \frac{1}{2}$. A possible solution proposed by Haldane and Smith (1947) is to use as a test statistic the average value $\bar{T}$ of the likelihood ratio between 0 and $\frac{1}{2}$. For this test statistic, too, inequality (3.6) holds when $T(\theta_1)$ in (3.5) is replaced by $\bar{T}(\theta_1)$, but, presumably, a test based on $\bar{T}$ is not very powerful and will often miss a true linkage.

In the general LR test, the LR criterion $T = L(H_1)/L(H_0)$ is constructed, where the likelihoods are evaluated at the MLEs of the parameter values considered. The n parameters estimated under H_1 may be viewed as spanning an n-dimensional space. H_0 generally represents a subspace of H_1, formed by a number d of linear restrictions. Most tests in general use (e.g., t-test, F-test) are LR tests. Asymptotically, the random variable $2\ln(T)$ follows a chi-square distribution with d degrees of freedom (df) (Rao 1973).

Tests of a hypothesis H_0: $\theta = r_0$ may be carried out in a one-sided or two-sided fashion. The test is two-sided when deviations from H_0 in either direction (low or high values of θ) can be significant. In linkage analysis, the test of H_0: $\theta = \frac{1}{2}$ is carried out in a one-sided manner; one usually does not even look at estimates of θ larger than $\frac{1}{2}$ (but see sections 4.6 and 5.9).

In the tests considered thus far, the number of observations is a fixed constant. In the *sequential probability ratio test* (SPRT), which was developed by Wald (1947) in connection with acceptance sampling, data are accumulated until a stopping criterion is met. The number of observations is thus a random variable. With this test, one tries to discriminate between two simple hypotheses, H_0: $\theta = \theta_0$ (e.g., $\theta_0 = \frac{1}{2}$) and H_1: $\theta = \theta_1$ (e.g., $\theta_1 = 0.2$). Observations are gathered one at a time. After each new observation, the likelihood ratio $T = L(\theta_1)/L(\theta_0)$ is formed for all observations and one of the following three actions is taken:

1. Continue sampling if $B < T < A$
2. Accept H_1 (reject H_0) if $T \geq A$
3. Accept H_0 (reject H_1) if $T \leq B$,

where A and B are suitably chosen constants, for example, $A = 1{,}000$ and $B = 0.01$ (see section 4.1). Approximately, for A large ($A \gg 1$) and B small ($B \ll 1$), the following relationships hold between the constants A, B and the error probabilities α, β defined above:

$$A \approx (1 - \beta)/\alpha, \quad B \approx \beta/(1 - \alpha).$$

Setting $A - B \approx A$, $1 - B \approx 1$, and $A - 1 \approx A$ leads to

$$\alpha \approx 1/A, \qquad \beta \approx B. \tag{3.7}$$

3.5. The Likelihood Method

The support (log likelihood) function may be used for finding an MLE (section 3.2), in which case only its properties at the MLE of the parameter are of interest. LR testing also makes use of the support function. In the so-called likelihood method, however, one uses likelihoods for inference directly (Edwards 1984). The whole support function is meaningful, not just its maximum.

No significance test is carried out in the likelihood approach; rather, hypotheses (or parameter values) are compared with respect to their associated relative likelihoods. In general likelihood ratio testing, only the null hypothesis is relevant for the distribution of the test statistic; in the likelihood method, however, the likelihood under either of the hypotheses to be compared is evaluated. A further difference between the various approaches is that, in maximum likelihood estimation, estimates for the same quantity obtained from different sources are combined by forming a weighted mean, the weights usually being the inverse of the variances. In the likelihood method, on the other hand, support functions are pooled (Edwards 1984).

Each of these approaches has advantages and disadvantages. The results of significance testing can be formulated in terms of probabilities, which is not possible in the likelihood method. On the other hand, hypotheses can be compared by the significance testing method only when they have a hierarchical structure (the null hypothesis must correspond to a subspace of that of the alternative hypothesis), whereas no such restrictions exist in the likelihood method.

As we will see in chapter 4, human linkage analysis uses elements from more than just a single method.

3.6. Interval Estimation

A *confidence interval* is a statistical construct that is intimately tied to the concept of significance tests (Rao 1973). Its definition is more complex than is generally appreciated by nonstatisticians, the reason being that confidence intervals refer to a set of parameter values, but one cannot make simple direct probability statements about parameters (they are not random variables). Imagine a statistical test of the hypothesis, $H_0: p = p_0$, that some parameter p has the value p_0. Further assume that an estimate, $\hat{p}$, of p has been obtained which may or may not have resulted in a significant result of the test of H_0. Generally, consider a set of hypotheses, $H_i: p = p_i$, each of which may be tested using the same estimate $\hat{p}$ of p. The confidence interval of p is now defined as consisting of all those points of p_i for which the corresponding hypothesis H_i is nonsignificant (Fisher 1960; Chotai 1984). When the hypothesis tests are carried out under a significance level α, the associated confidence interval is said to have a confidence coefficient of $100(1 - \alpha)$ percent.

As an example, given an estimate, $\hat{p} = k/n$, constructing an exact confidence interval for the parameter, p, of the binomial distribution may proceed as shown below (Pfanzagl 1966; see also section 4.7 in Armitage and Berry 1987). The test shall be two-sided, resulting in a lower (p_L) and an upper (p_U) bound of the confidence interval, where the two bounds are associated with the respective (one-sided) significance levels, α_L and α_U. These define an associated overall confidence coefficient of $100(1 - \alpha_L - \alpha_U)$ percent. Consider now a value, $p_L < \hat{p} = k/n$. The test of the hypothesis, $p = p_L$, against $p > p_L$ will be significant for large values of k, that is, the critical region of the test consists of all those values, $k \leq i \leq n$, whose probability of occurrence is (less than or) equal to α_L. Therefore, p_L is obtained as the solution of the equation,

$$\alpha_L = \sum_{i=k}^{n} \binom{n}{i} p_L^i (1 - p_L)^{n-i}. \tag{3.8}$$

Analogously, solving

$$\alpha_U = \sum_{i=0}^{k} \binom{n}{i} p_U{}^i (1 - p_U)^{n-i} \tag{3.9}$$

for p_U will yield the upper endpoint of the desired confidence interval. The BINOM program, which solves (3.8) and (3.9) numerically, may be used to determine confidence intervals for binomial proportions. For example, assume that, in a count of recombination events, two recombinants and eighteen nonrecombinants were observed, furnishing an estimate of the recombination fraction of $\hat{\theta} = \frac{2}{20} = 0.10$. Disregarding any considerations of prior probability of linkage (see section 4.2), the 99 percent confidence interval on the (true but unknown) recombination fraction is (0.005, 0.387), and the 95 percent confidence interval is (0.012, 0.317).

For $k = 0$ and $k = n$, equations (3.9) and (3.8) may be solved analytically as follows: When $k = 0$ is observed, the $100(1 - \alpha)$ percent confidence interval for the proportion p consists of all those values for which the probability of the observations, $(1 - p)^n$, is larger than α. The endpoint of the confidence interval is thus obtained by solving $(1 - p)^n = \alpha$ for p (equation [3.9]) so that the confidence interval is given by $(0, 1 - \alpha^{1/n})$. For example, with $\alpha = 0.05$ and $n = 100$, the 95 percent confidence interval associated with $k = 0$ is equal to (0, 0.03). Analogously, for $k = n$, solving $p^n = \alpha$ for p yields the confidence interval $(\alpha^{1/n}, 1)$.

As we will see later, in linkage analysis, determining a proper confidence interval on θ is usually impossible because the distribution of the MLE is unknown. Often, "approximate" p-values are calculated on the basis of the asymptotic distribution of the LR criterion, but in many applications (such as multipoint linkage analysis) the accuracy of this approximation is unknown and may be quite unsatisfactory. Possible solutions may be obtained using computer simulation (see chapter 8).

Another route often taken is to construct *support intervals*. For a unimodal likelihood curve with an interior maximum, the *m*-unit support limits for a parameter are the two parameter values astride the estimate at which the support is *m* units less than the maximum (Edwards 1984). Generally, for *n* parameters, the *m*-unit support region is that region in the parameter space bounded by the $n - 1$ dimensional region on which the support is *m* units less than the maximum. The value $m = 2$ has been recommended (Edwards 1984). In linkage analysis, it is customary to construct a similar support interval. The "1-unit-down" method defines a support region as that (possibly disjoint) region of the parameter space consisting of points with an associated $\log_{10}$ likelihood of $Z_{max} - 1$ or more (Conneally et al. 1985). Figure 4.3 shows the construction of such an interval for one parameter, the recombination fraction. Often, unfortunately, such support intervals are referred to as confidence intervals—another instance of the misuse of a technical term.

3.7. Bayes Theorem

Consider two nonindependent events, E and F, for example, the genotype E and phenotype F of an individual. It is often easy to specify the conditional probability, $P(F|E)$, and difficult to find $P(E|F)$, but the latter is what may be of interest. For example, models of inheritance spell out the penetrance $P(\text{phenotype}|\text{genotype})$, but often one would like to draw inferences on an underlying genotype, given an observed phenotype. Bayes theorem allows the calculation of "inverse" probabilities as follows:

$$P(E|F) = \frac{P(F|E)\ P(E)}{P(F)} = \frac{P(F|E)\ P(E)}{P(F|E)\ P(E)\ +\ P(F|E^c)\ P(E^c)} \qquad (3.10)$$

where E^c stands for the complement of E, "not E." Expression (3.10) may be generalized to a set of mutually exclusive events, E_i, whose conditional probabilities of occurrence are to be calculated, given that an observation F has been made. In analogy to (3.10), the conditional probability of the kth event E_k is then given by

$$P(E_k|F) = \frac{P(F|E_k)\ P(E_k)}{\Sigma_j P(F|E_j)\ P(E_j)}. \qquad (3.11)$$

A streamlined form of the Bayes theorem is often presented in a table with columns that correspond to the different events E_i of interest, the rows being formed by the various unconditional and conditional probabilities (Murphy and Chase 1975; Conneally and Rivas 1980). Some of the rows are often labeled "prior" and "posterior," but this is not done here, as no connection to bayesian inference shall be implied. As an example, consider a rare dominant disease with population frequency p of the disease allele. Two parents, one of whom is affected, have a number of children, and the two events of interest are E_1 and E_2 denoting homozygous and heterozygous disease status of the affected parent, respectively. Barring phenotypic differences between heterozygous and homo-

Table 3.3. Example of Calculation of Inverse Probabilities Using the Bayes Theorem (Probabilities P Explained in Text)

	E_1	E_2	Sum
Unconditional P	$p/(2 - p)$	$2(1 - p)/(2 - p)$	1
Conditional P	1	$(\frac{1}{2})^n$	—
Joint P^a	$p/(2 - p)$	$\dfrac{(1 - p)(\frac{1}{2})^{n-1}}{2 - p}$	$\dfrac{p + (1 - p)(\frac{1}{2})^{n-1}}{2 - p}$
Inverse cond. P^b	$\dfrac{2^{n-1}p}{2^{n-1}p + 1 - p}$	$\dfrac{1 - p}{2^{n-1}p + 1 - p}$	1

^{a} Multiply the two columns above.
^{b} Divide column above by sum on its right.

zygous affected individuals, the unconditional (sometimes called "prior") probability that the affected parent is homozygous is given as follows: The population frequency of homozygous affecteds is p^2 and that of heterozygous affecteds is $2p(1 - p)$. The relative frequency of the former is thus $P(E_1) = p^2/[p^2 + 2p(1 - p)] = p/(2 - p)$, and that of the latter is $P(E_2) = 2(1 - p)/(2 - p)$. These two probabilities are unconditional with respect to our observation F, but they are, of course, conditional on that parent's being affected. Assume now that all n children are affected, which represents the observation F. What is then the conditional (sometimes called "posterior") probability $P(E_1|F)$ that the affected parent is homozygous?

Table 3.3 shows the relevant calculations. On top one lists the set of mutually exclusive events E_i, for which "inverse" conditional probabilities shall be computed. The first line simply gives the relative unconditional probabilities of these events. On the second line, one computes the probabilities of the observation F ("n affected children") given each of the events E_i. In this case, for $E_1 = $ "affected parent is homozygous," all children are affected with probability 1. For $E_2 = $ "affected parent is heterozygous," each of the children is affected with probability ½. The answer to our question is obtained as the first expression in the last line. For example, given three affected children, the affected parent has an "inverse" conditional probability of $4p/(3p + 1)$ of being homozygous as compared with the unconditional probability of $p/(2 - p)$. For small p (disease rare), the two probabilities are approximately equal to $4p$ and $\frac{1}{2}p$, respectively, so that having three affected children increases the chances of the affected parent being homozygous by a factor of 8.

Problems

For problems 3.1–3.3, assume a gene with two alleles, *A* and *a*, and gene frequency $p = P(A)$, where the genotypes A/A and A/a determine the phenotype A +, and a/a determines the phenotype A −. (This example was used at the beginning of section 3.1.) Genotypes are assumed to be in Hardy-Weinberg equilibrium.

Problem 3.1. For an individual with phenotype A + who has no children, how could we be certain that he or she has genotype A/a? Hint: Consider the parents' phenotypes.

Problem 3.2. Assume two parents with phenotypes A + each, where the parents of these two individuals are unknown. What is the probability of their having a child with phenotype A +? Does this probability stay the same for each subsequent child, irrespective of the known phenotypes of children already born?

Problem 3.3. In the example of the three children with phenotypes A +, A +, and A −, whose parents both have genotypes A/a, the likelihood (probability of children's phenotypes) was calculated as $L_1 = (\frac{3}{4}) \times (\frac{3}{4}) \times (\frac{1}{4}) = \frac{9}{64}$. Another way of looking at this situation is to compute the probability that, of three children, two have phenotype A + and one has phenotype A − (only these two phenotypes are possible). According to the binomial formula, this probability is given by $L_2 = 3 \times (\frac{3}{4})^2 \times (\frac{1}{4}) = \frac{27}{64}$. Why are L_1 and L_2 different? What is the significance of this difference? Which is the correct likelihood?

Problem 3.4. Assume that, in ten opportunities for recombination, no recombination has been found such that $\hat{\theta} = 0$. What is the 90 percent confidence interval for the true recombination fraction based on this result?

4.

Methods of Linkage Analysis

This chapter is intended to introduce the reader to the basic principles of human linkage analysis as currently carried out involving two loci (methods involving more than two loci are introduced in chapter 6). A brief historical review is provided below, but it is by no means complete and only touches upon some of the earlier approaches to linkage analysis. For the novice in linkage analysis, it will be important to carefully follow the analysis presented for the pedigree shown in figure 4.1.

4.1. A Brief Historical Review

The so-called *direct method* of linkage analysis proceeds by directly observing and counting recombinants and nonrecombinants. The total of these recombination events is often referred to as the number of opportunities for recombination, n. If the number of observed recombinations is denoted by k, then a "natural" estimate of the recombination fraction is given by $\hat{\theta} = k/n$.

The direct method is appealing because one can see all recombination events. Many researchers, particularly in the past, have trusted no other method. However, with unknown phase, incomplete penetrance, and other factors clouding the direct view of genotypes through phenotypes, the direct method often extracts only a limited amount of information from the data, sometimes even in a biased manner. A pedigree in which the direct method extracts all linkage information is shown in figure 4.1. The estimate $\hat{\theta} = k/n$ is then the maximum likelihood estimate of the recombination fraction.

In figure 4.1, the dark symbols represent individuals affected with the autosomal dominant trait Charcot-Marie-Tooth neuropathy (CMT1), also called hereditary motor and sensory neuropathy type 1. On the left side of figure 4.1, the ABO blood types are shown. The first step in this analysis is to find out as much as possible about the genotypes, which may proceed as follows (results are shown on the right side of fig. 4.1): Individuals 2.1 and 3.2 are both homozygous normal, that is, they have the genotype d/d at the trait locus, whereas 3.1 must be heterozygous, D/d, since he inherited a normal allele from his mother and a disease allele from his father. As the disease is rare, the grandfather may be assumed to be heterozygous at the disease locus, but this assumption is not crucial for the present analysis. At the ABO locus, by his phenotype, 3.1 could be A/A or A/O, but the presence of O children as well as the O genotype of the grandmother excludes the A/A genotype, so that 3.1 must be doubly heterozygous. Furthermore, knowing that the alleles d and O came from his mother determines his phase, which is thus dO/DA, as shown on the right side of figure 4.1. Since 3.2 is doubly homozygous, each of the four children carries a dO haplotype. The remaining haplotypes must be DA in 4.1 and DO in each of 4.2 through 4.4. The father has therefore produced one nonrecombinant (DA) and three recombinant gametes, leading to the estimate $\frac{3}{4} = 0.75$ for the recombination fraction. As the true value of the recombination fraction is assumed to range from 0 through $\frac{1}{2}$, the $k/n = \frac{3}{4}$ is usually interpreted as $\hat{\theta} = \frac{1}{2}$.

Scoring recombination events in figure 4.1 is carried out by inspection of the children's phenotypes. A child is thus usually called a "recombinant" or a "nonrecombinant" depending on whether or not recombination occurred. One must keep in mind, however, that the events scored have taken place in one of the parents at the time of meiosis, preceding formation of the gametes.

Knowing the parental genotypes (including phase) is a necessary condition for direct linkage analysis. It is, however, not sufficient in all cases. For example, as will be seen later, two phase-known doubly heterozygous parents can have children who do not unequivocally reveal recombination events in the parents. The direct method is particularly useful for loci on the X chromosome, where the alleles in males are always in coupling (except for loci in the pseudoautosomal region).

Consider now the situation that the grandparents in figure 4.1 are unknown. This leaves the phase in the father (3.1) unknown so that the children cannot unequivocally be scored as recombinants or nonrecombinants. Each child is either a recombinant, given one of the phases, or a nonrecombinant, given the other phase. Early geneticists were under the impression that such pedigrees did not yield any information on linkage. The German physician Bernstein (1931) was the first to point out a possible type of indirect analysis, using the following approach: When k is the number of recombinants, given one of the phases in the doubly hetero-

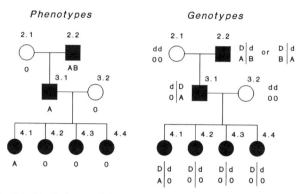

Figure 4.1. Kinship L (adapted from fig. 2 in Dyck et al. 1983). Phenotypes of the dominant disease CMT1 and the ABO blood types are shown on the *left*; genotypes are shown on the *right*.

zygous parent, then k may be small or large depending on the assumed phase. However, the product $y = k(n - k)$ is the same in either phase. Furthermore, the average value of this y statistic depends on the recombination fraction and is largest for $\theta = \frac{1}{2}$ and zero for $\theta = 0$. For several types of matings, Bernstein (1931) published the mean values of y for different sibship sizes and values of the recombination fraction. One of these tables is reproduced in Stern 1973. Later, R. A. Fisher showed that y statistics are less efficient than maximum likelihood estimates; that is, they waste some of the information contained in the data.

For the linkage analysis of two-generation families, Fisher (1935a) implemented a systematic scheme of the maximum likelihood method in the form of u *statistics*. These are functions of the observed frequencies of offspring phenotype classes such that, with a transformation of the recombination fraction, the likelihood (probability of occurrence of the observations) can be represented in a particularly simple form, although this involves some approximations. The whole procedure is quite elaborate, taking into account various mating types and modes of ascertainment. It was later extended by Finney but will not be pursued here any further. The interested reader is referred to Smith 1953 or Bailey 1961. As this method is applicable to two-generation data only, it is no longer in use.

Bell and Haldane (1937) analyzed known multigenerational pedigrees segregating hemophilia and color blindness by computing the likelihood with respect to gene frequency, recombination fraction between the two loci, and mutation rate at the hemophilia locus. They even discussed such modern concepts as germline mosaicism, although not under this name.

Ten years later, Haldane and Smith (1947) calculated the likelihood for seventeen pedigrees with hemophilia and color blindness, a task judged "very laborious" by the authors, although calculation of the likelihood is simpler in X linkage than in autosomal linkage. Based on the likelihood, these authors applied several analysis techniques. The maximum likelihood estimate of the recombination fraction between hemophilia and color blindness was equal to 9.5 percent.

Morton (1955) put forward the use of *sequential test procedures* in the linkage analysis between two loci, recognizing that the typical method of sampling small families was in fact sequential. Applying Wald's (1947) sequential probability ratio test (see section 3.4) of the null hypothesis $\theta_0 = \frac{1}{2}$ versus a fixed alternative value, $\theta_1 < \frac{1}{2}$, and postulating a power of 0.99 and a significance level of 0.001, he proposed to keep sampling families as long as

$$Z_1 < Z(\theta) < Z_0 | Z_0 = 3, \; Z_1 = -2, \tag{4.1}$$

where $Z(\theta)$ is Barnard's (1949) *lod* or *lod score*, $\log_{10}[L(\theta_1)/L(\theta_0)]$, summed over all families in the sample (for a simple step-by-step introduction of lod scores, see section 4.3). Sampling is terminated when either of the two bounds in (4.1) is reached or exceeded. When $Z(\theta)$ is equal to or larger than the upper bound, $Z_0 = 3$, the hypothesis of free recombination is rejected, and when $Z(\theta)$ reaches or drops below the lower bound, $Z_1 = -2$, the hypothesis of free recombination (absence of linkage) is accepted. The values of the two bounds in (4.1) are a consequence of Morton's (1955) requirement of a power of 0.99 at $\theta = \theta_1$ and a significance level of 0.001 in the sequential test (see section 3.4). The significance level was chosen to be this small because of the low prior probability of linkage for autosomal loci. For X-linked loci, as outlined in section 4.4, a less stringent critical lod score limit $Z_0 = 2$ is deemed sufficient.

Morton (1955) also defined a "posterior type I error,"

$$P(H_0|s) = \frac{P(s|H_0)P(H_0)}{P(s|H_0)P(H_0) + P(s|H_1)P(H_1)}, \tag{4.2}$$

where s stands for the event that the test is significant (Z_{max} exceeds 3), $P(s|H_0) = 0.001$ is the significance level, $P(s|H_1)$ is the average power for different values of θ, and $P(H_1) = 0.05$ is the approximate prior probability of linkage. Morton's (1955) choice of power and significance level was dictated by the aim that the rate of false-positive results (4.2) stay below 5 percent. For example, assuming an average power of 0.50, equation (4.2) yields $P(H_0|s) = 0.04$.

Statistically, the sequential test is no longer carried out in its original form (the current procedures are described in section 4.3). In particular, one no longer tests for linkage under a fixed value of the recombination fraction. Several of Morton's (1955) original recommendations, however, are still in current use.

In addition to proposing a sequential test for linkage, Morton (1955) streamlined its application by recommending that researchers accumulate and publish results of linkage analyses in the form of lod scores at a fixed set of θ values covering the range from 0 through $\frac{1}{2}$. This simple concept proved to be very effective. For two-point analyses, it is still in general use today. For many types of two-generation families, Morton (1955) and others published lod score tables that are reminiscent of the tables of y published by Bernstein (1931). The ease with which Morton's lod score concept could be applied represented a breakthrough in linkage analysis.

A very general approach to the analysis of pedigree data, proposed by Elston and Stewart (1971), set the stage for the currently used maximum likelihood estimation and likelihood ratio test procedures. Although not restricted to linkage analysis, this area is the one in which it probably proved most fruitful. This approach allows the representation of the likelihood, or lod score, for pedigrees with any number of generations and for qualitative as well as quantitative data. Missing information is dealt with in a very elegant manner. Furthermore, Elston and Stewart (1971) presented a recursive method, the *Elston-Stewart algorithm* (see section 8.2), for fast and exact calculation of pedigree likelihoods.

Based on the Elston-Stewart (1971) algorithm, I developed the *LIPED* computer program (for *li*kelihood in *ped*igrees) for linkage analysis between pairs of loci (Ott 1974a). Although it is restricted to two-point analysis, it is still in common use worldwide. Details of the program are discussed in section 8.3.

In the 1970s, methods of somatic cell genetics and of cytogenetics became widely available, allowing the localization of genetic markers to single chromosomes and to specific chromosome segments. Towards the end of the decade, the seemingly old-fashioned "family method" seemed doomed to disappear. The introduction, at the beginning of the 1980s, of molecular genetics methods made genetic linkage analysis suddenly very interesting again and led to an ever-increasing importance of these techniques.

The increasing availability of DNA polymorphisms as genetic markers called for the introduction of multipoint analysis methods, by which more than just two loci can be analyzed jointly (see chapter 6). One of the most general multipoint analysis programs is the *LINKAGE* program package (Lathrop et al. 1984), but various other programs exist, which are discussed in chapter 6.

Methods of linkage analysis other than those based on the pedigree likelihood have been proposed. They are discussed in section 4.8.

4.2. Prior and Posterior Distribution of θ

As will be seen in section 4.3, in this book the recombination fraction is treated as an unknown parameter that is to be estimated by maximum likelihood techniques. Other approaches exist, however, and one of them is briefly discussed here (for a "rough and ready" determination of the posterior probability of linkage, see section 4.4). It assumes that the recombination fraction θ (or the event that two loci are a distance θ apart) is a random variable with a prior density function, $f(\theta)$. The prior density is then modified by the observations, F, leading to a posterior density, $f(\theta|F)$. This approach is generally referred to as the bayesian method of linkage analysis. Related questions of prior probability of linkage and the number of markers required to span the human genome were discussed in section 2.7. The mathematically less inclined reader may want to skip the derivation presented in the subsequent paragraph and turn directly to the example in the next paragraph.

Smith (1959) assumed a mixed prior density for θ, which is uniform $f(\theta) = \frac{1}{11}$ on $\theta < \frac{1}{2}$, and a point mass of $\frac{21}{22}$ at $\theta = \frac{1}{2}$. The prior probability of linkage, therefore, is taken to be $\frac{1}{22} \approx 0.05$. With F standing for the observed family data, for $0 \leq \theta < \frac{1}{2}$, the posterior density of θ is obtained by the Bayes theorem as

$$f(\theta|F) = \frac{f(F|\theta)\,f(\theta)}{\int_{0 \leq t < 1/2} f(F|t)\,f(t)\,dt + f(F|\frac{1}{2})\,P(\theta = \frac{1}{2})}. \tag{4.3}$$

In this expression, $f(F|\theta)$ is the pedigree likelihood, $L(\theta)$, for a given value of θ. Dividing it by $L(\frac{1}{2})$ leads to the likelihood ratio, $L^*(\theta) = L(\theta)/L(\frac{1}{2})$, which is the antilog of the lod score, $Z(\theta)$. With this, equation (4.3) can be written as

$$f(\theta|F) = \frac{L^*(\theta)\,f(\theta)}{\int_{0 \leq t < 1/2} L^*(t)\,f(t)\,dt + P(\theta = \frac{1}{2})}. \tag{4.4}$$

If numerator and denominator in (4.4) are divided through by the prior probability of linkage, $P(0 \leq \theta < \frac{1}{2}) = \frac{1}{22}$, then the integral in the denominator becomes the expectation of $L^*(\theta)$, that is, the average height, Λ, of the (observed) likelihood ratio curve. Thus, one has $f(\theta|F) =$

$22\ L^*(\theta)\ f(\theta)/(\Lambda + 21)$. Integrating this over the range $0 \le \theta < \frac{1}{2}$ furnishes the posterior probability of linkage,

$$P(\theta < \tfrac{1}{2}) = \Lambda/(\Lambda + 21). \tag{4.5}$$

In practice, one divides the interval $0 \le \theta < \frac{1}{2}$ into a number of segments, depending on the number of θ values at which lod scores were calculated. The ith segment, of length b_i, then contains the likelihood ratio, $L^*(\theta_i)$, where $b_i = \frac{1}{2}(\theta_{i+1} - \theta_i) - \frac{1}{2}(\theta_i - \theta_{i-1})$, $\Sigma b_i = 0.5$. The average height of the likelihood ratio is then approximated by

$$\Lambda \approx 2 \sum L^*(\theta_i)\ b_i, \tag{4.6}$$

that is, the area underneath the likelihood curve divided by the length, $\frac{1}{2}$, of the θ axis.

As a numerical example, assume that, in a linkage analysis between two loci, one recombinant was observed out of twelve opportunities for recombination, so that the antilog of the lod score is given by $L^*(\theta) = 2^{12}\theta(1 - \theta)^{11}$. Using the values shown in table 4.1, the average height of the likelihood ratio, approximated by (4.6), is then obtained as 52.672, resulting in a value of 0.71 for Smith's (1959) posterior probability of linkage (4.5). Although a priori the chance that the two genes are located on the same chromosome is only about 5 percent, after only one recombinant in twelve opportunities is observed, this "chance" or belief is increased to 72 percent. For definite evidence of linkage, this method usually requires a posterior probability of linkage of 95 percent or higher.

The mathematically inclined reader may be interested in the exact solution to the calculations approximated above. Since the likelihood ratio is known analytically, one need not divide the θ axis into segments; rather, one solves the beta integral, $\int_{0 \le \theta < 1/2} \theta(1 - \theta)^{n-1}\ d\theta = [1 - (n + 2)(\frac{1}{2})^{n+1}]/[n(n + 1)]$. With the appropriate adjustments, this leads

Table 4.1. Lod Score $Z(\theta_i)$, Likelihood Ratio $L^*(\theta_i)$, and Interval Width b_i at Selected Values of θ_i for the Calculation of the Posterior Probability of Linkage

i	θ_i	b_i	$Z(\theta_i)$	$L^*(\theta_i)$
1	0.01	0.030	1.56	36.7
2	0.05	0.045	2.07	116.5
3	0.10	0.075	2.11	128.5
4	0.20	0.100	1.85	70.4
5	0.30	0.100	1.38	24.3
6	0.40	0.150	0.77	5.9

to a figure of 0.73 for the posterior probability of linkage. The approximate method of computation is thus quite reliable.

4.3. The Lod Score Method

In this section, the lod score method of linkage analysis for pairs of loci is introduced with as little mathematical statistics as possible. For the statistically minded reader, I would like to point out that the statistical techniques used in current linkage analysis are mostly based on maximum likelihood estimation and likelihood ratio testing. Occasionally, methods from other fields are also used, which may be irritating to the reader looking for a methodologically pure approach, but I am trying to present linkage analysis the way it is actually carried out. Statistical properties of the various procedures, where known, will be dealt with in later chapters. A scholarly review from a statistical viewpoint of the lod score method and some of its predecessors was given by Chotai (1984).

Under favorable circumstances, the phenotypes in a pedigree imply the underlying genotypes in such a way that recombination events can be scored unambiguously. An example is shown in figure 4.1, in which the phase of the doubly heterozygous father is known. In that example, one counts three recombinants and one nonrecombinant, leading to an estimate of the recombination of $\frac{3}{4}$, which is usually interpreted as $\hat{\theta} = \frac{1}{2}$.

A complication arises when parental phase is unknown. As an example, consider family 79 in Bodmer et al. (1987) segregating the autosomal dominant disease familial adenomatous polyposis (APC, adenomatosis polyposis coli, chromosomal location 5q21-q22). The family is displayed on the left side of figure 4.2. The phenotypes are affection statuses (filled symbols for affected, open symbols for unaffected) and typing results (allele numbers) for a chromosome 5 marker gene identified by the probe C11p11. In the parental generation, the two rightmost individuals are identical (monozygotic) twins. Genetically, they represent two independent expressions of a single zygote so that, for this marker, only one typing result is shown (in the analysis, they count as one individual). The affected females' spouse is unknown and is thus not shown—a customary abbreviation. Presumably, that spouse was unaffected.

The genetic interpretation of family 79 in Bodmer et al. (1987) is shown on the right side of figure 4.2. The grandmother is dead but is known to have been affected. Since she has unaffected offspring, she must be heterozygous F/f at the disease locus, where F stands for the disease allele and f for the normal allele. The grandfather is homozygous for both

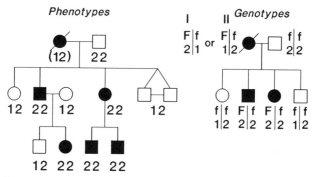

Figure 4.2. Family 79 (adapted from fig. 1 in Bodmer et al. 1987). Phenotypes of familial adenomatous polyposis (dominant) and a chromosome 5 gene identified by the probe C11p11 are shown on the *left*; the relevant genotypes are shown on the *right*.

the disease and the marker genes and thus always passes an *f 2* haplotype (gamete) to his children. The grandmother is untyped but her marker type can be inferred to be *1 2*, since some children received a *1* allele and others a *2* allele from her. Genotypes that can be unambiguously inferred are generally given in parentheses. However, her phase is unknown, the two possible phases being indicated by *I* and *II*. The two affected parents in the parental generation (middle generation on the left side of fig. 4.2) are both homozygous at the marker locus so that they are uninformative for linkage, that is, their children cannot reveal recombination events between marker and disease in the parents (for a formal demonstration of this fact, see section 5.1) and are thus not shown on the right side of figure 4.2.

If the grandmother's phase is *I*, her offspring reveal four nonrecombinations, and, if it is *II*, there are four recombinations, the two cases having equal a priori probabilities. Therefore, one cannot count recombinants and nonrecombinants in this family. Estimating the recombination fraction is then carried out by the method of maximum likelihood (see section 3.2). In this method, one calculates the likelihood (i.e., the probability of occurrence of the data) for a variety of assumed values of θ and selects that θ value associated with the highest likelihood as the best estimate. It is designated by the symbol $\hat{\theta}$.

In abbreviated form, the likelihood for this family is calculated as follows: Given phase *I*, there are four nonrecombinants, each of which occurs independently with probability $1 - \theta$, so that the likelihood for the four nonrecombinants is equal to $(1 - \theta)^4$. Analogously, given phase *II*, the likelihood is θ^4. Combining these results and allowing for the fact that each phase has a probability of occurrence of ½ lead to the likelihood for family 79 in Bodmer et al. (1987) of

$$L(\theta) = \frac{1}{2}[(1 - \theta)^4 + \theta^4]. \tag{4.7}$$

For any value assumed for θ, the corresponding likelihood can be calculated. The result is always between 0 and 1, but the numerical value of $L(\theta)$ is not generally of interest because it very much depends on the size of the family—the larger the family, the smaller the likelihood.

A more relevant quantity is the likelihood ratio that is obtained by dividing $L(\theta)$ by its value under free recombination,

$$L^*(\theta) = L(\theta)/L(\frac{1}{2}). \tag{4.8}$$

This likelihood ratio has loosely been called odds for linkage as it indicates, for a given value of $\theta < \frac{1}{2}$, how much higher the likelihood of the data is under linkage than under absence of linkage. Generally, however, the term *odds* refers to a ratio of probabilities and not of likelihoods (Armitage and Berry 1987). Notice that, by construction, $L^*(\frac{1}{2}) = 1$. For family 79, one obtains $L^*(\theta) = 8[(1 - \theta)^4 + \theta^4]$.

It is usually convenient to work not with the likelihood ratio but rather with its logarithm (to the base 10), the so-called *lod* or *lod score* (Barnard 1949),

$$Z(\theta) = \log_{10}L^*(\theta) = \log_{10}[L(\theta)/L(\frac{1}{2})]. \tag{4.9}$$

By construction, $Z(0.50) = 0$. Now, our estimate of the recombination fraction is that value of θ at which $Z(\theta)$ is highest. For family 79, the lod score is given by the expression $\log(8) + \log[(1 - \theta)^4 + \theta^4]$. For example, at $\theta = 0, 0.01, 0.05$, and 0.10, one obtains the respective lod scores $0.903, 0.886, 0.814$, and 0.720. The θ estimate is thus $\hat{\theta} = 0$, the same as if phase *I* has been assumed to be known, but this is not generally the case (see problem 4.2). Phase *I* is more plausible than phase *II* in the following sense: Under phase *I*, the offspring (four nonrecombinants) have probability of occurrence $(1 - \theta)^4$ which, at $\hat{\theta} = 0$, is equal to 1. Under phase *II*, the offspring (four recombinants) occur with probability θ^4 which, in the range $0 \le \theta \le \frac{1}{2}$, attains its maximum value of $(\frac{1}{2})^4 = 0.0625$ at $\theta = \frac{1}{2}$. The conditional likelihood, given phase *I*, is thus considerably higher than that given phase *II*.

Because of a variety of complicating factors such as incomplete penetrance, missing information, unequal male and female recombination fractions, etc., lod scores are rarely calculated analytically as in the model case discussed above. Instead, one has computer programs carry out this arduous job (see chapter 8).

In section 1.2, parents were said to be potentially informative for linkage when they are doubly heterozygous. A family or set of families is called *informative for linkage* when the lod score $Z(\theta)$ is different from zero for any value of $\theta < \frac{1}{2}$. Similarly, offspring are termed informative for linkage when their phenotype reveals linkage information.

As the observations in different families are statistically independent, lod scores at a fixed θ value can simply be added over families (assuming homogeneity; see heterogeneity in chapter 9). In publications, linkage analysis results are usually presented in a table with rows referring to different families and columns referring to different θ values. The body of such a table then contains the lod scores for the ith family at the jth θ value. The bottom row usually contains the sum of the lod scores for the different families at the corresponding θ values.

As is pointed out in chapter 8, linkage programs permit relatively easy calculations of lod scores. However, in addition to computing lods, one should also inspect the data for any unusual features that may not be reflected in the lod score. A case in point is skewed segregation. For example, the sex distribution among children is expected roughly to follow a binomial distribution with mean $\frac{1}{2}$, or a parent is expected to pass each of his or her two alleles to an offspring with probability $\frac{1}{2}$. Marked deviations from these expectations can be indicative of errors in the data. These deviations strongly reduce the likelihood of the data, but the reduction occurs both in the numerator and in the denominator of the likelihood ratio and thus cancels, so that skewed distribution does not show in the lod score. I vividly remember a case in which a parent seemingly had passed the same allele to all of her eight offspring; after many days of deliberations, a mix-up of samples in the laboratory was detected and retesting that nuclear family no longer resulted in any unusual segregation. On the other hand, cases of irregular segregation are known to occur and to have a biological basis (see section 11.9).

It has been recommended (Conneally et al. 1985) that one report two-point lod scores (i.e., between pairs of loci) at the following fixed set of θ values: 0, 0.001, 0.05, 0.1, 0.2, 0.3, and 0.4. Generally, lod scores are calculated at values of θ between 0 and $\frac{1}{2}$, but some computer programs (e.g., ILINK in the LINKAGE program package) find the maximum of the log likelihood for the whole range, $0 \leq \theta \leq 1$, the reason being that a value of $\theta > \frac{1}{2}$ with a high associated lod score may be indicative of problems in the data, which it is valuable to know.

Another of the recommendations issued at the Helsinki workshop (Conneally et al. 1985) was to report lod scores with an accuracy of two decimal places. This accuracy is certainly sufficient to represent the maximum lod score as evidence for linkage. However, some analyses such as tests for heterogeneity and computation of standard errors of the recombination estimate employ lod scores for further calculations, in which case two decimal places for the lod scores are insufficient for good accuracy of the final result. Lods should therefore be published with (at least) three decimal places.

4.4. Testing for Linkage

In the previous section, the maximum likelihood method of estimating the recombination was described, where the particular form of that method used in human genetics is known as the lod score method. Here, questions of significance of the result of a linkage analysis are addressed.

Positive lod scores indicate evidence for linkage, and negative lods indicate absence of linkage. When linkage in fact exists, as one accumulates more families, lod scores tend to become larger and larger. The maximum of the lod score, denoted by $Z(\hat{\theta})$ or Z_{max} or $\hat{Z}$, serves as a measure for the weight of the data in favor of the hypothesis of linkage. When that maximum reaches or exceeds a certain critical value, Z_0, the data are said to convey *significant evidence for linkage*. The critical value generally adhered to is the one originally proposed by Morton (1955), $Z_0 = 3$, for autosomal loci, and $Z_0 = 2$ for X-linked loci.

Declaring a linkage result significant when $Z_{max} > 3$ amounts to carrying out a likelihood ratio (LR) test with fixed sample size, which is conceptually quite different from Morton's (1955) sequential test procedure. The theory of LR tests predicts that asymptotically, under the null hypothesis of absence of linkage, $4.6 \times Z_{max}$ follows a chi-square distribution with 1 degree of freedom (df). Consequently, owing to the critical level of $4.6 \times 3 = 13.8$ for chi-square, the asymptotic significance level, α, of this likelihood ratio test for linkage is equal to 0.0001 (one-sided). Depending on the family type, however, the null distribution of Z_{max} can be quite different from chi-square (see section 4.6 for some examples).

For tests against a single alternative value of θ, inequalities (3.5) and (3.6) provide an upper bound for the significance level. Morton (1978) stated that these inequalities also hold in the generalized likelihood ratio test (where θ is estimated rather than fixed in advance), that is,

$$\alpha = P[Z_{max} \geq Z_0 | H_0] \leq 10^{-Z_0}. \qquad (4.10)$$

A heuristic explanation for this statement might be that power and significance level are highest in fully informative matings when the true recombination fraction is zero. In this case, as shown in section 4.6, equation

(4.10) with equality between the left and right sides provides the exact significance level. Chotai (1984) showed that inequality (4.10) indeed holds in the generalized likelihood ratio test. Consequently, the critical lod scores, $Z_0 = 3$ and $Z_0 = 2$ (in the X-linked case), have associated significance levels of no more than $10^{-3} = 0.001$ and $10^{-2} = 0.01$, respectively. Analogously, an observed maximum lod score, Z_{max}, has an associated empirical significance level, which is at most equal to $10^{-Z_{max}}$.

The significance level of the test for linkage is much smaller than the significance levels of 0.05 or 0.01 customarily used in statistical tests. The reason for the low value of α was given by Smith (1953) along the lines of arguments given below (more formal considerations follow from equation [4.2], above). Assume that one tests for linkage at a significance level of 5 percent. This means that, when no linkage exists, one will nonetheless declare the test for linkage significant at the (false-positive) rate of 5 percent. Consider now a test with 100 percent power, one that will detect every linkage whenever it is present. As the a priori chance that a pair of loci will be on the same chromosome is about 5 percent, our perfect test will "detect" as many nonexistent linkages as real ones (true positives). With less than perfect power, of course, the situation is even worse. The remedy lies in lowering the significance level to the much smaller values currently used.

Another way of interpreting the low formal significance level is in terms of a somewhat loosely defined "posterior probability of linkage." Although the prior probability of two random loci being on the chromosome is about 0.05, the chance that two loci are within measurable distance of each other is only $P(H_1) = 0.02$ (Elston and Lange 1975). The posterior probability of linkage is then expressed as

$$P(H_1|F) = \frac{P(F|H_1)P(H_1)}{P(F|H_1)P(H_1) + P(F|H_0)P(H_0)}$$

$$= 0.02R/(0.02R + 0.98),$$

where $R = P(F|H_1)/P(F|H_0)$ is the likelihood (odds) ratio. The conventional critical odds ratio, $R = 1000$, is then seen to correspond to a posterior probability of linkage of 95 percent.

In human linkage analysis, the accuracy of the estimate $\hat{\theta}$ is assessed by constructing a specific support interval. An example is graphically depicted in figure 4.3, which shows the lod score curve for eight recombinants out of forty recombination events. The curve reaches its maximum, $Z_{max} = 3.348$, at $\hat{\theta} = 8/40 = 0.20$. As recommended by Conneally et al. (1985), the $Z_{max} - 1$ *support interval* is obtained by drawing a horizontal

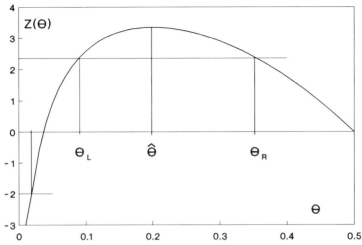

Figure 4.3. Lod score curve for eight recombinants in forty recombination events showing construction of support interval.

straight line at 1 unit of lod score below Z_{max} (here at $Z = 2.348$), provided that $Z_{max} \geq 3$ (otherwise, no support interval is constructed). The points of intersection of this line with the lod score curve, when projected onto the θ axis, mark the endpoints θ_L and θ_R of the support interval. Of course, when the lod score curve keeps increasing towards $\theta = 0$, only the upper bound of the support interval is defined in this way, the lower bound being at $\theta = 0$.

Testing a null hypothesis, $\theta = \theta_0$, such that the test is significant when chi-square exceeds 4.6 (1 lod score unit converted into chi-square units by multiplying it by 4.6) corresponds to an asymptotic significance level of 0.032. Therefore, the support interval defined in the last paragraph is sometimes interpreted as an asymptotic confidence interval, for it consists of all those points θ_0 which render the test nonsignificant. The asymptotic confidence coefficient of said confidence interval is better than 95 percent. According to inequality (4.10), the actual confidence coefficient is at least 90 percent.

A point of logical inconsistency should be noted in applying the $Z_{max} - 1$ support intervals. Generally, in statistical tests, there is a one-to-one correspondence between confidence intervals and test results in that the test is nonsignificant when the confidence interval contains the parameter value specified by the null hypothesis. In linkage analysis, the null parameter value is $\theta = \frac{1}{2}$, which would be included in the confidence interval only when $Z_{max} < 1$. On the other hand, the test is declared significant when $Z_{max} \geq 3$. As pointed out above, this discrepancy has been resolved by the recommendation (Conneally et al. 1985) that a confidence (support) interval should not be constructed while Z_{max} stays below the critical limit of 3. The logically consistent solution, however, is to construct a confidence interval as consisting of all those points with log likelihood larger than $Z_{max} - 3$—when this confidence interval contains $\theta = \frac{1}{2}$, the customary test for linkage is not significant.

In Morton's (1955) sequential test for linkage, the null hypothesis of free recombination ($\theta = \frac{1}{2}$) is not rejected when the lod score at the predetermined value $\theta = \theta_1$ dips below -2. In today's likelihood ratio test approach, that concept is sometimes invoked for constructing a set of "excluded" θ values, although it is incompatible with the support interval defined above. Specifically, all values of θ at which $Z(\theta) < -2$ are said to be definitely excluded. For the case of eight recombinants in forty recombination events shown in figure 4.3, values smaller than 0.015 are excluded by this criterion. This method of defining regions of exclusions or implausibility for θ is used particularly when all lod scores are negative and in the process of mapping a disease gene by testing it against many marker genes and thereby excluding one chromosomal segment after another (see section 11.6 on exclusion mapping).

4.5. Equivalent Observations

For an observed number of known recombinants and nonrecombinants, the corresponding lod score curve is known to have one single maximum, which may be interior (inside the bounds, $0 < \theta < \frac{1}{2}$) or at the boundary points. For family data with missing information, unknown or partially known phase, and other complicating factors, however, the lod score curves may have unusual shapes not seen with known recombination events. The lod score may also have more than one maximum, occasionally even in the interval $[0, \frac{1}{2}]$ (for an example, see Ott 1977b).

In their analysis of color blindness and hemophilia, Bell and Haldane (1937) approximated the likelihood of different families by a function, $\theta^k(1 - \theta)^{n-k}$, where n and k are not necessarily integers, and interpreted n as the number of gametes investigated and k as the number of crossovers found. Edwards (1971, 1976) extended this concept in the manner outlined below.

Generally, the lod score curve for large pedigrees has no simple interpretation. For a rough comparison of an observed lod score curve with that for known recombination events and for an intuitive interpretation of the information content of family data, Edwards (1976) suggested equating the observed Z_{max} with that corresponding to known recombination events and deducing an equivalent number of recombinants and nonrecombinants. If k denotes the number of recombinants out of n opportunities, then $\hat{\theta} = k/n$ is the maximum likelihood estimate of the recombination fraction, and the maximum of the lod score is known to be equal to

$$Z_{max} = \begin{cases} n[\log(2) + \hat{\theta} \log(\hat{\theta}) + (1 - \hat{\theta})\log(1 - \hat{\theta})] & \text{if } \hat{\theta} > 0 \\ n \log(2) & \text{if } \hat{\theta} = 0. \end{cases} \quad (4.11)$$

Working backward from these expressions, one obtains the equivalent numbers

$$n = \begin{cases} Z_{max}/[\log(2) + \hat{\theta} \log(\hat{\theta}) + (1 - \hat{\theta})\log(1 - \hat{\theta})] & \text{if } 0 < \hat{\theta} < \frac{1}{2} \\ Z_{max}/\log(2) & \text{if } \hat{\theta} = 0, \end{cases}$$

and

$$k = n\hat{\theta},$$

where $Z_{max} > 0$ is the maximum lod score obtained for the family data investigated and $\hat{\theta}$ is the θ value at which the maximum of the lod score occurred. This method is not applicable for recombination estimates of $\frac{1}{2}$ as this leads to $n = 0$. The equivalent number n of opportunities for recombination may serve as a measure of information content in the data. The equivalent numbers, n and k, may be obtained in this way from the EQUIV program.

As an example, consider the analysis of familial adenomatous polyposis (APC) discussed in the previous section. In six families, testing APC versus the gene identified by probe C11p11, Bodmer et al. (1987) obtained $Z_{max} = 3.26$ at $\hat{\theta} = 0$. This result corresponds to equivalent numbers of $k = 0$ and $n = 10.83$. Inspection of the data showed that in some matings phase was known and in others phase was unknown. Assigning the most probable genotypes in all cases, the data were consistent with an interpretation of no recombinants among twenty-four meioses (Bodmer et al. 1987). As twenty-four is much higher than the equivalent number of meioses of about eleven, assigning plausible phases and genotypes when these are only partially known is seen to overestimate the amount of information in the data. Looking at this situation from a different angle, the difference between the number of meioses (24) and the equivalent number of meioses (10.83) reflects the loss of information through not having data on phase (Edwards 1971). The maximum lod score, 3.26, of course, properly reflects all of the information in the data to the extent that gene frequencies and linkage disequilibrium are known and specified.

Edwards' equivalent number n of observations is useful for comparing observed lod score maxima with those expected for known recombination events at the same θ values. In comparisons of lod score maxima at different θ values, as is outlined in section 5.1, n has no easy interpretation. Also, of course, k does not give the number of known recombinants in a pedigree, and the numbers k and n must be used only for illustration purposes and *not*, for example, in chi-square or other statistical tests as if they corresponded to actual numbers of observations.

4.6. Exact Tests in Simple Family Types

The lod score method as outlined above serves two purposes: (1) estimation of the recombination fraction, θ, and (2) carrying out of a statistical test of the null hypothesis of free recombination ($\theta = \frac{1}{2}$) versus the alternative hypothesis of linkage ($\theta < \frac{1}{2}$). Important characteristics of a statistical test are its significance level and its power. In this section, these characteristics are briefly investigated for a few small families of a simple structure. The results will be relevant for sample size considerations, but questions of sample size are covered in a more general setting in section 5.10. The statistically less interested reader may want to skip the remainder of this section.

As outlined in section 3.4, the significance level (or type I error or rate of false positive results) is the probability, $\alpha = P(s; \theta = \frac{1}{2})$, that the test is significant (indicated by s) when there is no linkage. The rate of false negative results or type II error, $\beta = P(\text{not } s; \theta < \frac{1}{2})$, is the probability that the test is not significant although there is linkage. Its complement is the power, $1 - \beta = P(s; \theta < \frac{1}{2})$, that is, the probability of detecting linkage when it exists. By convention, as outlined above, the test for linkage is declared significant when the maximum, Z_{max}, of the lod score exceeds the bound $Z_0 = 3$. For X-linked loci, a less stringent criterion, $Z_0 = 2$, is appropriate.

Two family types are investigated here, (1) the phase-known double backcross and (2) the phase-unknown double backcross (see section 5.7). In either family type, one has a pair of parents, one being doubly homozygous and the other being heterozygous at both loci considered, and a number m of offspring per family. The number of families is denoted by n.

The phase-known double backcross allows unambiguous counting of recombination events. It is thus unimportant how the offspring are distributed over the different families, the only relevant quantity is the total number, nm, of recombination events. For simplicity, it will be assumed in the derivation of the formulas that n families with one offspring each are available.

With n phase-known families, there are $n + 1$ possible outcomes, $k = 0 \ldots n$, where k is the number of families with a recombinant offspring. Each outcome has a probability of occurrence, $P(k; \theta)$, which may be obtained from the binomial formula, θ being the true recombination frequency. Furthermore, for each outcome, the associated maximum lod score Z_{max} may be obtained from equation (4.11). The probability, $P(s; \theta)$, of a significant result is thus given by the sum of the probabilities of all of those outcomes, k, for which $Z_{max} \geq Z_0$, and depends on the true recombination fraction. Notice that $P(s; \theta)$ is the significance level for $\theta = \frac{1}{2}$ and the power for $\theta < \frac{1}{2}$.

For $Z_0 = 3$ and phase-known families, one finds that for $n < 10$, Z_{max} never reaches or exceeds 3. For $n = 10 \ldots 15$, $k = 0$ is the only outcome leading to $Z_{max} \geq 3$. Therefore, $P(s; \theta) = P(k = 0; \theta) = (1 - \theta)^n$, $n = 10 \ldots 15$. Similarly, when $n = 16 \ldots 19$, Z_{max} exceeds 3 when either 0 or 1 family contains a recombinant child so that $P(s; \theta) = (1 - \theta)^n + n\theta(1 - \theta)^{n-1} = (1 - \theta)^{n-1}[1 + (n - 1)\theta]$. For selected values of θ, numerical values are shown in the second and third columns of table 4.2. For $n = 10$ and $n = 16$, the respective significance levels ($\theta = \frac{1}{2}$) associated with the critical limit $Z_0 = 3$ are 0.001 and 0.00026.

Table 4.2. Probability, $P(Z_{max} > Z_0; \theta)$, of a Significant Linkage Result When n Double Backcross Families with m Offspring Each are Investigated and Probability, $P = P(H_0|s; \theta = 0.1)$, That a Significant Linkage Result is a False Positive

| | $Z_0 = 3$ | | | | $Z_0 = 2$ | | |
| | Phase Known | | Phase Unknown ($n = 10$) | | Phase Known | Phase Unknown | |
θ	$nm = 10$	$nm = 16$	$m = 2$	$m = 3$	$nm = 7$	$n = 7$, $m = 2$	$n = 4$, $m = 3$
0	1	1	1	1	1	1	1
0.01	0.904	0.989	0.819	0.966	0.932	0.869	0.886
0.05	0.599	0.811	0.369	0.572	0.698	0.497	0.541
0.10	0.349	0.515	0.137	0.202	0.478	0.249	0.284
0.20	0.107	0.141	0.021	0.015	0.210	0.067	0.073
0.30	0.028	0.026	0.004	0.001	0.082	0.022	0.019
0.40	0.006	0.003	0.001	0.00008	0.028	0.010	0.006
0.50	0.001	0.00026	0.001	0.00003	0.008	0.008	0.004
P	0.05	0.01	0.12	0.00	0.24	0.37	0.21

The empirical significance level p associated with an observed maximum lod score, Z_{max}, is the probability of obtaining a result as extreme or more extreme than the one observed. For counts of recombination events, with k observed recombinants in n informative meioses, the empirical significance level is given by the binomial probability $p = P(x \leq k; r = \frac{1}{2})$, where x denotes the possible number of recombinants (binomial random variable) and r denotes the assumed true recombination fraction. For any k and n, p can easily be calculated using the BINOM program. For example, $k = 2$ recombinants in $n = 20$ meioses represent an empirical significance level of 0.0002. With no recombinants observed, $k = 0$, one obtains $p = (\frac{1}{2})^n$. In this case, the maximum lod score occurs at $\theta = 0$ and attains a value of $Z_{max} = n \times \log(2)$. Applying equation (4.10) with this value of Z_{max} leads to $p = (\frac{1}{2})^n$, that is, in this case the significance level attains the upper bound predicted by (4.10). For $k > 0$, the upper bound of the significance level is not reached (see problem 4.4).

The last line in table 4.2 shows Morton's (1955) posterior type I error defined by equation (4.2), evaluated under the assumption of an a priori probability of linkage of 5 percent. It is then calculated as

$$P(H_0|s) = 19\alpha/(19\alpha + \phi), \tag{4.12}$$

where H_0 refers to the null hypothesis of no linkage, α is the significance level, and ϕ is the power at some value of θ. In table 4.2, ϕ is evaluated at $\theta = 0.10$. $P = P(H_0|s)$ thus is the conditional probability that a significant linkage result is a false positive. For example, in the second to last column of table 4.2, one has $\alpha = 0.008$ and $\phi = 0.249$ (at $\theta = 0.10$) so that $P = 0.37$ (the calculations are based on a larger number of significant digits than shown in the table).

For phase unknown families, one must keep track of the number m of offspring per family. For example, as outlined in section 5.9, families with $m = 3$ offspring fall into two distinct classes, a class 1 family occurring with probability $3\theta(1 - \theta)$. Evaluation of all possible outcomes and associated values of Z_{max} in $n = 10$ families shows that $Z_{max} > 3$ when the number of class 1 families is either 0 or 1. This leads to $P(s; \theta) = [1 - 3\theta(1 - \theta)]^9[1 + 27\theta(1 - \theta)]$.

One can read off table 4.2 that ten recombination events are sufficient for detecting linkage with a power of 90 percent, but only when the linkage is very tight ($\theta \leq 0.01$). With sixteen recombination events available, one is able to detect a slightly looser linkage although, at $\theta = 0.05$, the power has already dropped to 80 percent. Generally, it is much harder (requires more observations) to detect loose as opposed to tight linkage.

To show the effect of a less stringent criterion for linkage, table 4.2

also gives the power $P(s; \theta)$ for the critical limit $Z_0 = 2$ of the maximum lod score. Lowering Z_0 increases power considerably. For example, with phase-unknown matings of $m = 2$ offspring each (section 5.8), $n = 7$ families have greater power under $Z_0 = 2$ than do $n = 10$ families under $Z_0 = 3$. On the other hand, of course, the type I error (significance level) is also increased so that one tends to find more significant results although linkage is absent. It is thus not generally a good idea to consider a linkage significant when the maximum lod score exceeds 2 but not 3 (exception: X-linked loci).

Table 4.2 also shows that the significance level depends very much on the type of family and ranges from 0.001 down to 0.00003. Computing it for increasing numbers n of phase-known families with one offspring each, one finds that α oscillates around the limiting value of $0.0001 = 10^{-4}$, the deviations quickly becoming small; for $n > 10$, $0.3 \times 10^{-4} < \alpha < 2.6 \times 10^{-4}$.

Thus far, the tacit assumption has been that recombination in male parents occurs with the same frequency, θ_m, as that in female parents, θ_f. A possible difference between the two rates will be discussed more fully in section 9.1; it represents a particular test situation that is best covered in the present context. Consider the three hypotheses, $H_0: \theta_m = \frac{1}{2}$, $\theta_f = \frac{1}{2}$; $H_1: \theta < \frac{1}{2}, \theta_m = \theta_f = \theta$; $H_2: \theta_m < \frac{1}{2}, \theta_f < \frac{1}{2}, \theta_m \neq \theta_f$. Assume that tests are declared significant if the maximum lod score Z_{max} exceeds 3. Asymptotically, in the test of H_0 against H_2, $4.6 \times Z_{max}$ follows a chi-square distribution on 2 df if H_0 is true, where Z_{max} is the maximum lod score, $Z(\hat{\theta}_m, \hat{\theta}_f)$. The asymptotic (two-sided) significance level of this test is thus equal to 0.0010 as compared with the significance level of 0.0002 of H_0 versus H_1. When the same critical limit for Z_{max} is applied, allowing for different recombination rates in males and females is thus somewhat less conservative than assuming $\theta_m = \theta_f$. Exact significance levels may be seen in the subsequent example.

Consider two phase-known matings of a doubly heterozygous and a doubly homozygous parent each. In family 1 the father is informative for linkage, whereas in family 2 it is the mother who is doubly heterozygous. Let $n_1 = 8$ and $n_2 = 7$ be the respective numbers of offspring in these two families, and let k_i denote the number of recombinants in the n_i recombination events. In the test of H_0 versus H_1, there are in effect $n = 15$ recombination events. Significance ($Z_{max} \geq 3$) is reached only for $k = k_1 + k_2 = 0$, leading to a maximum lod score of 4.52. A significant result thus occurs with probability $P(s; \theta) = (1 - \theta)^{15}$, so that with $\theta = \frac{1}{2}$, the significance level of this test is equal to $\alpha_1 = (\frac{1}{2})^{15} = 0.00003$. On the other hand, when testing H_0 versus H_2, the lod score is given by $Z(\theta_m, \theta_f)$

$= Z_1(\theta_m) + Z_2(\theta_f)$, where Z_1 and Z_2 are the lod scores in families 1 and 2, respectively. The highest lod score is then just the sum of the individual maxima, $Z_1(\hat{\theta}_m)$ and $Z_2(\hat{\theta}_f)$, with possibly different recombination estimates in the male and female parents. Evaluation of all possible outcomes of k_1 and k_2 shows that a significant result is obtained for the three pairs of values, $(k_1, k_2) = (0, 0)$, $(0, 1)$, and $(1, 0)$. For example, $k_1 = 1$ yields a maximum lod score of 1.10 at $\hat{\theta}_m = \frac{1}{8}$, and $k_2 = 0$ yields a maximum lod score of 2.11 at $\hat{\theta}_f = 0$. The total resulting lod score thus exceeds the limit of 3. The three possible outcomes leading to a significant result occur with probability $P(s; \theta) = (1 - \theta_m)^7 (1 - \theta_f)^6 [1 + 7\theta_m(1 - 2\theta_f) + 6\theta_f]$, so that with $\theta_m = \theta_f = \frac{1}{2}$, the significance level is obtained as $\alpha_2 = 16(\frac{1}{2})^{15} = 16\alpha_1 = 0.00049$.

The results of the previous paragraph have the following interpretation: Allowing for different recombination fraction estimates in males and females increases the type I error. In the example given, the increase is sixteen-fold, but the higher of the two significance levels (H_0 versus H_2) is still smaller than 0.0005. According to the increase in significance level, the power is also increased when in the analysis θ_m is allowed to be different from θ_f, even if in reality they are the same (see problem 4.3).

4.7. Multiple Comparisons

In many linkage investigations, the relation between a test locus and a number, g, of marker loci is analyzed. If the markers form a linkage group (genetic map) (i.e., if they are linked with each other), one would usually carry out a multipoint linkage analysis (see chapter 6). If they are unlinked with each other, pairwise (two-point) linkage analyses are performed, test locus versus each of the marker loci. The test result is then considered significant when at least one of the comparisons exhibits a maximum lod score $Z_{max} \geq 3$. Questions have occasionally been raised whether a critical limit higher than 3 should be applied. The discussion below will show why multiple comparisons in the test for linkage do not generally warrant a higher critical lod score.

Generally, in biostatistics, multiple comparisons lead to an increased type I error because there is in each comparison a certain probability, α_1, that the test is significant even though the effect to be tested for may be nonexistent. Let α_1 be the significance level for an individual comparison. If the overall type I error (significance level) in g comparisons should be no higher than α_g, a rigorous solution is to choose

$$\alpha_1 = \alpha_g / g \tag{4.13}$$

for the significance in each individual test (Anderson and Sclove 1986). If one makes the assumption that the comparisons are mutually independent (which often is not quite true but represents a useful approximation), the probability that at least one comparison leads to a significant result, when the null hypothesis is true, is given by $\alpha_g = 1 - (1 - \alpha_1)^g$, where α_g is the overall significance level associated with carrying out the g comparisons. Solving this equation for α_1 leads to

$$\alpha_1 = 1 - (1 - \alpha_g)^{1/g}. \tag{4.14}$$

Equations (4.13) and (4.14) often yield very similar results, particularly when the values for α are small. For example, assume that $g = 10$ comparisons should be carried out and the overall significance level should be no greater than $\alpha_g = 0.05$. Each individual comparison must then be tested at a smaller significance level which is obtained from (4.13) as $\alpha_1 = 0.005$ and from (4.14) as 0.0051.

Formally, the increase of α_g over α_1 has been translated into an increase of the critical lod score limit as follows (Kidd and Ott 1984): Applying equation (4.10) to the overall significance level, $\alpha_g = g\alpha_1$, reads $g\alpha_1 \leq 10^{-Z_0}$ or $\alpha_1 \leq 10^{-[Z_0 + \log(g)]}$. To preserve the overall significance level corresponding to Z_0 in a single comparison, one would thus have to raise the critical limit for Z_{max} to

$$Z_c = Z_0 + \log_{10}(g), \tag{4.15}$$

where Z_0 is usually taken to be equal to 3. For example, with $g = 100$ markers, any of these 100 comparisons to a test locus would only then be considered significant when the maximum lod score exceeded $Z_0 + \log(100) = 3 + 2 = 5$.

An important aspect of multiple comparisons which has thus far been neglected is that an increase in the number of markers increases the prior probability of linkage. The criterion, that an observed linkage be declared significant when $Z_{max} \geq 3$, is associated with an asymptotic significance level of around 0.0001 in regular cases (sections 4.3 and 4.5). This stringency is required by the low prior probability of 0.05 of linkage (Smith 1953; Morton 1955). An increased prior probability of linkage will thus permit us to use a less stringent criterion for significance, that is, a higher overall significance level. This effect and the one discussed in the previous paragraph work in opposite directions and approximately cancel each other, which may be seen from the arguments given below.

If P_1 is the prior probability that a test locus is within a certain fixed distance from one marker locus, then the prior probability that the test locus is within that distance from at least one of g markers is given by

$P_g \approx gP_1$, assuming independence between the comparisons of the test locus and the different marker loci. Now consider Morton's (1955) posterior type I error (4.2), which may be written as

$$P(H_0|s) = \left[1 + \frac{\phi}{\alpha_1} \frac{P_1}{(1 - P_1)} \right]^{-1},$$
(4.16)

where P_1 is the prior probability of linkage to one marker, α_1 is the corresponding significance level, and ϕ is the power of the test. For g markers, P_1 is replaced by $P_g = gP_1$ (overall prior probability of linkage) and α_1 by $\alpha_g = g\alpha_1$ (overall significance level). Then, one g cancels in the numerator and denominator of (4.16), while $(1 - gP_1)$ and thus $P(H_0|s)$ decreases with increasing g, assuming constant power ϕ. Therefore, if anything, an increase in the number of markers leads to a decrease in the posterior type I error so that there is no need to set a higher critical limit for the maximum lod score.

The approximate treatment of multiple comparisons is presumably good for up to $g = 100$ markers, at which point the overall significance level has approximately reached 0.01. With that many or more markers, however, the appropriate threshold for Z_{max} has to be investigated by methods taking the whole gene map into account. Lander and Botstein (1989) investigated this question and concluded that, when the chance of a false positive occurring anywhere in the genome is at most 5 percent (overall significance level), the appropriate critical level for Z_{max} typically is between 2 and 3.

In summary, it is customary to declare single and multiple two-point linkage analyses significant when $Z_{max} \geq 3$ and the question of the empirical significance level associated with a particular observed maximum lod score is generally not raised. In particular cases, notably some practices of linkage analysis in complex traits (section 11.3) and in some types of multipoint linkage analysis, the conventional criterion for significance may no longer be appropriate. A possible solution is then to find an approximation to the empirical significance level by computer simulation techniques (see section 8.7).

4.8. The Likelihood of Family Data

As introduced in section 4.3, the lod score is a suitably scaled and transformed likelihood, where the likelihood is defined as the probability of the family data when certain values for the unknown parameters are assumed (thus far, only one parameter—the recombination fraction—has been taken into account). In the examples given above, likelihoods were calculated in an ad hoc manner. Here pedigree likelihoods are discussed more formally (for a more general discussion of pedigree likelihoods, see Thompson 1986).

Consider a human pedigree of size m and let x_i denote the phenotype of the ith pedigree member, where x_i refers to the two phenotypes at two loci jointly (more general cases are covered in section 8.2). The likelihood, being the probability of the observations, is then $L = P(x_1, x_2, \ldots, x_m)$. In classical statistical analysis generally, observations are mutually independent so that $L = \Pi P(x_i)$. Pedigree data are nonindependent so that such a simple representation of the likelihood is not possible. In most cases, however, they are conditionally independent, given genotypes:

$$P(x_1, x_2, \ldots, x_m | g_1, g_2, \ldots, g_m) = \Pi P(x_i | g_i).$$

The unconditional likelihood is then expressed as

$$L = P(x) = \sum_g P(x, g) = \sum_g P(x|g) \, P(g), \qquad (4.17)$$

where $x = (x_1, \ldots, x_m)$ is the array of phenotypes, $g = (g_1, \ldots, g_m)$ is an array of genotypes, and the sum is taken over all sets of genotype assignments to family members. The total number of these sets can be large. With two alleles at each of the two loci, there are $H = 4$ haplotypes so that potentially each individual has $H(H + 1)/2 = 10$ genotypes (section 1.1). With m family members, there are thus 10^m different sets of genotype arrays. For example, all individuals may have genotype A_1/A_1, or individual 1 has genotype A_1/A_2 and the other individuals have genotypes A_1/A_1, etc. Not all of these genotype arrays have to be considered, however, for many of them are incompatible with the mendelian laws. In addition, an individual's phenotype may preclude some of his or her genotypes. For example, in each of the pedigrees on the right side of figures 4.1 and 4.2, the genotypes in all but one individual are known, and in the single individual with an equivocal genotype there are just two possibilities. Therefore, the total number of genotypes compatible with the mendelian laws and the phenotypes is just two in each family.

A systematic approach to evaluating likelihoods and example calculations are given in chapter 8.

4.9. Nonparametric Approaches

In linkage analysis, the mode of inheritance of the loci must be specified exactly. For some conditions, however, several modes of inheritance may appear equally plausible. This problem is addressed in more detail in chapter 11. Here, I briefly discuss particular types of linkage analysis which require no assumptions about mode of inheritance of one of the two loci (here called the *trait*) to be studied.

The sib-pair method of Penrose (1935) is based on the relative frequencies of pairs of sibs to be alike or unlike for two traits whose linkage is to be investigated. It thus analyzes single-sibship data. For two phenotypes at each of two loci, the sib pairs are tabulated in a 2×2 table such that rows refer to locus *1* and columns to locus *2*. Each sib pair contributes one entry to the table. When the two sibs are alike with respect to their phenotype at the first locus, the pair is entered in the first row; otherwise it is entered in the second row. Analogously, a sib pair is entered in the first column when the sibs are alike at the second locus and in the second column when they are unlike. It can be shown (section 5.8) that, in the presence of linkage, the upper left and lower right cells of the table will preferentially be filled, so that linkage can be tested for by a chi-square analysis of the table. Since the parental phenotypes are disregarded, many uninformative matings fill the table with much useless data so that the power of this sib-pair analysis is rather low. Nonetheless, it was by this method that the first autosomal linkage was found in humans (Mohr 1954; see end of section 2.3, above). In the 1930s and 1940s, Penrose's sib-pair method evidently was *the* linkage analysis method and it was applied to numerous traits such as the presence or absence of cross-eyes, the ability to curl the tongue, the occurrence of warts, etc. (Kloepfer 1946).

The modern form of the sib-pair method focuses on *affected* siblings. These affected sib-pair methods rest on the hypothesis that a marker locus is closely linked to a disease locus so that the disease gene is transmitted to different offspring always with the same marker allele, that is, the one in coupling with the disease allele. Attention is, thus, focused on affected offspring who are known to have received a disease gene. This elegantly circumvents problems of incomplete penetrance but hinges on the assumption of absence of nongenetic cases—the occurrence of phenocopies severely reduces the power of the affected sib-pair methods (Bishop and Williamson 1990). The relevant observation in these methods is how frequently two affected offspring share copies of the same parental marker allele—such copies are said to be inherited "identical by descent," IBD (Fishman et al. 1978; Suarez 1978). For example, consider an autosomal recessive trait and a sufficiently polymorphic marker so that the parents show four different marker alleles. The number of alleles shared IBD among two affected sibs is 0, 1, or 2. In the absence of linkage, these numbers occur in the expected proportions of $1:2:1$; with linkage, however, one expects a deviation towards higher numbers of alleles shared IBD. One may then simply determine the mean number of alleles shared IBD in two affected sibs and determine whether the observed mean differs significantly from the expected mean of 1. When more than two affected siblings are present in a sibship, one may form all possible pairs of affected sibs and treat them as if they were independent (Hodge 1984; Suarez and Van Eerdewegh 1984). Various test statistics have been used, for example, Green and Woodrow's (1977) repeats statistic. The statistical power of three currently used forms of the affected sib-pair test was investigated by Blackwelder and Elston (1985). Problems of heterogeneity in the application of these tests were also addressed (Chakravarti, Badner, and Li 1987; Goldin and Gershon 1988).

Pairs of relatives other than siblings may be used in such analyses (Risch 1990). Often, identity by descent (IBD) cannot unequivocally be established. Then, one must rely on identity by state (Lange 1986), which reduces informativeness (Bishop and Williamson 1990). An extension from pairs to sets of affected relatives was developed by Weeks and Lange (1988) in the affected relative member (ARM) method. An easy to understand description of it may be found in Weeks and Lange (1990). For several diseases, deviation from random allele or haplotype sharing at the *HLA* loci has been observed, for example, for diabetes. Most of these deviations are interpreted as indicative of close linkage. They might, however, also be interpreted as a consequence of epistatic association (Hodge 1981).

Several other nonparametric methods for linkage analysis have been described. For example, Haseman and Elston (1972) based inference on the regression of the squared sib-pair trait difference on the estimated proportion of alleles IBD, where the trait may be quantitative or qualitative. Other approaches were proposed by Hill (1975) and Smith (1975).

In classical (parametric) linkage analyses, it is recommended to collect families such that pairs of affected siblings are available. In addition to the planned lod score analysis, these pairs can profitably be used for alternative analyses using nonparametric methods. Care will have to be taken to apply similarly strict criteria for significance to those in the lod score method. For example, a significance level of no higher than 0.001 should be used in these nonparametric test procedures.

A nonparametric mapping strategy was developed by Lalouel (1977). It combines pair-wise recombination data using Guttman multidimensional scaling and is referred to again in section 6.4.

4.10. Some Special Methods

For linkage analyses between a locus anywhere on a chromosome and a chromosomal variant located around the centromere, the term centromere or centromeric linkage has been used (Bailey 1961; Ferguson-Smith et al. 1975). Genetically very different from this is *centromere mapping* by means of ovarian teratomas (Ott et al. 1976). In ovarian teratomas, the proportion of second-division segregants, a quite different quantity from the recombination fraction, is estimated. The use of human ovarian teratomas for this type of centromere-related mapping rests on the assumption that these benign tumors originate parthenogenetically from a single germ cell by suppression of the second meiotic division (Linder, Kaiser McCaw, and Hecht 1975). Newer developments of this mapping approach take into account the varied origin of ovarian teratomas (Chakravarti and Slaugenhaupt 1987; Halloran and Chakravarti 1987).

Molecular genetics techniques allow the recognition of alleles of suitable genetic marker loci in *individual sperm cells* of a man (see review by Arnheim, Li, and Cui 1990). This method has the potential to score dozens or even hundreds of meioses in a single individual, and appropriate statistical analysis methods have been proposed for it (Boehnke et al. 1989). The analysis of single sperm may also be achieved using regular linkage programs. One way of doing this would be to define an artificial mate of the man, whose sperm has been investigated, where that mate is taken to be homozygous at each marker locus. Each sperm is then treated as a child of the man and his mate.

Problems

Problem 4.1. In the analysis of the pedigree shown in figure 4.1, recombination events were counted based on the children in the last generation only. Shouldn't one include in the analysis the offspring of the grandparents?

Problem 4.2. In the example family with a phase-unknown parent presented in section 4.3 (right side of fig. 4.2), the estimate of θ obtained assuming the more plausible phase is the same as the maximum likelihood estimate. Convince yourself that this is not generally the case. Consider the same mating as the one shown on the right side of figure 4.2 but assume different offspring such that, for parental phase I, there are k recombinants out of n opportunities for recombination. For each of the two cases, (1) $k = 1$, $n = 5$, and (2) $k = 1$, $n = 4$, derive the estimates of

θ (1) by assuming phase I to be known and (2) by maximizing the lod score for unknown phase.

Problem 4.3. For the example covered at the end of section 4.6, compute the power for the two test strategies, (1) H_0 versus H_1 and (2) H_0 versus H_2. Evaluate the power for the case $\theta = \theta_m = \theta_f = 0.01$. You need not derive any new formulas; you can simply manipulate the equations given in the text.

Problem 4.4. For $n = 20$ informative meioses in phase-known double backcross families, calculate (1) the empirical significance level (section 4.6) and (2) its upper bound (equation [4.10]) associated with $k = 1, 2, 3, 4,$ and 5 observed recombinants. Convince yourself that the significance level stays below its upper bound.

Problem 4.5. Assume that, in a linkage analysis between a disease and a marker, a lod score of -7.16 was observed at $\theta = 0$. How do you interpret this result?

5.

The Informativeness of Family Data

This chapter is of a somewhat technical nature and introduces the concept of informativeness for linkage. It requires some familiarity with calculus and may be skipped by the less mathematically minded reader, with the exception of the last section on number of individuals required for linkage analysis, which is of general interest. This chapter provides detailed instructions, for example, on how to calculate offspring genotype probabilities and measures of informativeness. The reader who wants to carry out serious statistical work should find useful guidance in it. An interpretation of the differences between expected lod scores and Fisher's expected information is given at the end of section 5.6.

The discussion of mating types in this chapter is rather general and explores informativeness of family data based only on mating types and relationships among family members. The more complicated problem of calculating expected lod scores conditional on observed phenotypes at one locus will be covered in chapter 8.

5.1. Measures of Informativeness

The amount of data collected and the pedigree structure generally determine how well one is able to discriminate between different hypotheses or different parameter values. For a given set of observations on family data, several measures of informativeness with respect to genetic linkage are available. Three such measures are considered here: (1) the maximum of the lod score, (2) Fisher's (1925) statistical *information*, and (3) Edwards' (1976) number of equivalent meioses. The latter was discussed in section 4.5 and is a measure for the number of opportunities for recombination if a count of recombination events were possible for the given family data. The maximum lod score was introduced in section 4.3 and measures the evidence for linkage versus absence of linkage. By definition, it is equal to zero for $\hat{\theta} = \frac{1}{2}$. When recombination events can be counted, k being the number of recombinants in n events, the maximum lod score is given by equation (4.11). Fisher's (estimated) information measures the precision of the recombination estimate by assessing how fast the log likelihood (or lod score) curve falls off from its peak at $\hat{\theta}$. Specifically, the degree of curvature is determined as minus the second derivative of the natural log likelihood, evaluated at $\hat{\theta}$,

$$\hat{I}(\hat{\theta}) = -d^2\ln L(\hat{\theta})/d\theta^2, \qquad (5.1)$$

where $\hat{I}(\hat{\theta})$ is called the estimated total amount of information. Note that $\hat{\theta}$ must be an *analytical* maximum (the first derivative of the log likelihood must be zero at $\theta = \hat{\theta}$). For an unbiased estimate, $1/\hat{I}(\hat{\theta})$ is the approximate sample variance of the recombination estimate. For counts of recombination events, the likelihood is equal to $\theta^k(1 - \theta)^{n-k}$, and evaluation of (5.1) yields $\hat{I}(\hat{\theta}) = n/[\hat{\theta}(1 - \hat{\theta})]$. In statistics, information is a technical term with a specific definition (see equation [5.1] and section 5.3).

The three types of measure of informativeness do different things and thus have different properties. In figure 5.1, they are graphed for counts of recombination events (for convenience, one countable recombination event is assumed). (1) Edwards' equivalent number of meioses is not shown—it is simply a horizontal straight line because of the assumption that recombination events can be counted. The other two measures are highest for $\hat{\theta} = k/n = 0$. (2) The maximum lod score gradually decreases towards $\hat{\theta} = \frac{1}{2}$, at which point it is zero, since that estimate conveys no evidence for linkage. (3) Fisher's estimated information initially decreases much faster than the maximum lod score (but then levels off faster) and reaches a minimum (>0) at $\hat{\theta} = \frac{1}{2}$, where the log likelihood curve (not shown) is least curved. For known recombination events, the lod score curve is not completely flat at $\hat{\theta} = \frac{1}{2}$, which is why the information is positive at $\hat{\theta} = \frac{1}{2}$.

Fisher's information and the lod score may be computed for a set of observations, as above, or averaged over all possible outcomes for some data or family type. When averaged, they measure the expected informativeness that the data set considered is capable of furnishing (sections 5.2 and 5.3). These measures can be used to compare the informativeness of different bodies of data or different mating types. In the first edition of this book, Fisher's expected information was preferentially used, in part because it measures accuracy of recombination estimates even at $\hat{\theta} = \frac{1}{2}$. (An application to the number of observations required in linkage analysis is given in section 5.10.) The expected lod score, being a measure of information content for detecting linkage, is always zero at $\theta = \frac{1}{2}$ but,

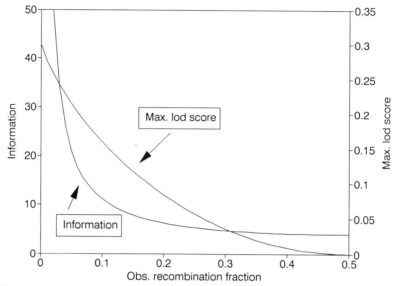

Figure 5.1. Maximum lod score and observed information for an estimated recombination fraction from counts of recombination events (n is set to 1).

as pointed out later, its limiting value for θ close to ½ may be different from zero.

A good measure of informativeness is additive over different data sets. Both the expected lod score (section 5.2) and Fisher's expected information (section 5.3) possess this additivity property. A few nonadditive measures are in current use, for example, the probability that the maximum lod score exceeds a certain threshold. They will also be discussed in section 5.2.

5.2. Expected Lod Score

In comparing different family types, one is interested in the expected evidence for linkage that a particular family type is able to provide. One then needs to know all of the possible phenotype constellations for that family type and their probability of occurrence, this probability typically depending on the true value, r, of the recombination fraction. The ith outcome is associated with the lod score, $Z_i(\theta)$, which is a function of the unknown parameter θ (the recombination fraction). For some fixed value of θ the expectation of the lod score function, also called expected lod score or ELOD, $E[Z(\theta)]$, is the weighted average of the $Z_i(\theta)$ over all possible outcomes, with the weights being the probabilities of occurrence of each outcome. In these calculations, one must carefully distinguish between the formal parameter value, θ, used as the argument of the lod score function, and the true value, r, of the recombination fraction assumed for the computation of the outcome probabilities.

For example, when $n = 3$ recombination events can be scored, there are four possible outcomes, $k = 0 \ldots 3$, where k denotes the number of recombinants. The probability of each outcome is given by the binomial formula, $P(k; r) = \binom{n}{k} r^k (1 - r)^{n-k}$, which depends on the true value r of the recombination fraction. The lod score $Z_k(\theta)$ for the kth outcome can be calculated using expression (3.2). For any given value of θ, the weighted average of the $Z_k(\theta)$ then yields the expected lod score,

$$E[Z(\theta)] = \sum_{k=0}^{n} P(k; r) \, Z_k(\theta), \tag{5.2}$$

the weights being given by the $P(k; r)$. For $n = 3$, table 5.1 demonstrates these calculations. The bottom row, in the columns labeled "$Z(\theta)$," shows the resulting expected lod scores. As pointed out in section 3.3, when the maximum likelihood estimate is consistent, the maximum of the ELOD curve occurs at the value $\theta = r$. In table 5.1, the maximum of the ELOD curve is 0.480 (at $\theta = r = 0.10$). Most often, in practice, the term ELOD refers only to the maximum, $E[Z(r)]$, or $E[Z(\hat{\theta})]$ in the case of an asymptotic bias (section 10.1), of the expected lod score curve rather than to the expected lod score function as a whole. This ELOD is closely related to Shannon's entropy (Shannon and Weaver 1949) and the Kullback-Leibler information (Kullback and Leibler 1951; Kullback 1959). The relations among these quantities were described by Akaike (1985).

Table 5.1. Calculation of Expected Lod Score, $E[Z(\theta)]$ = Weighted Average of $Z(\theta)$, and Expected Z_{max} under the True Recombination Fraction, $r = 0.1$

		$Z(\theta)$ at $\theta =$				
k	$P(k)$	0.01	0.09	0.10	0.11	Z_{max}
0	0.729	0.890	0.780	0.766	0.751	0.903
1	0.243	-1.106	-0.224	-0.188	-0.157	0.074
2	0.027	-3.101	-1.229	-1.143	-1.065	0
3	0.001	-5.097	-2.234	-2.097	-1.973	0
Average		0.291	0.479	0.480	0.479	0.676

Note: k, n, and $P(k)$ are as in table 3.1, and the average is a weighted mean with $P(k)$ as weights.

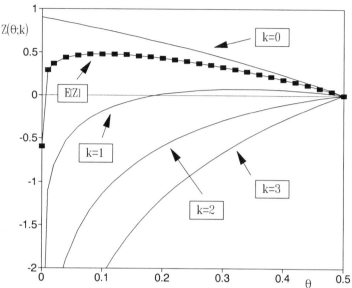

Figure 5.2. Graphs of the lod score curves associated with k observed recombinants in three recombination events.

Graphs of the lod score curves associated with the different outcomes, $k = 0 \ldots 3$, are shown in figure 5.2. Each of these curves depends only on θ and on the phenotypes of the data, but not on r. The weighted average of these curves (i.e., the expected lod score function) is also shown. Depending on the true value r of the recombination fraction, the weight attached to each lod score function is different, leading to a different expected lod score. It is only the weighing of the individual lod score functions that depends on r.

For a fixed value of θ, lod scores can simply be added over different family data to obtain the total lod score for all families combined (section 4.3); therefore, the ELOD, $E[Z(r)]$, is also additive over families (assuming r fixed). In fact, the ELOD of 0.48 in table 5.1 could have been obtained simply by just such an addition: Each recombinant occurs with probability r and contributes $\log(2\theta)$ to the lod score, and each nonrecombinant occurs with probability $1 - r$ and contributes $\log(2 - 2\theta)$. At $\theta = r$, the ELOD may be obtained as $E[Z(r)] = n[r\log(2r) + (1 - r)\log(2 - 2r)]$ which, for $n = 3$ and $r = 0.1$, is equal to 0.48, as in table 5.1. As an application of this additivity property, one may want to compute the number of families of size $n = 3$ referred to in table 5.1 that are required for the total expected lod score to be at least 3 (assuming $r = 0.10$). The answer is obtained by calculating

$3/0.48 = 6.25$, that is, seven such families are required (for six families, ELOD $= 2.88$).

In addition to the ELOD, a related yet different quantity is often used to assess information content. It is based on the distribution of Z_{max} (a single value for each outcome) rather than on the expectation of the lod score function and is defined as the probability, $P(Z_{max} \geq Z_0)$, that the maximum of the expected lod score (at whatever θ it occurs) reaches or exceeds a certain threshold, Z_0. Conventionally, $Z_0 = 3$ but, for comparison purposes, a lower limit may have to be used for some family types. This information measure is computed by evaluating all possible outcomes of a set of data and their probabilities of occurrence and by determining for each outcome whether the associated Z_{max} (at any θ) reaches or exceeds Z_0. The sum of the probabilities of all those outcomes for which $Z_{max} \geq Z_0$ is the desired information measure. For the example data in table 5.1, $P(Z_{max} \geq 3) = 0$, $P(Z_{max} \geq 0.5) = 0.729$, and $P(Z_{max} \geq 0.05) = 0.972$. This information measure has the advantage that it has a direct intuitive interpretation that lends itself for prediction of rates of success of linkage analyses. Its disadvantage is that it is not additive over different sets of family data because the maximum of the lod score for each outcome is evaluated at different θ values. The overall Z_{max} for the total of several sets of family data combined cannot be obtained from the Z_{max} values of the component family data.

In contrast to $P(Z_{max} \geq Z_0)$, the ELOD, $E[Z(r)]$, has no direct probabilistic interpretation. Very roughly, however, for large data sets, $P(Z_{max} > \text{ELOD}) \approx 1/2$, that is, the maximum lod score exceeds the ELOD with about a 50 percent probability (assuming an approximate equality between mean and median).

In addition to the two measures for informativeness discussed above, $E[Z(r)]$ and $P(Z_{max} > Z_0)$, a third quantity is sometimes used for measuring linkage information. It is the expected maximum lod score, $E(Z_{max})$, which, for our example data, is obtained as follows: In table 5.1, each outcome is associated with a lod score curve, which is shown in figure 5.2. Instead of averaging these curves at $\theta = r$ to find the maximum of the expected lod score, one may for each curve look at its maximum, wherever it occurs (for counts of recombination events, that maximum is given by equation [4.11] or may be obtained from the EQUIV program). The weighted average of these maximum values is the expected maximum lod score, $E(Z_{max}) = E[\max_\theta Z(\theta)]$, which should be carefully distinguished from the maximum of the expected lod score, $E[Z(r)] = \max_\theta E[Z(\theta)]$ (the ELOD), discussed above. Its construction is demonstrated in the last column of table 5.1 and leads to a value of 0.676.

$E(Z_{max})$ is always larger than or equal to the ELOD. As Z_{max} is never negative, its distribution is generally expected to be positively skewed. Since the Z_{max} values are obtained at different θ values, $E(Z_{max})$ is not additive over families (see problem 5.7). As it neither has a direct probabilistic interpretation nor is additive, it should not be used as a measure for informativeness for linkage.

Later in this book, to determine the consistency of an estimate in a particular situation, it will be necessary to calculate analytically at what value of θ the expected lod score has its maximum. This can be done by computing the first derivative, $dE[Z(\theta)]/d\theta$, setting it equal to zero, and solving the resulting equation for θ. In these calculations, one must be careful to distinguish between θ and r; the derivative is taken only with respect to θ, not r (r is a constant when taking derivatives with respect to θ). For example, when recombinants and nonrecombinants can be counted directly, the expected lod score function per recombination event is given by

$$E[Z(\theta)] = r \log(2\theta) + (1 - r) \log[2(1 - \theta)]$$
$$= 0.4343[r\ln(2\theta) + (1 - r)\ln(2 - 2\theta)]. \qquad (5.3)$$

With this, one calculates $dE/d\theta = 0.4343[2r/(2\theta) - 2(1 - r)/(2 - 2\theta)]$. Setting this equation equal to zero and solving it for θ yields $\theta = r$. After verification that the second derivative at $\theta = r$ is negative, one concludes that $E[Z(r)]$ is a maximum.

In this section, the ELOD was covered for general types of family data. For pedigrees with a specific observed structure and unknown phenotypes, the ELOD usually has to be approximated by computer simulations, and this is covered in section 8.7. A special case will be the determination of the ELOD conditional on phenotypes already observed at one locus.

5.3. Expected Information

In section 5.1, Fisher's estimated total amount of information, $\hat{I}(\hat{\theta})$, was introduced (equation [5.1]). For example, consider a family with one recombinant and three nonrecombinant offspring. The corresponding log likelihood is given by $\ln[L(\theta)] = \ln \theta + 3 \ln(1 - \theta)$ with a maximum at $\hat{\theta} = \frac{1}{4}$. The second derivative is computed as $[\ln(L(\theta))]'' = -1/\theta^2 - 3/(1 - \theta)^2$, so that one obtains $\hat{I}(0.25) = 1/(0.25)^2 + 3/(0.75)^2 = 21.3$. It is customary to use the symbol I for the total information over all observed data and i referring to a single observation or a single pedigree (a sampling unit), where the caret identifies *estimated* information.

In contrast to the estimated information, the *expected information* is evaluated at the true value r of the recombination fraction. For categorical data falling independently into c different classes (Elandt-Johnson 1971; section 5g in Rao 1973), Fisher's expected information per observation (or per pedigree) is given by

$$i(r) = \sum_{\ell=1}^{c} q_\ell^2(r)/p_\ell(r), \tag{5.4}$$

where $q_\ell(r) = dp_\ell(r)/dr$ and $p_\ell(r)$ is the probability of occurrence of the ℓth class. In (5.4), $(dp_\ell/dr)^2/p_\ell$ may be called the contribution of the ℓth class to the expected information. For example, in counts of recombinant and nonrecombinant offspring, one has $c = 2$ classes, recombinants occurring with probability $p_1 = r$, and nonrecombinants occurring with probability $p_2 = 1 - r$. With $dp_1/dr = 1$ and $dp_2/dr = -1$, equation (5.4) yields

$$i(r) = 1/[r(1 - r)] \tag{5.5}$$

as the expected information per offspring. The total expected information for n such offspring is then equal to $I(r) = ni(r)$.

It was mentioned in section 3.3 that maximum likelihood estimates such as $\hat{\theta}$ are asymptotically (in large samples) normally distributed and unbiased. Their *asymptotic variance* is equal to the inverse of the expected information. Approximately, then, the standard error of $\hat{\theta}$ is given by

$$\sigma(\hat{\theta}) \approx 1/\sqrt{I(r)} = [n\, i(r)]^{-1/2}. \tag{5.6}$$

Equation (5.4) can be extended to the case of several parameters estimated simultaneously (Elandt-Johnson 1971). Here, only the case of two parameters, r_1 and r_2, is considered; these parameters are not necessarily recombination fractions. Let $p_\ell = p_\ell(r_1, r_2)$ be the probability of occurrence of the ℓth phenotype class, where this probability is determined by the two parameters. Then, the so-called information matrix is equal to

$$I(r_1, r_2) = n\, i(r_1, r_2) = n \begin{pmatrix} a & c \\ c & b \end{pmatrix}, \tag{5.7}$$

where $a = \Sigma(\partial p_\ell/\partial r_1)^2/p_\ell$, $b = \Sigma(\partial p_\ell/\partial r_2)^2/p_\ell$, and $c = \Sigma(\partial p_\ell/\partial r_1)(\partial p_\ell/\partial r_2)/p_\ell$, the sums extending from $\ell = 1$ through c. For two parameters estimated simultaneously, the number of phenotype classes must be equal to three or more, $c \geq 3$. The inverse of $I(r_1, r_2)$ yields the approximate variance-covariance matrix,

$$V(\hat{\theta}_1, \hat{\theta}_2) \approx \frac{1}{n(ab - c^2)} \begin{pmatrix} b & -c \\ -c & a \end{pmatrix}, \tag{5.8}$$

where a, b, and c are as in equation (5.7). From this, the approximate correlation between $\hat{\theta}_1$ and $\hat{\theta}_2$ (the estimates of r_1 and r_2) is obtained as

$$\rho(\hat{\theta}_1, \hat{\theta}_2) \approx -c/\sqrt{ab}. \tag{5.9}$$

Approximate *estimated* standard errors and correlation may be calculated when the true parameter values in the equations above are replaced by their estimates. In practice, estimated standard errors are often calculated directly from the curvature of the log likelihood curve or by assuming normality of the estimates, that is, a quadratic likelihood curve or surface (see chapter 8).

5.4. Mating Types

In experimental genetics, matings were given specific names—mating types—depending on the genotypes of the mates. Consider two parental populations, P_1 and P_2, where individuals in P_1 are all homozygous *AA* at some locus, and individuals in P_2 are homozygous *aa* for another allele at that locus. Crossing $P_1 \times P_2$ leads to a uniform population of all heterozygous *Aa* individuals, the so-called F_1 generation (filial generation no. 1). Crosses $F_1 \times F_1$ are called *intercrosses*, and their offspring form the F_2 generation (filial generation no. 2). A cross $F_1 \times P_1$ or $F_1 \times P_2$ is called a *backcross* (or testcross).

These mating types can be extended to more than one locus. For example, let one of the mates be a double heterozygote, phase being known or unknown. If the other mate is doubly homozygous, singly heterozygous, or doubly heterozygous, the mating is called a *double backcross*, a *single backcross*, or a *double intercross*, respectively. In human genetics, these terms are infrequently used as they are defined on the basis of only two alleles per locus. Many matings, particularly when highly polymorphic marker loci are used in linkage analyses, involve three or four different alleles per locus. The classical mating type designations are then no longer appropriate.

In the subsequent sections, I will calculate how much linkage information per offspring is provided by some important mating types. The main purpose is to demonstrate how to carry out such calculations rather than to compile an exhaustive list of mating types. Note that, for various classical mating types, their information content was given by Mather (1936).

The first step in calculating an information measure (ELOD or Fisher's expected information) for a given mating type is to list all possible haplotypes (gametes) each parent can produce. Each pair of haplotypes (one from each parent) will then constitute one offspring genotype. Depending on the polymorphism of the loci involved, some of the offspring genotypes will be undistinguishable and can be collected into a single class. This merging of genotypes represents a reduction in genetic variability. The genotype probabilities will generally depend on the true recombination fraction, r, which may be different in male (r_m) and female (r_f) parents. In this chapter, however, r_m and r_f are taken to be equal.

The next step consists of combining into a single class those genotypes leading to the same phenotype, which represents a further reduction of variability. It is these reductions in variability that lead to loss of information. Different mating types will be seen to lead to a larger or smaller reduction in the number of classes as one proceeds from pairs of haplotypes to genotypes to phenotypes. The offspring phenotype classes and their probabilities of occurrence then determine the amount of information, for example, through formula (5.4). In the subsequent section, this procedure will be demonstrated step by step.

Below, only two loci will be considered at a time. It is often convenient to characterize a locus by one letter and to distinguish the two different alleles at this locus by the lower case and upper case of that letter. However, as more than two alleles may occur, I will enumerate the alleles at one locus alphabetically and distinguish the alleles at the other locus by numbering them from 1 through n.

5.5. Double Intercross with Two Alleles

In this section, according to the general scheme outlined in the previous few paragraphs, detailed instructions are provided for calculating expected information and lod scores. Consider a mating *A1/B2 × A1/B2* (double intercross) and assume codominant inheritance at each locus. Phase is assumed known so that, for example, allele *A* at the first locus is in coupling with allele *1* at the second locus. To obtain a list of all possible offspring genotypes with their probabilities of occurrence, one must prepare an exhaustive list of the haplotypes (gametes) that each parent can produce, including the probabilities with which they are produced. In this mating, each parent can produce four haplotypes. For example, a haplotype contains the A allele with probability $\frac{1}{2}$. Given that it does, the other allele is a 2 when a recombination takes place, where a recombination occurs with probability r. Therefore, the probability of an $A2$ haplotype occurring is equal to $\frac{1}{2}r$.

In table 5.2, the haplotypes and their probabilities are given along the borders. To keep this table general, male and female recombination rates are distinguished as r_m and r_f, respectively. In the subsequent calculations, however, this distinction will be dropped. Gametes from the two parents combine to form genotypes, each pair of gametes yielding a genotype.

The parents are assumed to mate at random with respect to their genotypes. Therefore, offspring genotype probabilities are obtained simply by multiplying the probabilities of the parental haplotypes making up the genotypes. For example, haplotypes $A1$ from the mother (probability $\frac{1}{2}[1 - r_f]$) and $B1$ from the father (probability $\frac{1}{2}r_m$) combine to form the genotype $A1/B1$, which is identical to $B1/A1$. Its probability of occurrence is $\frac{1}{4}r_m(1 - r_f)$. In this mating, both parents produce an identical set of haplotypes; therefore, the haplotypes $A1$ and $B1$ could come from the father and mother, respectively, and lead to the same genotype as before. That genotype, $A1/B1$, thus has probability of occurrence $\frac{1}{4}[r_m(1 - r_f) + (1 - r_m)r_f]$ which, for $r = r_m = r_f$, is equal to $\frac{1}{2}r(1 - r)$. Inspection of table 5.2 reveals that the sixteen pairs of parental haplotypes give rise to ten unique genotypes.

Each genotype gives rise to a phenotype, but some genotypes may lead to the same phenotype. The probability of such a phenotype is then simply the sum of the probabilities of its component genotypes. So, based on the list of genotypes, one prepares a list of unique phenotypes because, in a linkage analysis, offspring will be distinguishable only through their phenotypes. As can be seen from table 5.3, the ten unique genotypes determine nine unique phenotypes.

Many but not all offspring phenotypes can be traced back to unequivocal recombination events in the parents. For example, a BB-11 individual occurs by a recombination in each parent. Also, an AA-12 offspring has received a recombinant haplotype from one parent and a nonrecombinant from the other, but it is unknown which parent passed on which haplotype. As an aside, if recombination rates were distinguished by the sex of the parents, such uncertainty in the parental origin of the haplotypes would lead to a correlation between the male and female recombination estimates. The most "uncertain" offspring phenotype is AB-12, a double heterozygote with unknown phase, which corresponds to four cells in table 5.2. It originates either from two recombinant or two nonrecombinant haplotypes.

Table 5.2. Offspring Genotypes from the Mating $A1/B2 \times A1/B2$

Haplotypes from Other Parent		$A1$ $\frac{1}{2}(1 - r_m)$	$B2$ $\frac{1}{2}(1 - r_m)$	$A2$ $\frac{1}{2}r_m$	$B1$ $\frac{1}{2}r_m$
			Haplotypes from one parent		
$A1$	$\frac{1}{2}(1 - r_f)$	$A1/A1$	$A1/B2$	$A1/A2$	$A1/B1$
$B2$	$\frac{1}{2}(1 - r_f)$	$B2/A1$	$B2/B2$	$B2/A2$	$B2/B1$
$A2$	$\frac{1}{2}r_f$	$A2/A1$	$A2/B2$	$A2/A2$	$A2/B1$
$B1$	$\frac{1}{2}r_f$	$B1/A1$	$B1/B2$	$B1/A2$	$B1/B1$

Table 5.3. Phenotypes of Offspring from the Mating $A1/B2 \times A1/B2$, with Associated Probability p_i of Occurrence

i	Phenotype	p_i
1	AA-11	$\frac{1}{4}(1 - r)^2$
2	AA-12	$\frac{1}{2}r(1 - r)$
3	AB-12	$\frac{1}{2}[r^2 + (1 - r)^2]$
4	AB-11	$\frac{1}{2}r(1 - r)$
5	AA-22	$\frac{1}{4}r^2$
6	AB-22	$\frac{1}{2}r(1 - r)$
7	BB-11	$\frac{1}{4}r^2$
8	BB-12	$\frac{1}{2}r(1 - r)$
9	BB-22	$\frac{1}{4}(1 - r)^2$
Total		1

The probabilities of occurrence of the nine offspring phenotypes are listed in table 5.3. Each of these nine classes will contribute to the expected information measure. Before proceeding to these calculations, it will be useful to find the number of degrees of freedom (df) (i.e., the number of linearly independent probabilities in that table); this will make the calculations easier and will also provide insight into the structure of the data. Two or more probabilities are linearly independent when they cannot be represented as linear combinations of a smaller number of parameters (see examples below). The number of degrees of freedom is the number of linearly independent parameters through which the table probabilities can be represented or, in other words, it is the number of table probabilities minus the number of independent linear equations that exist among them. Clearly, when two probabilities are the same they are linearly *de*pendent, so one can first of all collect equal table probabilities into one class without loss of degrees of freedom. This leads to four phenotype classes, as shown in table 5.4.

The four class probabilities, p_1 through p_4, in table 5.4 are not linearly

Table 5.4. Offspring Phenotypes with Equal Probabilities Combined into One Class Each, Mating $A1/B2 \times A1/B2$

ℓ	i^a	p_ℓ	q_ℓ	$Z_\ell(\theta)$
1	$1 + 9$	$\frac{1}{2}(1 - r)^2$	$r - 1$	$\log[4(1 - \theta)^2]$
2	$2 + 4 + 6 + 8$	$2r(1 - r)$	$2(1 - 2r)$	$\log[4\theta(1 - \theta)]$
3	$5 + 7$	$\frac{1}{2}r^2$	r	$\log(4\theta^2)$
4	3	$\frac{1}{2}[r^2 + (1 - r)^2]$	$2r - 1$	$\log[2\theta^2 + 2(1 - \theta)^2]$
	Total	1	0	

^{a}Refers to the index i used in table 5.3.

independent. In fact, as one can easily verify, they are connected through the following three linear equations, the last of which is the usual one saying that they sum to 1: $2p_1 + p_2 + 2p_3 = 1$, $p_1 + p_3 = p_4$, and $p_1 + p_2 + p_3 + p_4 = 1$. Therefore, table 5.4 contains only 1 df, which means that only one parameter can be estimated from these data. It would not, for example, be possible to obtain estimates for male and female recombination fractions from such data, except for a fixed combination of these parameters such as their sum.

Table 5.4 can be used to calculate observed lod scores, expected information, and expected lod scores as follows: If some linkage data consist of the data type considered here (phase-known double intercross matings) and n_ℓ is the number of offspring in the ℓth class, the total observed lod score for these data is simply equal to $\Sigma n_\ell Z_\ell(\theta)$.

Fisher's expected information per offspring is obtained from table 5.4 using equation (5.4). One finds

$$i(r) = \frac{2}{r(1 - r)} - \frac{4r(1 - r)}{r^2 + (1 - r)^2} - 2. \tag{5.10}$$

The general shape of the graph of $i(r)$ looks very much like the estimated information curve in figure 5.1: it is positive at $r = \frac{1}{2}$ and tends to infinity as r approaches 0. For small values of r, (5.10) is approximately equal to $2/r$, that is, twice as large as the corresponding value for the phase-known double backcross mating (section 5.7). Such comparisons will be investigated in section 5.6.

Expected lod scores are calculated from table 5.4 in analogy to equation (5.2),

$$E_r[Z(\theta)] = \Sigma p_\ell(r)Z_\ell(\theta). \tag{5.11}$$

The result is a function of the formal parameter θ, whose shape depends on the true value r of the recombination fraction. As outlined at the end of section 3.3, the maximum of the expected lod score, the ELOD, occurs at $\theta = r$. With this, one obtains as the ELOD per offspring in the data type considered here,

$$E[Z(r)] = (1 - r^2)\log[2(1 - r)] + r(2 - r)\log(2r)$$
$$+ \tfrac{1}{2}[r^2 + (1 - r)^2]\log[2r^2 + 2(1 - r)^2]. \qquad (5.12)$$

For any given true value r of the recombination fraction, the ELOD (5.12) provides a measure for the average linkage information per offspring in phase-known double intercross matings. It is zero at $r = \tfrac{1}{2}$ and rises to its maximum of 0.45 at $r = 0$. To obtain, for example, an expected lod score of 3 or more, assuming tight linkage, one needs to investigate seven ($\tfrac{3}{0.45} = 6.67$) offspring from matings $A1/B2 \times A1/B2$.

Equations (5.10) and (5.12) are easy to evaluate numerically on a calculator or in a spreadsheet program.

5.6. Double Intercross with More Than Two Alleles

The phase-known double intercross of the previous section was used as a model mating to introduce the calculation of expected information and the ELOD. That mating is also relatively common in gene mapping, particularly in the CEPH reference families (Dausset et al. 1990), the phase in the parents being known owing to knowing the grandparents. The marker systems used in actual family data may have more than two alleles but, because of chance, only two specific alleles happen to segregate. In this section, the two-allele mating type will be extended to a type involving more polymorphic markers, and resulting increases of expected information and ELOD will be interpreted. Also, the practically important case of a recessive disease versus genetic markers will be covered.

Consider two very polymorphic genetic markers such that, with high probability, four different alleles segregate in a family at each marker locus. Specifically, consider the phase-known mating $A1/B2 \times C3/D4$. Going through the same steps as in the previous section shows that all of the sixteen offspring genotypes are distinct. Since the parental origin of each allele is unequivocally known, all of the phases in the offspring are known (each offspring is a double heterozygote). Inspection of the sixteen phenotypes (genotypes in this case) reveals that only three different phenotype probabilities occur, $\tfrac{1}{4}(1 - r)^2$, $\tfrac{1}{4}r(1 - r)$, and $\tfrac{1}{4}r^2$. Combining phenotypes with equal probabilities into one class each leads to three class probabilities of $(1 - r)^2$, $2r(1 - r)$, and r^2. These are binomial probabilities corresponding to counts of $k = 0$, 1, or 2 recombinants in $n = 2$ recombination events, so that these data, too, contain only 1 df.

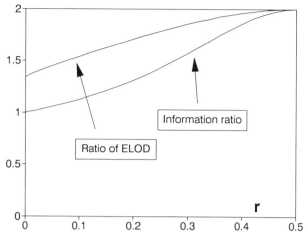

Figure 5.3. Ratios of ELOD and expected information for mating *A1/B2* × *C3/D4* over those for mating *A1/B2* × *A1/B2*.

Offspring from the mating *A1/B2* × *C3/D4* are maximally informative in that each exhibits two known recombination events. According to equation (5.5), Fisher's expected information for two recombination counts is equal to $2/[r(1-r)]$, and the corresponding ELOD is obtained from equation (5.3) as $2r\log(2r) + 2(1-r)\log[2(1-r)]$. The expected information (5.10) and the ELOD (5.12) obtained above for the mating *A1/B2* × *A1/B2* are smaller than those obtained here, the differences being entirely due to an increase in the degree of marker polymorphism. The ratio of the ELOD for the four-allele case over that for the two-allele case is shown in figure 5.3 (upper curve). Also shown is the analogous ratio of the expected information (lower curve). For example, with a recombination fraction of $r = 0$ between the two loci, the ELOD equals $E[Z(0)] = 0.601$ in the four-allele case and 0.451 in the two-allele case, leading to a ratio of 1.33. On the other hand, the expected information tends to infinity in both cases as $r{\rightarrow}0$, but in the limit the corresponding ratio is 1.

The ELOD measures informativeness for detecting linkage, whereas the expected information is a measure for the precision of the recombination fraction estimate, the latter being important in gene mapping given that linkage is established. Thus, for linkage detection, under tight linkage, families with highly polymorphic markers are more powerful than those segregating less polymorphic markers—for the mating types considered here, 100 offspring in the four-allele case yield as high an ELOD as do $100 \times 0.601/0.451 = 133$ offspring in the two-allele case. On the other hand, under tight linkage, the precision of the recombination fraction estimate (expected information) is practically the same for four or two alleles. With looser linkage, as r approaches ½, offspring in the four-allele case tend to be twice as informative as those in the two-allele case, both for linkage detection and for estimation of the recombination fraction—then, only half as many offspring of four-allele matings as two-allele matings are needed on average. At r = ½, the ratio of ELODs is undefined 0/0, but the limiting value for $r{\to}$½ is as shown in figure 5.3.

A particular type of phase-unknown mating of two doubly heterozygous individuals is represented by the parents of children, some of whom are affected with a recessive disease, when linkage to a highly polymorphic marker is investigated. Calculations of the ELOD, conditional on number of affected and unaffected offspring, will be presented at the end of section 11.3.

5.7. Phase-known Double Backcross

The phase-known double backcross mating, $A1/B2 \times A1/A1$, has already been referred to at various places in this book. It allows a direct estimate of the recombination fraction, $\hat{\theta} = k/n$, where k is the number of recombinants among the n offspring. Fisher's expected information is given in equation (5.5). The ELOD per offspring is obtained from equation (5.3) as $E[Z(r)] = r\log(2r) + (1 - r)\log[2(1 - r)]$. At r = 0, since $0^0 = 1$ and $\log(1) = 0$, one finds $E[Z(0)] = \log(2)$. The phase-known double backcross often serves as a standard against which informativeness of other mating types is compared, for each offspring is equivalent to one recombination event.

For this mating, as well as for all other matings with known parental genotypes (including phase), n families with one offspring each provide the same information as, for example, $n/2$ families with two offspring each or as one family with n offspring. This simple relationship no longer holds when parental genotypes are not unambiguously known, as will be seen in the subsequent sections.

The observed lod score for k recombinants in n recombination events (opportunities for recombination) is given by equation (3.2).

5.8. Phase-unknown Double Backcross with Two Offspring

As was pointed out in section 4.1, one needs at least three generations of individuals to be able unequivocally to count recombinants and nonrecombinants. Two-generation families also yield information on linkage but not in a direct way (see y statistics, section 4.1). A typical such family is the phase-unknown double backcross—a mating between a double heterozygote and a double homozygote. Specifically, assume that the possible genotypes of the double heterozygote are *A1/B2* (I) and *A2/B1* (II), where I and II identify the two phases. The other parent is taken to have genotype *A1/A1*.

For a single offspring, the probability of an observed phenotype (the likelihood) is calculated as demonstrated below. Consider, for example, an offspring with phenotype $x = A1/A1$. One can easily calculate the probability of occurrence of x once phase is known. Therefore, one conditions on the phases and computes the offspring probability as $P(x) = P(x|\text{I})P(\text{I}) + P(x|\text{II})P(\text{II}) = \frac{1}{2}(1 - r) \times \frac{1}{2} + \frac{1}{2}r \times \frac{1}{2} = \frac{1}{4}$, where r is the (true) recombination fraction and, according to population genetics, the phases occur with probabilities of $\frac{1}{2}$ each (assuming linkage equilibrium, see section 11.4). As $P(x)$ does not depend on r, the lod score associated with such an observation is zero. Carrying out these calculations for each possible offspring genotype shows that none of them is informative for linkage. Consequently, the phase-unknown double backcross with a single offspring is not useful for linkage analysis. It was previously mentioned that a parent must be doubly heterozygous to be potentially informative for linkage. This condition is thus seen to be necessary but not sufficient.

Consider now two offspring from the mating type assumed above, for example, both offspring with phenotypes $x_1 = x_2 = A1/A1$. The likelihood for these two observations is given by $P(x_1, x_2) = P(x_1, x_2|\text{I})P(\text{I}) + P(x_1, x_2|\text{II})P(\text{II})$. For given phase, the two observations are conditionally independent so that one obtains $P(x_1, x_2) = \frac{1}{4}(1 - r)^2 \times \frac{1}{2} + \frac{1}{4}r^2 \times \frac{1}{2} = [(1 - r)^2 + r^2]/8 \equiv f_1$. Similarly, for $x_1 = A1/A1$ and $x_2 = A2/A1$, one obtains $P(x_1, x_2) = \frac{1}{4}r(1 - r) \equiv f_2$. When one carries these calculations through for all possible pairs of offspring genotypes, it turns out that each has either probability f_1 or f_2, which is shown in table 5.5. According to the principle used in section 5.5, one can collapse equal genotype probabilities into a single class so that one is left with a table of two rows and two columns (table 5.6). The first row and column each correspond to an offspring who is a nonrecombinant given phase I—call this a type 1 phenotype. The second row and column correspond to a recombinant given phase I—call this a type 2 phenotype. The result is shown in table 5.6. For example, the table entry in the first row and first column is simply the sum of the corresponding uncollapsed four terms, $4f_1 = \frac{1}{2}[(1 - r)^2 + r^2]$. The margins reflect the result obtained in the previous paragraph, namely, that a single offspring is uninformative for linkage.

Table 5.5. Joint Genotype Probabilities of Two Offspring from a Mating $[A1/B2$ or $A2/B1] \times A1/A1$, $f_1 = [(1 - r)^2 + r^2]/8$, $f_2 = r(1 - r)/4$.

	Child 2			
Child 1	*A1/A1*	*B2/A1*	*A2/A1*	*B1/A1*
A1/A1	f_1	f_1	f_2	f_2
B2/A1	f_1	f_1	f_2	f_2
A2/A1	f_2	f_2	f_1	f_1
B1/A1	f_2	f_2	f_1	f_1

Table 5.6. Joint Offspring Genotype Probabilities from a Phase-unknown Double Backcross Mating (Table 5.5 Collapsed)

	Child 2		
Child 1	Type 1	Type 2	Total
Type 1	$[(1 - r)^2 + r^2]/2$	$r(1 - r)$	$\frac{1}{2}$
Type 2	$r(1 - r)$	$[(1 - r)^2 + r^2]/2$	$\frac{1}{2}$
Total	$\frac{1}{2}$	$\frac{1}{2}$	1

Table 5.6 demonstrates the important general fact that offspring genotypes are not mutually independent when the parental genotypes are equivocal. In this case, the nonindependence arises because, for example, $P(x_1 = \text{type 1}, x_2 = \text{type 2}) \neq P(x_1 = \text{type 1}) \, P(x_2 = \text{type 2})$, or $\frac{1}{2}[(1 - r)^2 + r^2] \neq \frac{1}{2} \times \frac{1}{2}$, where x_1 and x_2 are phenotypes of child 1 and child 2, respectively. The correlation coefficient for table 5.6 is calculated as $\rho = (1 - 2r)^2$. The quantity $1 - 2r$ is known as the *linkage parameter*. The correlation between the offspring genotypes is zero only when there is absence of linkage, $r = \frac{1}{2}$; otherwise, it is positive. This is, of course, the basis for the sib-pair method referred to in section 4.9.

The list of joint genotypes of offspring pairs in table 5.6 shows that only two probabilities occur (binomial situation) so that, again, genotypes with equal probabilities can be combined into a single class. Phase-unknown double backcross families thus occur in two classes with class probabilities of $p = 2r(1 - r)$ and $1 - p = r^2 + (1 - r)^2$. Class 1 with frequency p corresponds to offspring of unequal type (one offspring is type 1, the other is type 2), whereas class 2 with frequency $1 - p$ corresponds to offspring with equal type (both offspring are type 1 or both are type 2), these class frequencies being independent of the population allele frequencies as long as the two loci are in linkage equilibrium (see

Table 5.7. Phenotype Classes of Pairs of Offspring from a Phase-unknown Double Backcross Mating

Phenotype	ℓ	p_ℓ	q_ℓ	$Z_\ell(\theta)$
Type unequal	1	$2r(1 - r)$	$2(1 - 2r)$	$\log[4\theta(1 - \theta)]$
Type equal	2	$r^2 + (1 - r)^2$	$-2(1 - 2r)$	$\log[2\theta^2 + 2(1 - \theta)^2]$
Total		1	0	

section 11.4). If they are not, the two phases in the informative parent are not equally frequent and their frequency depends on the allele frequencies.

Knowing the offspring phenotype (genotype) distribution allows calculation of expected information and ELOD per unit of observation which is, in this case, a pair of offspring. The relevant quantities are shown in table 5.7 and lead to the expected information of

$$i(r) = \frac{2}{r(1 - r)} \frac{(1 - 2r)^2}{1 - 2r(1 - r)}. \tag{5.13}$$

In the limit of zero recombination, the two offspring from the phase-unknown double backcross carry the same amount of information as two offspring from a phase-known double backcross. Thus, at $r = 0$, not knowing phase does not lead to a loss of precision of the θ estimate. It does, however, as r increases. At $r = \frac{1}{2}$, in contrast to the phase-known double backcross, there is even no information left for estimating r, that is, the expected lod score curve is completely flat at $r = \frac{1}{2}$.

The ELOD is calculated as $\Sigma_\ell p_\ell(r)Z_\ell(\theta)$ and evaluated at $\theta = r$,

$$E[Z(r)] = 2r(1 - r)\log[4r(1 - r)]$$
$$+ [r^2 + (1 - r)^2]\log[2r^2 + 2(1 - r)^2]. \tag{5.14}$$

For $r = 0$, note that $0^0 = 1$ so that the first term is equal to zero. One then obtains $E[Z(0)] = \log(2)$, which is only half as much as the ELOD for *two* offspring from a phase-known double backcross. This result has been interpreted to mean that, for detecting linkage, one loses one offspring because of not knowing phase. But one generally loses even more than that. Consider the ratio R of the ELOD for two offspring from a phase-known mating over the ELOD for two offspring from a phase-unknown mating. At $r = 0$ we have $R = 2$ but, with increasing recombination fraction, R increases until it becomes infinite in the limit as $r \rightarrow \frac{1}{2}$. For example, at $r = 0.1$, 0.2, and 0.3, one obtains $R = 3.32$, 5.82, and 12.80, respectively.

While the recombination fraction is generally estimated by maximizing the lod score, for a number n of phase-unknown double backcross families with two offspring each, a direct estimation is possible. Let k denote the number of families of class 1 (the two offspring are of unequal type), where each such family occurs with probability $p = 2r(1 - r)$. Since the maximum likelihood estimate of p is equal to k/n, solving for r leads to the following estimate of the recombination fraction:

$$\hat{\theta} = \begin{cases} \frac{1}{2}[1 - \sqrt{1 - 2k/n}] & \text{if } k < \frac{1}{2}n \\ \frac{1}{2} & \text{if } k \geq \frac{1}{2}n. \end{cases} \qquad (5.15)$$

From (5.13), the approximate standard error of $\hat{\theta}$ is obtained as $1/[n \times i(r)]^{1/2}$ when r is known, and an estimated approximate standard error is obtained by substituting $\hat{\theta}$ for r.

5.9. Phase-unknown Double Backcross with More Than Two Offspring

If parental genotypes are not unequivocal (e.g., phase unknown), then the offspring genotypes are statistically dependent (see previous section) so that the number of offspring per family becomes important. Let m denote the number of offspring of a phase-unknown double backcross mating and n the number of such families. Offspring phenotypes are of two kinds: type 1 is a recombinant under one of the parental phases (phase I, say) but a nonrecombinant under the other, and for type 2 the situation is reversed. Given phase I, a type 1 offspring occurs with probability r, and a type 2 offspring occurs with probability $1 - r$, r being the true recombination fraction. The conditional probability that i type 1 individuals out of m offspring are observed is thus $P(i|\text{I}) = \binom{m}{i}r^i(1 - r)^{m-i}$ for phase I and $P(i|\text{II}) = \binom{m}{i}(1 - r)^i r^{m-i}$ for phase II. The unconditional probability of i type 1 individuals is then $P(i) = \frac{1}{2}[P(i|\text{I}) + P(i|\text{II})]$, $i = 0 \ldots m$. Now, for any i, $P(i)$ is equal to $P(m - i)$ so that two such probabilities each can be combined into one class (for $i = m - i$, only a single probability exists). The resulting class probability is then equal to $P(i) + P(m - i) = \binom{m}{i}[r^i(1 - r)^{m-i} + r^{m-i}(1 - r)^i]$, $i \neq m - i$, while $P(i) = \binom{m}{i}r^i(1 - r)^i$ for $i = m - i$. The number of distinct classes for a phase-unknown double backcross family is given by

$$c = \begin{cases} \frac{1}{2}(m + 1) & \text{if } m \text{ is odd} \\ 1 + \frac{1}{2}m & \text{if } m \text{ is even}. \end{cases} \qquad (5.16)$$

Generally, when $c > 2$, the probability distribution of m such families is multinomial.

The simplest case, $m = 2$, is binomial and was covered in the previous section. The case of $m = 3$ offspring each (referred to in section 4.6) again leads to $c = 2$ classes only: a family of class 1 consists of three offspring, some of which are of a different type than others, the corresponding probability of occurrence being $p = 3r(1 - r)$. The other family class (all or no recombinants) occurs with probability $1 - p = r^3 + (1 - r)^3$. From this, the expected information per family can be derived as

$$i(r) = \frac{3}{r(1 - r)} \frac{(1 - 2r)^2}{1 - 3r(1 - r)}. \tag{5.17}$$

The lod scores corresponding to the two family classes are $Z_1(\theta) = \log[4\theta(1 - \theta)]$ and $Z_2(\theta) = \log[4\theta^3 + 4(1 - \theta)^3]$, from which the ELOD may be obtained.

For $m > 3$, the formal derivation of expected information and ELOD becomes cumbersome. Generally, at $r = 0$, the expected information is the same for phase-known and phase-unknown families. At $r = \frac{1}{2}$, it is zero for phase-unknown families but positive for phase-known families. Consequently, phase-unknown families are not very informative for detecting loose linkage. For a phase-unknown family with m offspring, the ELOD at $r = 0$ turns out to be equal to $(m - 1)\log(2)$, which is the same as the ELOD for a phase-known family with $m - 1$ offspring. Therefore, as noted in the previous section, one tends with tight linkage to "lose" one offspring because of not knowing phase, but the loss is relatively larger at larger values of the recombination fraction. At $r = 0$, the "loss" of one offspring for not knowing phase may be explained heuristically as follows: In the absence of recombination, the phenotypes of the first offspring reveal the parental phase so that effectively phase is known for subsequent offspring. If some recombination occurs ($r > 0$), phase is not completely revealed so that, even after knowing the first offspring, information from the other offspring is not as good as in a phase-known situation.

The observed lod score for a phase-unknown double backcross family with k type 1 individuals among the m offspring is given by

$$\begin{aligned} Z(\theta) = {}& (m - 1)\log(2) \\ & + \log[\theta^k(1 - \theta)^{m-k} + (1 - \theta)^k\theta^{m-k}]. \end{aligned} \tag{5.18}$$

Figure 5.4 shows a comparison of the observed lod scores with the same values of $k = 1$ and $m = 7$ for a phase-known (equation [3.2]) and a phase-unknown family (equation [5.18]). The graphs are given for the whole range of values, $0 \leq \theta \leq 1$. Apart from the higher lod score for the

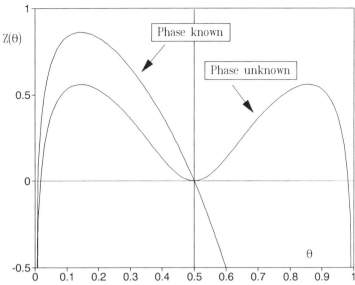

Figure 5.4. Observed lod scores for double backcross matings with seven offspring each (phase-known: one recombinant, phase-unknown: one type 1 individual).

phase-known family, a major difference between the two curves is that, in the phase-known case, the lod score has only one peak whereas in the phase-unknown case, it has two. The estimates are practically the same, $\hat{\theta} = 0.14$. In most linkage analyses, lod scores are calculated only for the range $0 \le \theta \le \frac{1}{2}$. However, when a large pedigree containing many different matings is analyzed or when several families are combined, inspecting the combined lod score at θ values higher than $\frac{1}{2}$ can show whether the data contain a sizeable proportion of phase-unknown matings. When the maximum at $\theta > \frac{1}{2}$ is close to the maximum at $\theta < \frac{1}{2}$, little phase-known information is present. In addition, when the maximum of the lod score is much higher for $\theta > \frac{1}{2}$ than for $\theta < \frac{1}{2}$, this warrants scrutiny for possible errors in the data; it is for this reason that the ILINK computer program of the LINKAGE package (section 8.3) computes estimates of $\theta > \frac{1}{2}$.

In equation (5.18), the two terms in the logarithm correspond to the two parental phases, whose unconditional (population) probabilities were assumed to be equal to $\frac{1}{2}$ each. Because of unknown phase, it was said above that counting recombinants and nonrecombinants among the offspring was not possible. In many cases, however, the conditional probability of phase I, say, given the observations, is so close to 0 or 1 that in practice the phase may be assumed to be known. Applying Bayes theorem, this conditional probability is calculated as $P(\text{phase I}|F) = P(F|\text{phase I}) P(\text{phase I}) / P(F)$, where F stands for the observations, $P(F)$ is the pedigree likelihood, and $P(\text{phase I}) = \frac{1}{2}$. Thus, one obtains

$$P(\text{phase I}|F) = \frac{\theta^k(1 - \theta)^{m-k}}{\theta^k(1 - \theta)^{m-k} + \theta^{m-k}(1 - \theta)^k} \qquad (5.19)$$

$$= \frac{1}{1 + [\theta/(1 - \theta)]^{m-2k}}.$$

Clearly, with small θ and k, it takes only a small number of offspring for the phase to have probability close to 1.

5.10. The Number of Observations Required to Detect Linkage

In planning a linkage analysis, an important question is how many individuals or families one reasonably needs. The answer will depend on various factors influencing informativeness such as penetrance, degree of phase knowledge, etc. A general approach is discussed in this section. A more specific approach is to determine numerically the conditional expected lod score for a given set of families with phenotypes observed at one locus. The latter approach is discussed in section 8.7.

As a starting point, consider known recombination events (offspring of phase-known double backcross matings). One may now ask what number, n, of these are required such that with high probability, ϕ (power), one will find a significant linkage ($Z_{max} \geq Z_0$) when the true recombination fraction is equal to r. The result may be obtained from the following approximate formula (Elandt-Johnson 1971, expression [13.69] modified):

$$n \approx [1.073\sqrt{Z_0} + x_\phi\sqrt{r - r^2}]^2/(r - \frac{1}{2})^2, \qquad (5.20)$$

where x_ϕ is the normal deviate associated with an upper tail probability ϕ, for example, $x_\phi = 0.84$ for a power of 80 percent and $x_\phi = 1.28$ for a power of 90 percent. Table 5.8 presents some numbers calculated using equation (5.20). To detect a recombination fraction of 5 percent or smaller using the customary criterion, $Z_0 = 3$, roughly twenty recombination events are required.

Depending on the informativeness inherent in different mating types, a larger or smaller number of observations are required for the total number of observations to carry the same overall degree of informativeness. One might use either Fisher's expected information or the ELOD as a measure of informativeness for linkage. As the latter is better known

Table 5.8. Number of Known Recombination Events Required to Find $Z_{max} \geq Z_0$ with Power ϕ, Given True Recombination Fraction r

Z_0	ϕ	True Recombination Fraction					
		0.01	0.05	0.10	0.20	0.30	0.40
2	0.80	11	14	20	38	91	373
	0.90	11	16	23	46	111	461
3	0.80	16	21	28	54	126	516
	0.90	16	22	31	62	150	618

among human geneticists and since its absolute value is better interpretable, it will preferentially be used throughout this book. Consider now two family types with respective ELODs of E_1 and E_2 per family. Assume that n_1 families of type 1 have been collected. The total ELOD for the type 1 families is thus equal to $n_1 E_1$. How many families of type 2 are required such that their total ELOD is the same as that furnished by the type 1 families? For an equal total ELOD from families of type 2, the equation $n_1 E_1 = n_2 E_2$ must hold so that the number of families of type 2 is obtained as

$$n_2 = R\, n_1, \quad R = E_1/E_2. \tag{5.21}$$

In later chapters, the ratio R will be calculated for various factors reducing informativeness. At the end of this book (section 11.10), such results will serve as a guide for deciding how many families are required in a given linkage study.

As a simple example, consider the following expected lod scores at $r = 0$: $\log(2) = 0.301$ for one known recombination event as well as for two offspring from a phase-unknown double backcross, $2\log(2)$ for three offspring from a phase-unknown double backcross, and $5\log(2)$ for six offspring from a phase-unknown double backcross. Take $n_1 = 16$ as the number of known recombination events needed for a linkage analysis (table 5.8). How many phase-unknown families with three offspring each are required for the same ELOD as the sixteen known recombination events? With $E_1 = \log(2)$ and $E_2 = 2\log(2)$, following equation (5.21), one finds $n_2 = (E_1/E_2)n_1 = \frac{1}{2} \times 16 = 8$ families.

In planning a linkage analysis one may ask what is more informative— a large number of small families or a small number of large families? An answer to this question depends on several factors such as problems of genetic heterogeneity. In terms of statistical informativeness, when phase-unknown double backcross matings are considered, results of the previous paragraph may be used to show that a small number of large families is better. Consider a total number of six offspring from a varying number of families of different sizes: (1) two offspring each in three families, (2) three each in two families, and (3) all six offspring in a single family. The corresponding total ELODs for these three cases are (1) 3log(2), (2) 4log(2), and (3) 5log(2).

Problems

Problem 5.1. Show formally that a mating in which no parent is a double heterozygote is not informative for linkage. Assume the mating $A1/B1 \times C1/C2$ and proceed in analogy to table 5.2. List all possible offspring genotypes.

Problem 5.2. In table 5.4, the first three phenotype classes identify known recombination events, whereas the fourth class represents ambiguous cases. Researchers sometimes analyze data by simply omitting the latter. Using the probabilities and lod scores given in the table, determine whether and to what extent discarding this information introduces an asymptotic bias in the recombination estimate. Hint: set the first derivative with respect to θ of the expected lod score function equal to zero and solve the resulting equation for θ as a function of r; this will yield the value of θ at which the expected lod score function has its maximum. Make sure that the conditional probabilities used sum to 1.

Problem 5.3. Show that a pair of offspring from a phase-unknown double backcross mating carries the same amount of linkage information (equation [5.13]) as one offspring from the double intercross mating $A1/B2 \times A2/B1$ (codominant inheritance at each locus). Hint: Show that, for both cases, the same number of phenotype classes and the same class probabilities occur.

Problem 5.4. Assume two trait loci with alleles T and t at locus 1 and alleles D and d at locus 2. Both traits follow a strictly dominant mode of inheritance, $T > t$ and $D > d$. For a phase-known mating $Td/tD \times Td/tD$, derive Fisher's expected information, $i(r)$, and the ELOD, $E[Z(r)]$, and evaluate these quantities numerically for a range of values, $0 \leq r \leq \frac{1}{2}$.

Problem 5.5. Compute the ELOD at recombination fraction r for the mating $A1/B2 \times A?/A?$. The second parent is untyped at the second locus, which has alleles *1* and *2* with the respective population gene frequencies p and $1 - p$.

Problem 5.6. Consider two parents and n children, all individuals being doubly heterozygous (*1/2*, *1/2*). Is this family informative for linkage? Hint: Derive the likelihood ratio $L(\theta)/L(\frac{1}{2})$ and check whether it is different from 1 for $\theta < \frac{1}{2}$. What is the likelihood ratio at $\theta = 0$?

Problem 5.7. Show in an example that the ELOD, $E[Z(r)]$, is additive over families but the expected maximum lod score, $E(Z_{max})$, is not (section 5.2). Hint: Use the data of table 5.1 for a phase-known double backcross family of size 3, carry out analogous calculations for two families of size 3 (which are the same as for one family of size 6), and compare the results. It is easiest to obtain $P(k)$ from the BINOM program and the $Z(0.10)$ and Z_{max} values from the EQUIV program.

6.

Multipoint Linkage Analysis

Traditionally in human genetics, linkage analyses have been carried out as a sequence of pairwise (two-point) comparisons between a trait locus and each of a number of marker loci. For each comparison, trait versus ith marker, or marker versus marker, lod scores are computed and combined over families and investigators. With the linkage map growing denser, the simultaneous analysis of several linked loci (multipoint analysis) became important. In practice, as a first step, two-point lod scores are still computed and reported in most studies.

Some theoretical aspects of multipoint analysis may be found in Bailey (1961). In human genetics, early approaches to multipoint analysis include those of Renwick and Bolling (1971), Cook et al. (1974), and Meyers et al. (1975, 1976). A few multipoint analyses in classical genetics will be quoted below as well (e.g., Fisher 1922). This chapter addresses theoretical and practical aspects of multipoint analysis. Although examples are provided, specific computational problems will be deferred to chapter 8. The first section of this chapter introduces some notation and terminology required for the joint analysis of several loci. Basic principles of multipoint analysis will then be addressed in sections 6.2 and 6.3, with section 6.2 containing examples demonstrating the increase in informativeness of multipoint over two-point analysis. Sections 6.4 through 6.6 cover more theoretical topics, and the later sections are again devoted to practical aspects.

6.1. Notation and Terminology

With many loci, linkage analysis is quantitatively as well as qualitatively different from two-point analysis. For one thing, the order of the loci now matters. Also, the number of parameters, haplotypes and genotypes, increases drastically with the number of loci considered. This section will introduce the notation and terms required in subsequent sections. If some of this seems too abstract, it may be best to skip this portion of the text and consult it only when required. Examples will be provided in the subsequent sections.

As pointed out in section 1.2, the total number of different haplotypes or gametes with respect to a number of loci is given by the product of the numbers of alleles at these loci, $H = \Pi\, n_i$. For example, the presence of three alleles at each of five loci defines $H = 3^5 = 243$ haplotypes. For any individual, the total number of different multilocus genotypes (pairs of haplotypes) is equal to $H(H + 1)/2$. With $H = 243$, one has 29,646 possible genotypes. The sheer size of this figure gives an impression of the computational problems that may be involved in the calculation of the likelihood (equation [4.16]). Calculation of genotype probabilities will be demonstrated in section 6.2.

Thus far a fixed order of the loci has been assumed. As will be seen below, genotype probabilities are generally different for different orders. It is thus important to consider the number, n_0, of different possible orders. It is simply equal to the number of possible permutations divided by 2, since two orders are considered the same if one is just the mirror image of the other, for example, 1243 and 3421. Therefore,

$$n_0 = \frac{n!}{2} = \frac{n(n - 1)(n - 2)\, \ldots\, (3)(2)(1)}{2}. \tag{6.1}$$

For example, $n = 3$ loci can occur in $n_0 = 3$ possible orders, and $n = 5$ loci in 60 orders. For large n, it may not be easy to enumerate all possible orders. A systematic method of listing these orders (Johnson 1963) is implemented in the PERMUTE program.

A collection of n loci define $n - 1$ intervals between adjacent loci. When the lengths of these intervals are known, this collection of loci is called a map. If, in addition, an interval is defined to the left of the leftmost locus and one to the right of the rightmost locus, $n + 1$ intervals are distinguished, which may be numbered as shown in table 6.1. The ith interval is denoted by I_i.

In two-point linkage analysis, support for linkage is customarily ex-

Table 6.1. Numbering System for Loci and Map Segments

Locus number	*1*	*2*	*3*	. . .	*n* − 1	*n*	
------- + ------- + ------- + ----- + ----- + --------- + -----
Interval number	0	1	2	3	. . .	*n* − 1	*n*

pressed in terms of the lod score, which is the logarithm of the likelihood ratio L_1/L_0, L_1 being the likelihood under linkage and L_0 referring to absence of linkage. With multiple loci, depending on the hypotheses considered, there are many different ways of expressing support. Following the International System for Human Linkage Maps, ISLM 1990 (Keats et al. 1991), three measures of statistical support are distinguished, each defined by $\log_{10}(L_1/L_2)$, with L_1 and L_2 being defined as shown below for the specific support measures. *Global support* measures the evidence that a locus belongs to a map of loci. It is calculated by taking L_1 as the maximum likelihood when the locus is inserted in the map and L_2 as the likelihood when the locus is not on the map. "Definite" linkage of the locus with the map is said to be established when global support is 3 or more. *Interval support* measures the evidence that the locus is in a particular interval of the map, where L_1 is the maximum likelihood with the locus being in that interval and L_2 is the highest likelihood obtained by placing the marker in any other interval. To express *support for a given order*, L_1 is taken as the maximum likelihood of the best supported order and L_2 is the maximum likelihood for the given order.

Loci with interval support of at least 3 are termed *framework loci*, and a map composed entirely of such loci is called a *framework map* (Keats et al. 1991). A map is called *comprehensive* if it aims to include all syntenic loci (no support requirements for a comprehensive map).

In addition to the three types of multilocus support mentioned above, a fourth type has customarily been used to designate the overall evidence that a set of loci form a linkage group. It is obtained as the maximum likelihood L_1 under the best supported order divided by the likelihood L_0 assuming all loci are unlinked,

$$\log(L_1/L_0) = \log\frac{L(\theta_{12}, \ldots, \theta_{n-1,n})}{L(\frac{1}{2}, \frac{1}{2}, \ldots, \frac{1}{2})}, \tag{6.2}$$

where θ_{ij} is the recombination fraction between loci i and j. The support defined by equation (6.2) has been called *generalized support* or generalized lod score. Calculating and reporting such lod scores may be meaningful during the initial stages of map construction as they measure the overall evidence that a set of loci is linked. However, interpreting a generalized multipoint lod score (6.2) is not straightforward as it may involve several estimated recombination fractions. Numerical examples of calculating generalized lod scores are provided in section 6.2. Clearly, the $n - 1$ recombination fractions in (6.2) cannot specify the probabilities of all joint recombination events occurring among the n loci—additional assumptions are required to do that (see section 6.6). In other words, a lod score such as (6.2) does not summarize all of the information in the data unless the probabilities of the joint recombination events are specified, for example, by assuming independent relationships between the θ values.

The four types of support considered above are all single numbers, obtained by maximizing likelihoods over portions of the genome. In analogy to the two-point situation, support for the various positions x of a single locus relative to a map of loci can be expressed as a *map-specific multipoint lod score*, $Z(x) = \log[L(x)/L(\infty)]$, where x is any map position of the locus in question on the fixed marker map and the infinite location $x = \infty$ indicates that the single locus is off the map ($\theta = \frac{1}{2}$ between the single locus and any of the marker loci on the map). For example, if x specifies a location of the locus in question in interval 0 of the map of markers and θ_{ij} denotes the recombination fraction between loci i and j, this map-specific multipoint lod score is given by

$$Z(\theta_{01}, \theta_{12}, \theta_{23}, \ldots, \theta_{n-1,n}) = \log \frac{L(\theta_{01}, \theta_{12}, \ldots, \theta_{n-1,n})}{L(\frac{1}{2}, \theta_{12}, \ldots, \theta_{n-1,n})}. \tag{6.3}$$

Another transformation of the likelihood ratio $L(x)/L(\infty)$ is the *location score*, $S(x) = 2 \ln[L(x)/L(\infty)]$ (Lathrop et al. 1984). It is a simple multiple of the lod score, $S(x) = 2 \times \ln(10) Z(x)$, where $2 \times \ln(10) \approx 4.6$. Obviously, it would not be meaningful to compute a generalized lod score when mapping a new locus to a known map of markers. The generalized lod score would not represent the evidence for the relation between the new locus and the map of markers, as the relation among the latter is known from other sources.

For the calculations outlined later in this chapter, it is useful to distinguish two types of multiple recombination probabilities (see also Liberman and Karlin 1984). When gametes are produced by a parent, in each interval a recombination (odd number of crossovers per strand, i.e., per chromatid) either does or does not occur. For example, on the right side of figure 6.1, a recombination occurs in interval 1 (top) but none occurs in interval 2. The probability, which specifies for each interval whether a recombination has occurred or not, is called an *n-fold recombination fraction* (Risch and Lange 1979) or a multilocus or *joint recombination probability*. Its notation may be formalized as follows: For n loci, consider an array $\varepsilon = (\varepsilon_1, \varepsilon_2, \ldots, \varepsilon_{n-1})$, in which $\varepsilon_i = 1$ if a recombination occurs in interval I_i and $\varepsilon_i = 0$ for no recombination in I_i. The joint recombination probability is then conveniently written as $G(\varepsilon)$. For example, with

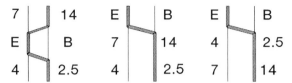

Figure 6.1. Crossover events leading to the haplotype received by individual 3.5 in figure 6.2 for different locus orders.

four loci, the fact that a recombination occurs in intervals I_1 and I_2 but not in I_3 is denoted by $\varepsilon = (1, 1, 0)$ and its probability of occurrence is $G[(1, 1, 0)]$ or g_{110}. As there are two possibilities in each of the $n - 1$ intervals, the possible number of arrays ε and thus of joint recombination probabilities is equal to 2^{n-1}. The joint recombination events are mutually exclusive, and the sum of the probabilities $G(\varepsilon)$ over all ε is equal to 1.

A recombination between two specific loci, which need not be adjacent, is the consequence of an odd number of crossovers between them. The probability of occurrence of such a recombination is just the regular two-point recombination fraction. A special case of it is the recombination fraction between two adjacent loci—one of the marginal probabilities of the $G(\varepsilon)$ defined in the previous paragraph. These recombination fractions may be generalized in the following way (Liberman and Karlin 1984): Consider a region W of a map of n loci such that W consists of some of the intervals, I_i, where the I_i need not be contiguous. Define an array $\boldsymbol{\delta} = (\delta_1, \delta_2, \ldots, \delta_{n-1})$, in which $\delta_i = 1$ if I_i belongs to W and $\delta_i = 0$ otherwise. The δ_i are thus indicator variables identifying W. The probability of an odd number of crossovers occurring in W is called the *recombination value* $R(\boldsymbol{\delta})$ (notice that the sum of the recombination values over all $\boldsymbol{\delta}$ is not generally equal to 1). When the I_i are contiguous, the recombination value R is identical with the two-point recombination fraction between the endpoints of W. $R(\boldsymbol{\delta})$ may also be denoted by $r_{ij\ldots k}$, where the subscripts indicate the intervals included in W. For example, for four loci A-B-C-D, the recombination fraction between loci A and C (over intervals 1 and 2) is denoted by r_{12} or $R[(1, 1, 0)]$, since $\boldsymbol{\delta} = (1, 1, 0)$. Since any interval between n loci may or may not be included in W, there are 2^{n-1} possible recombination values.

There is a one-to-one relationship between joint recombination probabilities and recombination values (Karlin and Liberman 1978):

$$G(\varepsilon) = \sum_{\delta} (-1)^s \frac{1 - 2R(\boldsymbol{\delta})}{2^{n-1}}, \qquad (6.4)$$

$$R(\boldsymbol{\delta}) = \tfrac{1}{2}\left[1 - \sum_{\varepsilon} (-1)^s\, G(\boldsymbol{\varepsilon}) \right], \tag{6.5}$$

where $s = \sum_{i=1}^{n-1} \delta_i \varepsilon_i$.

6.2. Three-Point Analysis

The basic data type for three-point linkage analysis consists of the n offspring from phase-known matings in which one parent is triply heterozygous and the other is triply homozygous (a triple backcross), $ABC/abc \times abc/abc$, where A and a are the two alleles at locus A, B and b those at locus B, and C and c those at locus C. A recombination between two loci was introduced in section 1.2 as that process occurring in a parent leading to the occurrence of two alleles (one at each locus) from different grandparents occurring on the same haplotype of a child (see fig. 1.1). As one has only two maternal and two paternal grandparents, any offspring cannot be recombinant for each of the three locus pairs, AB, BC, and AC. Rather, for example, a recombination for AB and BC implies nonrecombination for AC. On the other hand, no individual can be recombinant for only one pair of loci and not for any other; for example, recombination for AB and nonrecombination for BC implies recombination for AC. All of this holds irrespective of the particular order of loci.

For any number of loci, if haplotypes can be recognized in offspring, one may, for example, indicate grandmaternal origin of an allele by 0 and grandpaternal origin by 1. A haplotype is then characterized by a string of 0's and 1's, where a change from 0 to 1 or 1 to 0 identifies the occurrence of a recombination between the two corresponding loci (for examples, see table 2 in White et al. 1985).

With respect to recombination for AB and BC jointly, assuming locus

Table 6.2. Joint Recombination Fractions (g_{ij}) and Two-Point Recombination Fractions (θ) for Recombination (R) and Nonrecombination (NR) among Loci A, B, and C

	Loci B and C		
Loci A and B	R	NR	Total
R	g_{11}	g_{10}	θ_{AB}
NR	g_{01}	g_{00}	$1 - \theta_{AB}$
Total	θ_{BC}	$1 - \theta_{BC}$	1

order A-B-C, four classes of offspring can be distinguished whose probabilities of occurrence are listed in table 6.2: double recombinants with recombination for AB and BC, occurring with probability g_{11}; single recombinants with a recombination for loci AB but none for BC (probability g_{10}); single recombinants with a recombination for BC but none for AB (probability g_{01}); and nonrecombinants, occurring with probability g_{00}. Since $\Sigma\Sigma g_{ij} = 1$, there are three independent parameters, say, g_{11}, g_{10}, and g_{01}. The unrestricted maximum likelihood estimates of the multinomial parameters g_{ij} are simply the corresponding observed proportions of offspring, $\hat{g}_{ij} = n_{ij}/n$.

As a simple example, consider figure 6.2, which shows the most likely genotypes for three X-chromosomal marker loci in part of family 21 of Musarella et al. (1989). Let A, B, and C stand for the loci *DXS85*, *DXS255*, and *DXS14*, respectively. Following the gametes from parents

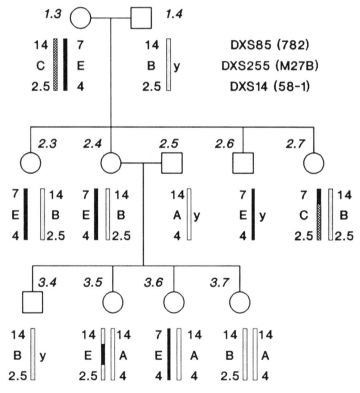

Figure 6.2. Portion of family 21 (adapted from fig. 7 in Musarella et al. 1989) showing segregation of haplotypes at three X-chromosomal marker loci.

to the children, one finds $n_{00} = 6$ cases of nonrecombinant haplotypes; $n_{10} = 1$ haplotype (received by individual 2.7) is recombinant for AB and nonrecombinant for BC, and $n_{11} = 1$ haplotype (received by individual 3.5) is recombinant for both AB and BC. No case of a single recombinant between B and C ($n_{01} = 0$) is observed in this small family segment. The total number of haplotypes counted is $n = 8$.

The recombination fractions are obtained from the joint recombination probabilities as follows: The probability of a recombination between loci A and B, irrespective of what happens between B and C, is $\theta_{AB} = g_{11} + g_{10}$ (table 6.2). Analogously, $\theta_{BC} = g_{11} + g_{01}$. Finally, the probability of a recombination between loci A and C is given by $\theta_{AC} = g_{01} + g_{10}$. For example, the data of the previous paragraph give the estimates $\hat{\theta}_{AB} = (1 + 1)/8 = \frac{1}{4}$, $\hat{\theta}_{BC} = 1/8$, and $\hat{\theta}_{AC} = 1/8$.

The relations leading from the g_{ij}'s to the θ's are easily inverted to yield the joint recombination probabilities in terms of the two-point recombination fractions, where the indicated restrictions ensure that the joint probabilities g_{ij} are nonnegative:

$$g_{11} = \frac{1}{2}(\theta_{AB} + \theta_{BC} - \theta_{AC}), \qquad \theta_{AC} \le \theta_{AB} + \theta_{BC} \qquad (6.6a)$$

$$g_{10} = \frac{1}{2}(\theta_{AB} - \theta_{BC} + \theta_{AC}), \qquad \theta_{BC} \le \theta_{AB} + \theta_{AC} \qquad (6.6b)$$

$$g_{01} = \frac{1}{2}(-\theta_{AB} + \theta_{BC} + \theta_{AC}), \qquad \theta_{AB} \le \theta_{BC} + \theta_{AC} \qquad (6.6c)$$

$$g_{00} = 1 - g_{11} - g_{10} - g_{01} = 1 - \frac{1}{2}(\theta_{AB} + \theta_{BC} + \theta_{AC}) \qquad (6.6d)$$

With the g's defined as in table 6.2, the equations (6.6a–d) do not depend on locus order (but see the locus-specific inequalities [6.11]). In practice, one usually works with yet another set of parameters involving the coefficient of coincidence, which will be introduced in section 6.4.

The log likelihood for three-point observations is given by

$$\log L(g_{11}, g_{10}, g_{01}) = \sum_i \sum_j n_{ij} \log(g_{ij}). \qquad (6.7)$$

When all two-point recombination fractions involving the three loci are equal to $\frac{1}{2}$, the g_{ij}'s become $\frac{1}{4}$ each. A generalized lod score may thus be obtained from (6.7) as

$$Z(g_{11}, g_{10}, g_{01}) = \sum_i \sum_j n_{ij} \log(4g_{ij}). \qquad (6.8)$$

For example, with the data of figure 6.2, $n_{00} = 6$, $n_{01} = 0$, $n_{10} = n_{11} = 1$, one finds $Z = 6\log(4g_{00}) + \log(4g_{10}) + \log(4g_{11})$. At the maximum likelihood estimates, $\hat{g}_{ij} = n_{ij}/n$, the maximum of the generalized lod score for the given observations is obtained as 2.26.

In practice, three-point data rarely occur as counts of haplotypes from phase-known double backcross matings. In many matings, only one of the two intervals is informative. For example, in figure 6.2, individual 2.7 is homozygous at marker *DXS14* and thus uninformative for recombination events between loci *DXS255* and *DXS14*. Her sons (not shown; she had no daughters) contribute information only for the recombination fraction θ_{BC} but not for joint recombination probabilities at both intervals. Therefore, the likelihood for the data shown in figure 6.2 plus the data contributed by the sons of individual 2.7 cannot be represented in the simple form of (6.7) or (6.8).

When, in a collection of families, each family is informative for the recombination fraction between two markers only, then the total lod score is simply the sum of the two-point lod scores,

$$Z(\theta_{AB}, \theta_{BC}, \theta_{AC}) = Z(\theta_{AB}) + Z(\theta_{BC}) + Z(\theta_{AC}). \tag{6.9}$$

A formula analogous to (6.9) applies to more than three loci. As a first step, linkage data are often analyzed in pairwise comparisons. However, the overall log likelihood cannot generally be represented as a sum of two-point log likelihoods as in (6.9) because of sample nonindependence of $\hat{\theta}_{AB}$, $\hat{\theta}_{BC}$, $\hat{\theta}_{AC}$. Some approximate analysis approaches are based on combinations of two-point lod scores (see section 6.7).

In several respects, three-point (and generally multipoint) analysis yields more information than does two-point analysis. As shown by Thompson (1984), "three-way data provide very much more information, particularly with regard to the problem of ordering the loci"; where individuals informative for all three loci are observed, information is lost (or overestimated) by summarizing the data in pairwise form. Lathrop et al. (1985) calculated the relative efficiency of three-locus versus two-locus estimates of recombination rates and found, for example, making no assumptions on interference, that three-point data can be over five times as efficient, thus requiring less than one fifth the number of observations than two-point data for the same precision of the estimates.

An illuminating example was given by Lathrop et al. (1985). In two parents, phase is known owing to grandparental genotypes. The parental genotypes are *ABc/abC* and *ABC/aBc*, respectively. An offspring has the respective genotypes *A/a*, *B/b*, and *C/C* at the three loci. The salient point here is that the offspring is completely uninformative for linkage between loci *1* and *2*. Parent 2 is homozygous *B/B*, and parent 1 either passed a recombinant or a nonrecombinant gamete to the offspring, the corresponding two probabilities adding to 1. However, when locus *3* is also considered, the offspring becomes informative for recombination between loci *1* and *2*, the reason being that, in parent 2, alleles *C* and *c* at locus *3* help discriminate between the two *B* alleles at locus *2* (a *C* allele is known to have been passed to the offspring by parent 2). When tight linkage between loci *2* and *3* is assumed, the relation between loci *1* and *2* is essentially carried by the relation between loci *1* and *3*, which specifies that either two recombinations or two nonrecombinations have occurred. The corresponding maximum lod score is equal to 0.301 as opposed to zero when locus *3* is disregarded.

As another instructive example, consider two parents and two children, each typed at three two-allele loci. The phase unknown genotypes are (*1/2*, *2/2*, *1/2*) for the mother and (*1/2*, *1/2*, *2/2*) for the father. The children's genotypes are (*2/2*, *1/2*, *2/2*) and (*1/2*, *2/2*, *1/2*). Any pairwise analysis is completely uninformative, but a three-point analysis reveals a known recombination between the flanking loci. This example is constructed in analogy to the situation of the first son of family A47, table 8.1, who is a recombinant under one parental phase and a nonrecombinant under another so that he becomes uninformative for linkage. The known recombination in the artificial family considered here may be seen as follows: The first child has phase known genotype *212/222*. Postulating absence of recombination, this child's genotype implies the parental genotypes *121/222* for the mother and *122/212* for the father. The second child has genotype *121/222* or *122/221*, each of which requires at least one recombination in the father or the mother.

The examples in the previous paragraphs are contrived, but they point out important aspects of multipoint analysis. A case found in real data was demonstrated by Scheffer et al. (1989), who reported a recombination in an offspring between Wilson's disease and a neighboring marker; the recombination was undetectable by two-point analyses and was only recognized in three-point analysis. In that family, the parents had genotypes *3 w 2/1 + 2* and *2 + 4/2 w 2*, respectively, *w* being the disease allele and *+* the normal allele (the flanking loci are *RB1* with alleles *1*, *2*, and *3* and *D13S12* with alleles *1* and *2*). The parental phases are the ones compatible with no recombination in children 2 through 4. The first child (with the recombination) had the respective genotypes *2/3*, *w/+*, and *2/2* at the three loci.

6.3. Phase-unknown Triple Backcross with Two Offspring

As will be seen below, for many multilocus problems explicit solutions are unavailable; they can be found analytically only for special cases such as phase-unknown triple backcross matings with two offspring each, which will be covered in this section. The results obtained will not be of much use in practice, but they give insight into several important theoretical aspects, for example, why maximum likelihood estimates in linkage analysis generally are biased. Readers less interested in theory may skip this section.

Consider three loci with two alleles each, where the alleles are designated as A,a; B,b; and C,c at loci A, B, and C, respectively. Assume a triply homozygous parent, abc/abc, and a triply heterozygous parent, $(A/a, B/b, C/c)$. In the latter, four phases are possible: (I) ABC/abc, (II) ABc/abC, (III) AbC/aBc, and (IV) Abc/aBC. Under regular conditions (linkage equilibrium, chapter 11), each of these phases occurs with probability ¼. Although the triply homozygous parent produces only one kind of haplotype, abc, potentially eight different haplotypes originate from the heterozygous parent, which are listed in table 6.3 along with their conditional probabilities of occurrence given parental phase. For example, under phase I, with no recombination in interval 1 but a recombination in interval 2, that is, with probability g_{01} (table 6.2), either an ABc or an abC haplotype occurs. The probability for each of these two possibilities is ½ so that, under phase I, the haplotype ABc is produced with probability $\frac{1}{2}g_{01}$, as is the haplotype abC.

Assuming dominance at each locus, the haplotype symbols in table 6.3 may be interpreted as offspring phenotype symbols. The figures in table 6.3 then give the conditional probabilities with which offspring phenotypes occur. Now, in analogy to the phase-unknown double backcross (section 5.8), assume two offspring in each family. Their joint probability of occurrence has to be computed as in the following example: Assume phenotype ABC (genotype ABC/abc, $i = 1$ in table 6.3) for child

Table 6.3. Conditional Haplotype Probabilities Given Phase, Produced by a Triply Heterozygous Parent (A/a, B/b, C/c)

		Phase			
i	Haplotype	I	II	III	IV
1	ABC	$\frac{1}{2}g_{00}$	$\frac{1}{2}g_{01}$	$\frac{1}{2}g_{11}$	$\frac{1}{2}g_{10}$
2	ABc	$\frac{1}{2}g_{01}$	$\frac{1}{2}g_{00}$	$\frac{1}{2}g_{10}$	$\frac{1}{2}g_{11}$
3	AbC	$\frac{1}{2}g_{11}$	$\frac{1}{2}g_{10}$	$\frac{1}{2}g_{00}$	$\frac{1}{2}g_{01}$
4	Abc	$\frac{1}{2}g_{10}$	$\frac{1}{2}g_{11}$	$\frac{1}{2}g_{01}$	$\frac{1}{2}g_{00}$
5	aBC	$\frac{1}{2}g_{10}$	$\frac{1}{2}g_{11}$	$\frac{1}{2}g_{01}$	$\frac{1}{2}g_{00}$
6	aBc	$\frac{1}{2}g_{11}$	$\frac{1}{2}g_{10}$	$\frac{1}{2}g_{00}$	$\frac{1}{2}g_{01}$
7	abC	$\frac{1}{2}g_{01}$	$\frac{1}{2}g_{00}$	$\frac{1}{2}g_{10}$	$\frac{1}{2}g_{11}$
8	abc	$\frac{1}{2}g_{00}$	$\frac{1}{2}g_{01}$	$\frac{1}{2}g_{11}$	$\frac{1}{2}g_{10}$
	Total	1	1	1	1

Table 6.4. Offspring Phenotype Classes in Phase-unknown Triple Backcross Families with Two Offspring

k	ij	P_k
1	11,22,33,44,55,66,77,88,45,36,27,18	$g_{11}^2 + g_{10}^2 + g_{01}^2 + g_{00}^2$
2	12,34,35,17,46,28,56,78	$2(g_{11}g_{10} + g_{01}g_{00})$
3	23,14,15,26,37,48,67,58	$2(g_{11}g_{01} + g_{10}g_{00})$
4	13,24,25,16,47,38,57,68	$2(g_{11}g_{00} + g_{10}g_{01})$
	Total	1

Note: i and j refer to the numbering of the haplotypes in table 6.3, interpreted here as phenotypes. Cases $i > j$ are not listed.

1 and phenotype AbC (genotype AbC/abc, $i = 3$) for child 2. Given phase I, the joint probability of occurrence of these two phenotypes is $(\tfrac{1}{2}g_{00}) \times (\tfrac{1}{2}g_{11})$; under phase II, it is $(\tfrac{1}{2}g_{01}) \times (\tfrac{1}{2}g_{10})$, and so on. The unconditional probability for the phenotype ABC in child 1 and AbC in child 2 is then calculated as $\tfrac{1}{4}(\tfrac{1}{2}g_{00})(\tfrac{1}{2}g_{11}) + \tfrac{1}{4}(\tfrac{1}{2}g_{01})(\tfrac{1}{2}g_{10}) + \ldots = \tfrac{1}{8}(g_{11}g_{00} + g_{10}g_{01})$. Disregarding the order of the two offspring, their joint probability of occurrence is given by $\tfrac{1}{4}(g_{11}g_{00} + g_{10}g_{01})$. In this manner, the probabilities for all $8 \times 9/2 = 36$ possible pairs of phenotypes can be calculated. It then turns out that, among the thirty-six probabilities, only four different values occur so that those pairs of phenotypes with the same probabilities can be combined into single classes (section 5.8). Offspring phenotypes with the same probabilities are listed in table 6.4, along with the probabilities p_k of the resulting phenotype classes. The lod score associated with the kth phenotype class is given by $\log(4p_k)$, since $g_{ij} = \tfrac{1}{4}$ under absence of linkage.

The offspring phenotype classes in table 6.4 are determined by three independent parameters (degrees of freedom), say, p_1, p_2, and p_3. Their maximum likelihood estimates are given by the multinomial proportions, $\hat{p}_k$, that is, the proportions of families with offspring phenotype class k. The p_k depend on the joint recombination probabilities, g_{ij}, or, equivalently, on the recombination fractions θ_{AB}, θ_{BC}, and θ_{AC}. Since the number of the latter parameters is also equal to 3, their MLEs can simply be obtained as functions of the $\hat{p}_k$. The equations for p_k in table 6.4 can easily be solved, for example, by writing $p_3 + p_4 = 2(g_{11}g_{01} + g_{10}g_{00} + g_{11}g_{00} + g_{10}g_{01}) = 2(g_{11} + g_{10})(g_{01} + g_{00}) = 2\theta_{AB}(1 - \theta_{BC})$, as pointed out by Dr. Paul Van Eerdewegh. Solving this quadratic leads to

$$\hat{\theta}_{AB} = \begin{cases} \tfrac{1}{2} - \tfrac{1}{2}\sqrt{1 - 2(\hat{p}_3 + \hat{p}_4)} & \text{if } \hat{p}_3 + \hat{p}_4 < \tfrac{1}{2} \\ \tfrac{1}{2} & \text{otherwise.} \end{cases} \quad (6.10)$$

In an analogous manner, $\hat{\theta}_{BC}$ is determined by $\hat{p}_2 + \hat{p}_4$, and $\hat{\theta}_{AC}$ by $\hat{p}_2 + \hat{p}_3$.

The multinomial proportions $\hat{p}_k$ are known to be unbiased estimates of the class probabilities p_k, that is, $E(\hat{p}_k) = p_k$. However, nonlinear functions of MLEs such as the recombination fractions (6.10) are generally biased. This suggests that, in practically all cases of practical importance, recombination estimates are biased, but this bias tends to disappear as the number of observations increases, since MLEs are generally consistent (see section 3.3).

The ranges of the estimates (6.10) are restricted by the inequalities in equations (6.6a–c), which do not depend on locus order. For a given order of the loci, *A-B-C*, one usually requires an additional restriction, namely that θ_{AC} be at least as large as either of θ_{AB} and θ_{BC},

$$\theta_{AC} \geq \theta_{AB} \quad \text{and} \quad \theta_{AC} \geq \theta_{BC}. \qquad (6.11)$$

This imposes limits on the ranges of the p_i so that often the θ_{ij} cannot be estimated directly using equation (6.10). For example, $\hat{p}_1 = 0.45$, $\hat{p}_2 = 0.10$, $\hat{p}_3 = 0.15$, and $\hat{p}_4 = 0.30$ lead to $\hat{\theta}_{AB} = 0.342$, $\hat{\theta}_{BC} = 0.276$, and $\hat{\theta}_{AC} = 0.146$. Such estimates are inadmissible, and the recombination fractions have to be estimated by numerical maximization of the likelihood under the restrictions (6.11) (for an example, see section 6.7).

6.4. Interference

In many species, a frequent observation is that in the different intervals between genes on a chromosome, recombinations do not occur independently of each other. This nonindependence is called *interference* and is defined below.

For three loci in the order *A-B-C*, the frequency of double recombinations (a recombination in each of the two intervals) has been denoted by g_{11} (see table 6.2). Under independence, a double recombination occurs with probability $\theta_{AB}\theta_{BC}$ where θ_{ij} is the recombination fraction between loci i and j. In genetics, the deviation from independence is measured by the *coefficient of coincidence* (Muller 1916),

$$c = \frac{g_{11}}{\theta_{AB}\theta_{BC}} = \frac{1}{2} \frac{\theta_{AB} + \theta_{BC} - \theta_{AC}}{\theta_{AB}\theta_{BC}}, \qquad (6.12)$$

and interference is defined as $I = 1 - c$ (Ayala and Kiger 1984). Thus, interference is absent ($I = 0$) for $c = 1$, negative ($I < 0$) for $c > 1$, and positive ($I > 0$) for $c < 1$.

It is often more convenient to work with c rather than with θ_{AC}. From (6.12), one obtains

$$\theta_{AC} = \theta_{AB} + \theta_{BC} - 2c\theta_{AB}\theta_{BC}. \tag{6.13}$$

Replacing θ_{AC} in (6.6a–d) by the right side of (6.14) leads to the new parametrization,

$$g_{11} = c\theta_{AB}\theta_{BC} \tag{6.14a}$$

$$g_{10} = \theta_{AB}(1 - c\theta_{BC}) \tag{6.14b}$$

$$g_{01} = \theta_{BC}(1 - c\theta_{AB}) \tag{6.14c}$$

$$g_{00} = 1 - \theta_{AB} - \theta_{BC} + c\theta_{AB}\theta_{BC}. \tag{6.14d}$$

The right side of equation (6.12) shows that, in principle, c can be negative, which is the case if $\theta_{AC} > \theta_{AB} + \theta_{BC}$, that is, if the recombination fraction across two intervals is larger than the sum of the recombination fractions in the two intervals. In genetics, this phenomenon is referred to as *map expansion* (Holliday 1964), but human geneticists sometimes use this term with different meanings.

In three-point analysis, the requirements that probabilities assume values between 0 and 1 and recombination fractions be between 0 and ½ puts limits on the possible range of c in equation (6.12). Assume fixed values of θ_{AB} and θ_{BC}. Then the lower limit of c is attained when no double recombinants occur, $g_{11} = 0$, in which case $c = 0$. In addition, one must have $\theta_{AC} \leq$ ½ so that, using (6.13), one obtains $c \geq (\theta_{AB} + \theta_{BC} - ½)/(2\theta_{AB}\theta_{BC})$. Therefore, the lower limit of c is given by $c \geq \max[0, (\theta_{AB} + \theta_{BC} - ½)/(2\theta_{AB}\theta_{BC})]$. From the right side of equation (6.12), one can see that the upper limit of c is given by the requirements that $\theta_{AC} = (g_{10} + g_{01}) \leq$ ½ and that each of g_{10} and g_{01} be nonnegative, which leads to an upper limit of c of $1/\theta_{AB}$ or $1/\theta_{BC}$, whichever is less. Put together, these limits read

$$\max[0, (\theta_{AB} + \theta_{BC} - ½)/(2\theta_{AB}\theta_{BC})] \leq c \leq \min(1/\theta_{AB}, 1/\theta_{BC}). \tag{6.15}$$

In some organisms, for tightly linked loci (sum of the recombination fractions in two intervals of 1 percent or less), instances of high negative interference are observed, and multiply recombinant chromatids are common. This phenomenon is related to gene conversion rather than to multiple crossing over occurring within a short distance (Ayala and Kiger 1984). In most species, however, interference seems to be positive ($I > 0$, $c < 1$) so that one usually assumes $c \leq 1$ and takes "interference" to mean "positive interference." Also, complete interference is usually taken to mean $c = 0$. The limitation to zero or positive interference sharpens the restrictions (6.11) on θ_{AC}. With $c \leq 1$, rearranging (6.12) leads to

$$\theta_{AB} + \theta_{BC} - 2\theta_{AB}\theta_{BC} \leq \theta_{AC} \leq \min(\theta_{AB} + \theta_{BC}, \frac{1}{2}). \tag{6.16}$$

For small distances and under the assumption of complete interference, map distances are equal to the recombination fractions (Morgan map function) so that, for three loci A-B-C, the recombination fraction between loci A and C is simply the sum, $\theta_{AC} = \theta_{AB} + \theta_{BC}$. For other cases, θ_{AC} may be obtained via the map functions. This may be done with the MAPFUN program by calculating map distances, x_1 and x_2 from θ_{AB} and θ_{BC}, adding them, and converting their sum back into a recombination fraction. For some of the map functions, *addition formulas* can be obtained analytically. Based on (6.13), setting $c = 1$ leads to the Haldane addition formula, $\theta_{AC} = \theta_{AB} + \theta_{BC} - 2\theta_{AB}\theta_{BC}$. For the Kosambi map function, the coefficient of coincidence is given by

$$c = 2\theta_{AC} = 2\,\frac{\theta_{AB} + \theta_{BC}}{1 + 4\theta_{AB}\theta_{BC}} \tag{6.17}$$

(Bailey 1961). Dividing (6.17) by 2 leads to the Kosambi addition formula,

$$\theta_{AC} = \frac{\theta_{AB} + \theta_{BC}}{1 + 4\theta_{AB}\theta_{BC}}. \tag{6.18}$$

Estimates of the coincidence coefficient c are obtained when the recombination fractions in (6.12) are replaced by their estimates. However, estimates of c have a large standard error (Elandt-Johnson 1971) so that distinguishing $c < 1$ from $c = 1$ (absence of interference) can be difficult, which is shown below. Consider three ordered loci A-B-C and two family types, the phase-known triple backcross with one offspring (section 6.2) and the phase-unknown triple backcross with two offspring (section 6.3). In each of these family types, four offspring phenotype classes occur with associated probabilities p_k. If the p_k are parametrized using equations (6.14a–d), the 3×3 information matrix with respect to the parameters θ_{AB}, θ_{BC}, and c is obtained by computing all partial derivatives of p_k. Its inverse is the approximate variance-covariance matrix. One of its diagonal elements is the variance, $\sigma^2(\hat{c})$. For simplicity, assume the same recombination rates in the two intervals, $\theta = \theta_{AB} = \theta_{BC}$. For selected values of θ, table 6.5 shows the standard errors of the estimates of the coincidence coefficients per family, which are seen to be very large. For information

Table 6.5. Asymptotic Standard Error $\sigma(\hat{c})$ for Coincidence Coefficient Estimates and Number n of Families Required to Detect Positive Interference

c	θ	Phase known[a]		Phase unknown[b]	
		$\sigma(\hat{c})$	n	$\sigma(\hat{c})$	n
0.04	0.01	19.99	34,826	74.27	56,452
0.20	0.05	8.85	2,327	17.81	3,872
0.38	0.10	5.92	1,013	10.96	2,056
0.55	0.15	4.52	847	9.05	2,334
0.69	0.20	3.56	949	8.65	4,024
0.88	0.30	2.28	2,285	11.59	38,711

[a] One offspring per family.
[b] Two offspring per family.

purposes, table 6.5 shows the coincidence coefficients (6.17) predicted by the Kosambi formula, but the calculations outlined above were made without assuming any mapping function. Also given in table 6.5 are approximate numbers n of families of each type (i.e., total number of offspring in phase-known families) required to detect a deviation from $c = 1$. The family numbers were calculated by

$$n = \frac{(1.64\sigma_0 + 0.84\sigma_1)^2}{(c - 1)^2} \tag{6.19}$$

(adapted from Elandt-Johnson 1971, 380), where $\sigma_0 = \sigma(\hat{c}; c = 1)$, $\sigma_1 = \sigma(\hat{c}; c < 1)$, and the constants 1.64 and 0.84 were chosen for a power of 80 percent and a significance level of 5 percent. The results indicate that testing for the presence of interference is most powerful for moderate values of θ. Even so, more than 800 offspring from phase-known triple backcross parents are required. It may thus be difficult to establish significant positive interference. The question of interference for ordering loci will be discussed in section 6.6.

As outlined in section 1.5, map functions $\theta = M(x)$ relate map distance x between two loci to the recombination fraction θ between them. One way of obtaining such map functions is to apply Haldane's method (for an overview, see Karlin 1984). For three ordered loci, *1-2-3*, assume map distance x and recombination fraction θ between loci *1* and *2*, and map distance Δx between loci *2* and *3*. Letting Δx go to zero, Haldane (1919) obtained the *marginal coincidence coefficient*,

$$c_0 = \frac{1 - d\theta/dx}{2\theta}, \tag{6.20}$$

where $d\theta/dx = M'(x)$ is the first derivative (the slope) of the map function, and c_0 is viewed as a function of θ (or of x when $M(x)$ is substituted for θ). Rearranging terms in (6.20) leads to the differential equation,

$$d\theta/dx = 1 - 2\theta c_0. \tag{6.21}$$

Solving (6.21) under specific assumptions on c_0 leads to various well-known map functions. For the map functions of Haldane (equation [1.2]), Morgan (1.1), Kosambi (1.3), Carter and Falconer (1.4), and Felsenstein (1.6), the respective marginal coincidence coefficients are given by $c_0 = 1, 0, 2\theta, (2\theta)^3$, and $K - 2\theta(K - 1)$. Kosambi interference, for example, tends to be complete ($c_0 = 0$) as θ tends towards zero and increases linearly with θ until it is equal to 1 at $\theta = \frac{1}{2}$.

The marginal coincidence coefficient (6.20) is often used as a convenient measure to characterize map functions regarding their interference properties. For given θ, it is proportional to minus the slope $M'(x)$ on the map function, that is, a larger slope indicates stronger marginal interference. However, as pointed out by Risch and Lange (1979), marginal coincidence does not necessarily give an accurate picture of coincidence as defined by (6.12) for two map lengths. Marginal coincidence may be less than one with coincidence being greater than one.

Since estimates of the coincidence coefficient from three-point data are very imprecise (see table 6.5), another avenue is sometimes taken to estimate interference. It makes use of the fact that different map functions incorporate different levels of interference. Particularly the Rao map function (section 1.5) has been fitted to observed data by varying its parameter p. Using linkage data for loci on chromosome 3 of *Drosophila*, Lalouel (1977) found an estimate for p of 0.56, which suggests interference operating approximately at the Kosambi level. He also reported suggestive evidence of nonuniformity of interference along the chromosome. Pascoe and Morton (1987) investigated data for the X chromosome of *Drosophila* and estimated p at 0.33, corresponding to an interference level between that predicted by the Kosambi and Carter-Falconer map functions.

6.5. Multilocus Map Functions

In this section, the relation between map functions and multilocus recombination probabilities G or recombination values R will discussed. Based on this relation, map functions will be investigated as to whether they yield valid gamete probabilities G, that is, values of G in the range between 0 and 1. If they do, they are suitable for use in computer programs and thus allow estimating interference using more than three loci.

The subject matter in this section is rather technical and may be skipped by the reader not interested in mathematical derivations. It is, however, noteworthy that most map functions in current use (e.g., the Kosambi, Falconer, and Rao functions) are invalid for multilocus analysis.

As was seen in section 5.5 and as will be discussed in more detail in chapter 8, one of the basic steps in evaluating the likelihood for family data is to calculate the probabilities of all possible gametes a parent is capable of producing. These gamete probabilities are exactly the joint recombination probabilities $G(\varepsilon)$ mentioned in section 6.1. For example, with four loci, $G[(1, 1, 0)]$ or g_{110} is the probability that a recombination occurs in each of the intervals 1 and 2 but not in interval 3. On the other hand, as shown by Liberman and Karlin (1984), map functions predict the recombination values, $R(\delta)$. For example, $R[(1, 1, 0)]$ is the probability that an odd number of crossovers (a recombination) occurs in the map region spanned by intervals 1 and 2, irrespective of what happens in interval 3, or $R[(1, 0, 1)]$ is the probability of an odd number of crossovers in the map region consisting of intervals 1 and 3. Through the relation (6.4), map functions can be used to specify gamete probabilities, as shown below.

A map function $\theta = M(x)$ translates a map distance x into a recombination fraction θ. For example, consider $n = 4$ ordered loci *A-B-C-D* with recombination fractions in the different intervals of $\theta_{AB} = 0.10$, $\theta_{BC} = 0.05$, and $\theta_{CD} = 0.20$, and assume the Kosambi map function. These recombination fractions thus correspond to interval lengths of $x_1 = 0.1014$, $x_2 = 0.0502$, and $x_3 = 0.2118$, as obtained by the inverse of the Kosambi function. Any map region W, made up of contiguous or noncontiguous intervals, has length $x(\delta) = \Sigma \delta_i x_i$, where $\delta_i = 1$ if the ith interval belongs to W, and the map function translates this length into the corresponding recombination value, $R(\delta) = M[x(\delta)]$. For example, to calculate the probability of a recombination (an odd number of crossovers) in the map region spanned by intervals 1 and 3 [$\delta = (1, 0, 1)$], one adds x_1 and x_3 and simply translates their sum into a recombination value. In this case, $x_1 + x_3 = 0.3132$, leading to $R[(1, 0, 1)] = 0.2778$. In this manner, as shown in the left half of table 6.6, all of the 2^{n-1} recombination values can be calculated. Their knowledge, in turn, allows the calculation through formula (6.4) of joint recombination probabilities, $G(\varepsilon)$, which are required in the calculation of multilocus likelihoods. To obtain, for example, the probability $G[(0, 0, 1)]$ of a gamete recombinant in interval 3 and nonrecombinant in the other two intervals, one forms the sum (6.4) over all $\delta = (\delta_1, \delta_2, \delta_3)$ (each row on the left side of table 6.6 corresponds to one such array). For each δ, one reads off $R(\delta)$ from table 6.6

Table 6.6. Recombination Values R under the Kosambi Map Function for Four Loci with Recombination Fractions $\theta_{12} = 0.10$, $\theta_{23} = 0.05$, and $\theta_{34} = 0.20$ and Joint Recombination Probabilities G Predicted by the Haldane and Kosambi Map Functions

δ in Interval					ε in Interval			$G(\varepsilon)$ under:	
1	2	3	$x(\delta)$	$R(\delta)$	1	2	3	Haldane	Kosambi
0	0	0	0	0	0	0	0	0.6840	0.6687
0	0	1	0.2118	0.2000	0	0	1	0.1710	0.1829
0	1	0	0.0502	0.0500	0	1	0	0.0360	0.0425
0	1	1	0.2620	0.2404	0	1	1	0.0090	0.0600
1	0	0	0.1014	0.1000	1	0	0	0.0760	0.0862
1	0	1	0.3132	0.2778	1	0	1	0.0190	0.0123
1	1	0	0.1516	0.1471	1	1	0	0.0040	0.0026
1	1	1	0.3634	0.3105	1	1	1	0.0010	−0.0012

and computes $\Sigma \delta_i \varepsilon_i = s$, where $\varepsilon_1 = 0$, $\varepsilon_2 = 0$, and $\varepsilon_3 = 1$. For $\delta = (0, 0, 0)$, one obtains $s = 0$, $(-1)^s = 1$, and the first term in the sum becomes $1 \times (1 - 2 \times 0) = 1$. For $\delta = (0, 0, 1)$, one obtains $s = 1$, $(-1)^s = -1$, and the second term in the sum becomes $-1 \times (1 - 2 \times 0.20) = -0.60$. For $\delta = (0, 1, 0)$, one obtains $s = 0$, $(-1)^s = 1$, and the third term in (6.4) becomes $1 \times (1 - 2 \times 0.05) = 0.90$, and so on. The final sum is then divided by $2^{(4-1)} = 8$ resulting in $G[(0, 0, 1)] = 0.1829$. As a check of the calculations, the G values must sum to 1. Also, for example, the sum of all $G[(\varepsilon_1, \varepsilon_2, \varepsilon_3)]$ with fixed $\varepsilon_3 = 1$ is the marginal probability of a recombination in interval 3, $r_3 = 0.20$. The right side of table 6.6 shows the results of these calculations for the Kosambi map function. For comparison, analogous results for the Haldane map function are also given (these are based on R values different from the ones in the table, of course).

A problem with many map functions is that they may not furnish valid gamete probabilities (Bailey 1961). Liberman and Karlin (1984) defined a map function as *multilocus-feasible* when it yields proper joint recombination probabilities, $0 \leq G(\varepsilon) \leq 1$, for any map distances, x_i, and any number of loci. They showed that a map function $\theta = M(x)$ is multilocus-feasible when

$$(-1)^k M^{(k)}(x) \leq 0, \qquad k = 1, 2, \ldots, \tag{6.22}$$

for all $x \geq 0$ (Liberman and Karlin 1984), that is, when all even numbered derivatives $M^{(2k)}(x) = d^{2k}M(x)/dx^{2k}$ are less than or equal to zero and all odd numbered derivatives are nonnegative.

Most map functions in current use, for example, the Kosambi, Carter-

Falconer, and Rao map functions, are not multilocus-feasible for more than three loci. An example is calculated in table 6.6 for the Kosambi map function resulting in a negative probability for triple recombinant haplotypes, $G(1, 1, 1) = -0.0012$. As another example, when the map distances between four loci are equal to 20 cM each, the Kosambi map function predicts a probability for triple recombinant gametes of -0.0023 and, for interval lengths of 25 cM, the Carter-Falconer map function predicts triple recombinants with a probability of -0.015. Therefore, these map functions are invalid for multilocus analysis and *unrealistic* in the following sense: Whatever the process by which gametes are produced, they occur according to some (unknown) probability distribution, $G(\varepsilon)$, which results in observed recombination fractions in the different intervals of a map. When a map function predicts $G < 0$ for some ε, it assumes a set of recombination values R that does not occur in nature.

Historically, many map functions have been derived based on specific assumptions on the functional form of the marginal coincidence coefficient (equation [6.20]). Most of them are not multilocus-feasible and are thus invalid for multilocus analysis. Hence, rather than obtaining gamete probabilities from predetermined map functions, it appears more meaningful to take the reverse approach, that is, to model the gamete probabilities $G(\varepsilon)$ and to derive the map function corresponding to the postulated distribution G. The map functions outlined in the remainder of this section are based on this approach. They are, of course, multilocus-feasible by construction.

The simple assumption that crossovers occur independently of each other according to the Poisson law leads to the Haldane (1919) map function (equation [1.2]). Interference is assumed absent under the Haldane map function. Gamete probabilities G could be obtained from map distances by the technique demonstrated above for the Kosambi map function, or they are simply calculated as the products of terms θ_i or $1 - \theta_i$ depending on whether $\delta_i = 1$ or 0, where θ_i is the two-point recombination fraction in interval i. Observations on experimental organisms suggest that absence of interference is an unrealistic assumption, but conclusive support for interference in the human genome is difficult to obtain. Furthermore, neglecting interference when it is present seems to lead to small errors only for map distance estimates (White and Lalouel 1987), although support for different locus orders can depend strongly on the level of interference assumed (see section 6.6).

Sturt (1976) assumed one obligatory crossover while additional crossovers occur independently of each other following the Poisson distribution. The resulting map function (1.7) contains a mapping parameter, the chromosome length, $L \geq \frac{1}{2}$, and map distances are restricted to the interval $0 \leq x \leq L$. For $L = \frac{1}{2}$, the Sturt map function coincides with the Morgan map function (1.1), and as $L \to \infty$ it tends towards the Haldane map function. The requirement of an obligatory crossover introduces interference. The limiting marginal interference for small x is given by $\lim(c_0)_{x \to 0} = 1 - 1/(4L^2)$ (Sturt 1976), which tends to zero (complete interference) as L approaches $\frac{1}{2}$ but is positive for larger L (for comparison, the Kosambi limiting marginal interference is always zero). For example, in a chromosome of length $L = 1M = 100$ cM, the marginal interference for small x is equal to $\frac{3}{4}$.

Risch and Lange (1979) and Karlin and Liberman (1978) presented a general class of map functions in which the nonrandomness of crossovers is in the numbers of crossovers that occur, not in their locations. The results of these authors can be summarized as follows: Let c_k denote the probability of occurrence of k crossovers. Then, $m = \Sigma_k k c_k$ is the mean number of crossovers. Let $f(s) = \Sigma c_k s^k$ be the probability-generating function (Feller 1968) of any distribution c_k of the number of crossovers. An associated map function can then be constructed by

$$\theta = M(x) = \tfrac{1}{2}[1 - f(1 - 2x/m)]. \tag{6.23}$$

The Sturt mapping function turns out to be a special case of (6.23) with c_k being specified by a truncated Poisson distribution.

As an application of (6.23), take the binomial distribution, $c_k = \binom{N}{k}p^k q^{N-k}$, $q = 1 - p$, which was also considered by Liberman and Karlin (1984). Its probability generating function is given by $f(s) = (ps + q)^N$, and its mean is $m = Np$. If $f(s)$ is evaluated at $s = 1 - 2x/m$ and inserted in (6.23), one obtains the map function (1.8). It introduces interference by restricting the number of crossovers, whose upper limit is given by the mapping parameter, N. Map distances are restricted to the interval $0 \leq x \leq N/2$, that is, total map length is $L = N/2$. For $N = 1$, the binomial map function coincides with the Morgan map function. The limiting marginal interference for small x is obtained as $\lim(c_0)_{x \to 0} = (N - 1)/N$. For $N = 2$ (map length of 100 cM), $(N - 1)/N$ becomes $\frac{1}{2}$, which suggests that the binomial map function has stronger interference than Sturt's.

To model multilocus recombination probabilities, Pascoe and Morton (1987) assumed absence of more than three crossovers and postulated that a crossover divides the chromosome into two segments between which there is no interference. This permits writing down the joint recombination probabilities G for the different gamete classes.

Goldgar and Fain (1988) proposed a chiasma-based model for joint recombination probabilities, G, which includes the relative positions of the different crossovers. The model contains an interference parameter that makes closely spaced crossovers unlikely. A maximum of three crossovers is permitted. The map function implied by Goldgar and Fain's (1988) parametrization is unavailable in explicit form. Applying this model to X-chromosome data of *Drosophila* results in a fit that is better than that achieved by other methods. For map distances up to about $x = 50$ cM, the graph of Goldgar and Fain's (1988) map function (full model) exhibits stronger marginal interference than that of the Rao map function and, for larger x, it exhibits smaller marginal interference.

An objection occasionally raised against some of the map functions discussed above is that interference is not complete at small map distances, as would be expected from empirical evidence. For that reason, the Kosambi or Carter-Falconer map functions are sometimes preferred. Unfortunately, as seen above, they are unrealistic in their predictions of gamete probabilities for more than three loci and thus are unsuitable for general use in linkage programs. This also applies to the Rao map function (except when it coincides with the Haldane map function) and the compound map function proposed by Haldane (equation [1.5]). The marginal coincidence for the Haldane compound map function (1.5) is obtained as $c_0 = p/[1 - 2\theta(1 - p)]$, which approaches p as θ tends to zero. Parameter values $p > \frac{1}{2}$ thus produce less limiting marginal interference than does the binomial map function with $N = 2$. Thus, the binomial map function appears to be a useful multilocus map function. Its incorporation in linkage programs would be a way of introducing interference in multipoint linkage calculations and would allow estimating interference from multipoint data based on more than three loci. In this approach one estimates map distances rather than recombination fractions between adjacent loci. A different method of jointly estimating recombination fractions and interference coefficients was recently published (Zhao, Thompson, and Prentice 1990).

6.6. Ordering Loci

The process of mapping a number of loci can be viewed as consisting of two main components: (1) determining gene order within a linkage group and (2) adding a locus to an established map of loci. Estimating map distances, given a locus order, represents a third component that is related to the other two because, as will be outlined below, the order of loci is defined by the map distances or recombination fractions among them. The main object of this section is to provide some of the theoretical background required for an appreciation of the "ordering problem." It will be easiest to present the salient features of different locus orders for the case of three loci, which will occupy most of this section and can be generalized to more than three loci. Practical aspects of ordering loci will be covered in section 6.8.

In principle, the order of three loci ABC is determined by the magnitude of the (true) recombination fractions θ_{AB}, θ_{BC}, and θ_{AC}, where θ_{ij} is the two-point recombination fraction between loci i and j. The largest of these indicates which of the three loci are farthest apart, as spelled out by the inequalities (6.11) for the order ABC. Another order, for example, ACB, is determined by analogous inequalities, $\theta_{AB} \geq \theta_{AC}$ and $\theta_{AB} \geq \theta_{BC}$. A geometric interpretation of the different restrictions among the recombination fractions imposed by gene order can be given as follows: Consider a three-dimensional space with coordinates θ_{AB}, θ_{BC}, and θ_{AC}. With $0 \leq \theta \leq \frac{1}{2}$, this parameter space is equal to a cube with three side lengths of $\frac{1}{2}$ each. In this cube, the different orders of the three loci A, B, and C represent particular three-dimensional regions as defined by the inequalities mentioned above. One should note that these regions are not subspaces in the statistical sense, since they are all of the same dimensionality.

In an analysis resulting in estimates $\hat{\theta}_{AB}$, $\hat{\theta}_{BC}$, and $\hat{\theta}_{AC}$, the best-supported order will be the one in which i and j are the flanking loci when $\hat{\theta}_{ij}$ is the largest estimated recombination fraction. This order may not correspond to the true, unknown order when by chance $\hat{\theta}_{ij}$ turns out largest, while in fact the true value of θ_{ij} might not be largest. It is thus useful to consider the plausibility of different locus orders, that is, to maximize the likelihood or the lod score under each gene order.

Different locus orders imply different interpretations of the observations. For example, consider the three loci $A = DXS85$, $B = DXS255$, and $C = DXS14$ in figure 6.2. For the order ABC, individual 3.5 was seen to be a double recombinant. The formation in individual 2.4 (parent of 3.5) of the relevant gamete is depicted on the left side of figure 6.1. For different assumed locus orders, however, figure 6.1 shows that the same individual is only a single recombinant. The relationships among the three orders may be formalized as shown below.

As an example, consider $n = 20$ offspring from a phase-known triple backcross mating. Assume that seventeen offspring are nonrecombinant. Further assume that among the three recombinant offspring, $n_{AB} = 1$ offspring is recombinant for AB, $n_{BC} = 2$ offspring are recombinant for BC, and $n_{AC} = 3$ offspring are recombinant for AC (the sum of these numbers exceeds three because a recombinant individual must be recombinant for two of the three possible relations; see second paragraph in section 6.2). Depending on the order of the three loci, these numbers of recombinants fall into different classes of gametes (table 6.2) received by the offspring. For a given order, let R_1 be the number of offspring who are recombinant for the first interval (irrespective of whether they are recombinant or not in the second interval), R_2 is the number of offspring recombinant in the second interval, and R_3 is the number of offspring recombinant over both intervals, that is, with recombination for the two flanking loci. Then, in analogy to equations (6.6a–c), the numbers of gametes in the different classes are given by

$$k_{11} = \frac{1}{2}(R_1 + R_2 - R_3), \qquad\qquad (6.24a)$$

$$k_{10} = R_1 - k_{11}, \qquad\qquad (6.24b)$$

$$k_{01} = R_2 - k_{11}, \qquad\qquad (6.24c)$$

$$k_{00} = n - k_{11} - k_{10} - k_{01} \qquad\qquad (6.24d)$$

where k_{11} is the number of doubly recombinant (in intervals 1 and 2) gametes, k_{10} those with recombination in interval 1 and nonrecombination in interval 2, k_{01} those with nonrecombination in interval 1 and recombination in interval 2, and k_{00} is the number of nonrecombinant gametes.

Table 6.7 shows the results of our example for the three locus orders (the probabilities for each of the 2×2 tables in table 6.7 are as in table 6.2). For example, under order *BAC*, interval 1 refers to the chromosome region between loci B and A, and interval 2 refers to the region AC. The sum across row R_1 reflects the one recombinant for AB, and the sum down column R_2 reflects the three recombinants for AC (interval 2). In the main diagonal of the table, the sum $2 + 0$ represents $R_3 = 2$ recombinants for BC (flanking loci). From these marginal numbers, the numbers of the gamete classes in the body of the table are obtained by (6.24a–c). For example, still under order *BAC*, the number of double recombinants is given by $\frac{1}{2}(1 + 3 - [2 + 0]) = 1$. For the assumed data, depending on the locus order, one has either 0, 1, or 2 double recombinants.

The next task is to calculate log likelihoods under each of the three locus orders. For this, one must specify the probabilities g_{ij} with which observations in each of the four cells in one of the 2×2 tables of table 6.7 occur. Parametrization may be carried out in one of two ways. One approach is to estimate directly the four gamete class frequencies, g_{ij}, subject to the restriction that the coefficient of coincidence (6.12) be between zero and one, $0 \le c \le 1$ (6.16). The multinomial class frequencies are estimated simply as $\hat{g}_{ij} = k_{ij}/n$. Under locus order ABC, one obtains

$\hat{g}_{11} = 0$, $\hat{g}_{10} = 1/20 = 0.05$, $\hat{g}_{01} = 0.10$, and $\hat{g}_{00} = 0.85$. The estimated coefficient of coincidence is $\hat{c} = 0$. The maximum of the generalized lod score (6.8) for order ABC is thus obtained as $Z = 1 \times \log(4 \times 0.05)$ $+ \ldots + 17 \times \log(4 \times 0.85) = 7.540$ (the zero class contributes nothing to this sum). For order BAC, the unrestricted estimate of the coefficient of coincidence is $(1/20) / [(1/20) \times (3/20)] = 20/3$, which exceeds the upper limit of 1. Thus, within $0 \leq c \leq 1$, the estimate is $\hat{c} = 1$, implying independence of recombination in the two intervals. Consequently, the gamete class frequencies are given by the products of the marginal frequencies, that is, by equations (6.14a–d) with $c = 1$. Thus, under locus order *BAC*, the frequency of double recombinant gametes is estimated as $\hat{g}_{11} = 1 \times (1/20) \times (3/20) = 0.0075$, $\hat{g}_{10} = 0.0425$, $\hat{g}_{01} = 0.1425$, and $\hat{g}_{00} = 0.8075$. With these estimates, the lod score (6.8) is calculated as 6.645. Formally, the drop in lod score from 7.540 is caused by restricting $\hat{c}$. Finally, under the order *BCA*, one finds again $\hat{c} = 1$ and the lod score is obtained as 5.546.

Another, more commonly used parametrization rests on the observation that estimates of the coincidence are very inaccurate (section 6.4). Rather than estimating c, one either assumes an appropriate value of c (most often $c = 1$) or a certain level of interference predicted by a map function. For the three loci considered here, define the map distance x_{AB} as a vector from A to B such that x_{AB} is positive for locus order AB and negative for the order BA. Analogously, define x_{BC} as a map distance vector from B to C. Then, $x_{AC} = x_{AB} + x_{BC}$ is the map distance from loci A to C. For the locus order ABC, x_{AB} and x_{BC} are both positive. For BAC, x_{AB} is negative but smaller in absolute value than x_{BC}, and for BCA, $-x_{AB} > x_{BC}$. The three locus orders can thus be represented as regions of a plane with coordinate axes x_{AB} and x_{BC}, as shown in figure 6.3. The

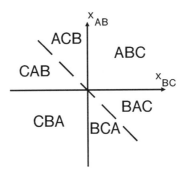

Figure 6.3. Regions of different locus orders with three gene loci A, B, and C. x = map distance.

Table 6.7. Offspring Numbers from Phase-known Triple Backcross Matings Interpreted under Three Locus Orders

	Order ABC			Order BAC			Order BCA		
	R_2	N_2	Σ	R_2	N_2	Σ	R_2	N_2	Σ
R_1	0	1	1	1	0	1	2	0	2
N_1	2	17	19	2	17	19	1	17	18
Σ	2	18	20	3	17	20	3	17	20

Note: R_i = recombination in interval i, N_i = nonrecombination in interval i.

graph of the lod score, $Z(x_{AB}, x_{BC})$, then forms a mountainous surface above the plane.

In table 6.7, observations for different locus orders are presented in 2×2 tables, in which rows correspond to recombination and nonrecombination in the first interval and columns correspond analogously to the second interval. To calculate lod scores $Z(x_{AB}, x_{BC})$, it will be more convenient to refer to a fixed 2×2 table, in which rows correspond to the interval AB and columns correspond to BC, irrespective of locus order. The observations in the four cells are then the same for the different orders, but their interpretation changes with order. For example, assume the same data as those used for table 6.7, that is, gamete numbers 0, 1, 2, and 17, when the leftmost 2×2 table is read row-wise. A given point (x_{AB}, x_{BC}) determines the order of the three loci as well as the absolute map distances among them. For instance, $x_{AB} = -0.32$ and $x_{BC} = 0.12$ imply the order BCA. Using a particular map function, one then translates the absolute map distances ($x_{AB} = 0.32$, $x_{BC} = 0.12$, $x_{AC} = 0.20$) into recombination fractions. For the given map distances, the Kosambi function furnishes $\theta_{AB} = 0.2824$, $\theta_{BC} = 0.1177$, and $\theta_{AC} = 0.1900$ (the MAPFUN program may be helpful here). From these recombination fractions, using equations (6.6a–d), one obtains gamete probabilities as $g_{11} = 0.10505$, $g_{10} = 0.17735$, $g_{01} = 0.01265$, and $g_{00} = 0.70495$, corresponding to the numbers of offspring $n_{11} = 0$, $n_{10} = 1$, $n_{01} = 2$, and $n_{00} = 17$ (notice that under the current order BCA, the $n_{01} = 2$ gametes are the double recombinants). The lod score at the assumed point (x_{AB}, x_{BC}) = (-0.32, 0.12) is then calculated by equation (6.8) as $Z = 0 + [1 \times \log(4 \times 0.17735)] + [2 \times \log(4 \times 0.01265)] + [17 \times \log(4 \times 0.70495)] = 4.91$.

For the Kosambi map function, table 6.8 presents the calculations of the previous paragraph for a grid of x_{AB} and x_{BC} values. The lod score surface appears as a mountainous surface with three hills separated by two crevices, each dipping down to $-\infty$. The hills correspond to the three

Table 6.8. Lod scores $Z(x_{AB}, x_{BC})$ under Kosambi Interference for the Observations in Table 6.7

x_{AB}	Map Distance, x_{BC}					
	0.05	0.10	0.15	0.20	0.25	0.30
0.10	7.22	7.38	7.29	7.09	6.84	6.57
0.05	7.35	7.53	7.44	7.25	7.01	6.75
0.01	6.98	7.17	7.10	6.92	6.69	6.43
0.00	$-\infty$	$-\infty$	$-\infty$	$-\infty$	$-\infty$	$-\infty$
-0.01	4.46	5.41	5.74	5.83	5.80	5.70
-0.05	$-\infty$	5.35	6.00	6.21	6.24	6.17
-0.10	3.34	$-\infty$	5.39	5.98	6.15	6.14
-0.15	4.17	3.86	$-\infty$	5.25	5.79	5.93
-0.20	4.50	4.57	4.01	$-\infty$	5.02	5.53
-0.25	4.61	4.83	4.65	4.00	$-\infty$	4.74
-0.30	4.60	4.89	4.86	4.58	3.89	$-\infty$
-0.40	4.42	4.76	4.83	4.77	4.60	4.26

locus orders (fig. 6.3), and the top of each hill defines the estimates of x_{AB} and x_{BC} under the given locus order. These estimates, accurate to two decimal places of x_i, are given on the right side of table 6.9, which also lists analogous results for other map functions. Under each map function, the best locus order is *ABC*. With increasing interference, the difference in maximum lod score between the best and second best locus order increases, the major reason being that different locus orders predict different numbers of double recombinants, which are less likely with increased interference. Hence, map functions with stronger interference permit better discrimination between locus orders and may be used for this purpose if there is clear evidence for the level of interference assumed in the analysis (otherwise, power for discrimination between orders is overestimated). In the limit of complete interference (binomial map function with at most $N = 1$ crossover or Sturt map function with map length $L = \frac{1}{2}$), the maximum lod score is 7.540 under locus order *ABC*, any other order having zero likelihood as it requires more than one crossover between the flanking loci.

The type of data considered thus far have been offspring of phase-known triple backcross matings, for which the likelihood under different locus orders can be calculated analytically. In practice, one may want to look at more than three loci. Also, matings are usually informative for some of the loci and uninformative for others so that generally the likelihood will have to be calculated with the aid of computer programs. Notice, however, that the techniques of the previous paragraphs can only be

Table 6.9. Maximum Lod Scores and Estimates of Absolute Map Distances x_1 and x_2 in the Two Intervals for Different Orders of Three Loci A, B, and C and for Different Map Functions (Observations as in Table 6.7)

	Haldane			Binomial ($N = 2$)			Kosambi		
Order	x_1	x_2	Z	x_1	x_2	Z	x_1	x_2	Z
A B C	0.05	0.11	7.493	0.05	0.11	7.515	0.05	0.10	7.527
B A C	0.05	0.18	6.645	0.05	0.16	6.382	0.06	0.18	6.247
B C A	0.11	0.18	5.546	0.11	0.17	5.022	0.12	0.20	4.912

directly extended to more than three loci if map functions are used, which are valid for multilocus analysis (see section 6.5).

There has been a continuing debate on what level of interference shall be incorporated in multipoint linkage analyses. Lathrop et al. (1985) offered the arguments for disregarding interference quoted below. While experiments with laboratory animals give evidence for positive interference, good estimates of interference in humans are extremely difficult to obtain (see section 6.4). If interference is absent, estimates of recombination rates are most efficient when independence of recombination in adjacent intervals is assumed. In the presence of interference, when recombination is estimated assuming absence of interference, these estimates are presumably biased, but their mean square error may still be smaller than the estimates obtained with the coincidence estimated simultaneously. For some data types, this is indeed the case (Lathrop et al. 1985) so that the biased estimates still have better precision for estimating genetic locations. The effects of ignoring interference on estimates of recombination fraction were studied in more detail by Bishop and Thompson (1988). These authors showed that, for gametes from phase-known triple heterozygotes, no bias in the recombination fraction for adjacent loci results from the assumption of lack of interference even if interference is present. However, for samples from pairwise informative data, there is bias introduced. Consequently, when data are analyzed jointly at multiple loci, the effect of disregarding interference on estimates of the recombination fraction can be expected to be negligible.

If interference is assumed in the analysis (not estimated), power for discriminating between locus orders increases somewhat with the level of interference (Ott and Lathrop 1987a). As pointed out by Goldgar, Fain, and Kimberling (1989), their work suggests that "restrictions in the numeric distribution of chiasmata is of greater significance for models of multilocus recombination than restrictions in locations of multiple chiasmata." The binomial map function might therefore be a good vehicle for estimating and using interference in multipoint analysis, should this be desired. Of course, interference should only be assumed in the analysis if there is clear evidence of its existence in the portion of the human genome under study. Currently, absence of interference is usually assumed, at least when more than three loci are analyzed.

Statistical tests for declaring one locus order "significantly" better than another cannot be carried out as customary likelihood ratio tests, since locus orders correspond to different regions of the same parameter space. One avenue might be to test for goodness of fit of different orders with the observations. All of those locus orders with good fit of the observations would then form a confidence space of locus orders. Although such tests have been developed for certain simple data types (Lathrop et al. 1987; Ott and Lathrop 1987a), they have not been extended to more general situations. For these, computer-based ad hoc tests appear more promising (section 8.7). However, the analytical tests reveal the following important properties of the locus ordering problem: Power for ordering loci is very small for closely linked loci and reaches an optimum value at recombination rates of about 20 percent between loci (Bishop 1985; Ott and Lathrop 1987a). An increasing density of marker loci is thus expected to lead to maps with well-supported order for not too closely spaced loci, but ordering neighboring loci may be difficult on purely genetic grounds. An interesting discussion of these points was given by Higgins et al. (1990), who reported a physical order of three closely spaced markers on chromosome 13 which contradicted the order found previously by genetic mapping.

Eventually, with a dense map of markers, one will presumably carry out gene mapping on the basis of observed crossovers (see section 6.7), which will obviate the need for estimating interference. Efforts are already under way to take up points of recombination in the human gene-mapping database.

6.7. Mapping under Complete Interference

In many applications, it is reasonable to assume the occurrence of at most one crossover in the map under study, which is equivalent to complete interference. Ordering loci can then be carried out in a simplified manner (Fain et al. 1989). For example, consider a set of loci in the order *A-B-C-D-E-F* and a multiple phase-known backcross mating *ABCDEF/ abcdef × abcdef/abcdef*. Assume now that an offspring receives a recombinant haplotype such as *ABCdef*, in which a crossover (recombination) occurred between the loci C and D. Looking at pairs of loci only, one recognizes that any pair of loci to the left of the crossover point (AB, AC, and BC) is nonrecombinant, and the same is true for pairs of loci to the right of the crossover (de, df, and ef). However, any locus on the left side of the crossover is recombinant with any locus on the right side of the crossover. Hence, the point of crossover divides the loci into two distinct groups. For unknown locus order, the argument may now be reversed. If a crossover has occurred, pairwise nonrecombinant loci form a group of (unordered) loci, which must be separated by the crossover from any other locus. A single crossover permits division of the loci into two separated groups. Another crossover at a different location will introduce a new point of separation such that three ordered groups of loci are present, with the loci in each group still unordered. Eventually, when a crossover has occurred in each interval, the order of all loci has been unequivocally established.

This method of mapping is also being used to place disease loci on a map of known markers. For an example, see figure 2 in Musarella et al. (1989).

At the end of the previous section, some of the difficulties of establishing order among closely linked loci were pointed out. Under complete interference, these difficulties can be roughly quantified as follows: To confirm the order of three closely linked loci, as pointed out above, the occurrence of at least one crossover in each of the two intervals is required. Assume a relative interval width of p each, for example, a width of 1 cM in a map of length 100 cM leading to $p = 0.01$. How many observations (gametes from a phase known triple backcross), n, does one need to be reasonably certain that at least one crossover falls into each of the two intervals? If crossovers are uniformly distributed over the length of the map, the probability of at least one crossover in one interval is equal to one minus the probability of no crossovers, $1 - (1 - p)^n$. The probability that this happens in each of the two intervals is equal to $\phi = [1 - (1 - p)^n]^2$, where ϕ is the power for ordering the three closely linked loci. Therefore, the number of gametes from phase-known triple backcrosses required for establishing order is equal to $n = \log(1 - \sqrt{\phi})/\log(1 - p)$. For a power of $\phi = 95$ percent, $n = 366$ gametes are required, and for $\phi = 99$ percent, $n = 527$ gametes must be investigated. These are relatively large numbers. The extended panel of sixty-one CEPH families contains 1036 potentially informative meioses (Dr. M. Lathrop, personal communication, December 1990) so that, with highly polymorphic markers, these families are capable of ordering loci with map distances of only 1 cM.

At the end of section 6.3 it was pointed out that, in multipoint analysis, combining independent two-point data may lead to inconsistent recombination estimates in the sense that, for example, the recombination rate between two loci is larger than the sum of the recombination rates in the intervals between these markers. Here is an interesting example, in which recombination rates can be estimated under complete interference in a relatively simple manner using iteration. Discussing the analysis of data from pairs of loci, J. H. Edwards (1989a) referred to this example of three loci in *Drosophila*, which had been analyzed by Fisher (1922) on the basis of pairwise counts of recombinants and nonrecombinants. (A thorough maximum likelihood analysis of these and additional loci was described by Smith 1989.) The three ordered loci in question are *scute* (locus *A*), *beaded* (locus *B*), and *rough* (locus *C*), with observed two-point recombination fraction estimates of $\hat{\theta}_{AB}$ = 4/279 (recombinants/ [recombinants + nonrecombinants]) = 0.0143, $\hat{\theta}_{BC}$ = 11/455 = 0.0242, and $\hat{\theta}_{AC}$ = 453/6388 = 0.0709. The estimated recombination rate between the flanking loci is seen to be larger than the sum of those in the two intervals between these loci. The coefficient of coincidence is thus estimated to be zero (complete interference). Under this condition, the iterative analysis (an example of the EM algorithm) shown below rapidly provides maximum likelihood estimates of the recombination rates.

Consider the layout of table 6.2 and assume absence of double recombinants, g_{11} = 0. Then, the gamete frequency g_{10} is equal to θ_{AB}, and g_{01} = θ_{BC}, where θ_{AB} and θ_{BC} are the recombination rates to be estimated, and $\theta_{AB} + \theta_{BC} = \theta_{AC}$ under complete interference. In addition to being a recombination rate, θ_{AB} is also the frequency of (multipoint) gametes recombinant for *AB* and nonrecombinant for *BC*, and θ_{BC} is the frequency of gametes recombinant for *BC* and nonrecombinant for *AB*. The frequency of nonrecombinant gametes is then given by $1 - \theta_{AB} - \theta_{BC}$. The number of observations is n = 7122, which is taken to be the total number of gametes in table 6.10, which has a layout analogous to that of table 6.2. Let k_{ij} be the number of recombinants and s_{ij} the number of nonrecombinants for each pair of loci; thus, k_{AB} = 4, s_{AB} = 275, k_{BC} = 11, s_{BC} = 444, k_{AC} = 453, s_{AC} = 5935. The object is now to count gametes by appropriating the two-point numbers of recombinants and nonrecombinants to the various gamete classes. Although one wants to *estimate* the proportions of gametes, θ_{AB} and θ_{BC}, for inference purposes, they are provisionally assumed to be known.

What is the number, $\theta_{AB}n$, of gametes recombinant for *AB* and nonrecombinant for *BC* (upper right cell in table 6.10)? First, they must comprise all of the k_{AB} = 4 recombinants for *AB*, since these contribute only

Table 6.10. Counts of Gametes Recombinant (R) and Nonrecombinant (NR) for Loci *AB* and *BC*

	Loci *BC*	
AB	R	NR
R	0	$4 + \dfrac{444\,\theta_{AB}}{1 - \theta_{BC}} + \dfrac{453\theta_{AB}}{\theta_{AB} + \theta_{BC}}$
NR	$11 + \dfrac{275\theta_{BC}}{1 - \theta_{AB}} + \dfrac{453\theta_{BC}}{\theta_{AB} + \theta_{BC}}$	$\dfrac{275(1 - \theta_{AB} - \theta_{BC})}{1 - \theta_{AB}} + \dfrac{444(1 - \theta_{AB} - \theta_{BC})}{1 - \theta_{BC}} + 5935$

to the first row of table 6.10, and double recombinants for *AB* and *BC* are lacking. Next, the $s_{BC} = 444$ nonrecombinants for *BC* are distributed over the two cells of the second column in table 6.10. The upper and lower cell probabilities are θ_{AB} and $1 - \theta_{AB} - \theta_{BC}$ (their sum is $1 - \theta_{BC}$), respectively, so that the respective relative cell probabilities become $\theta_{AB}/(1 - \theta_{BC})$ and $(1 - \theta_{AB} - \theta_{BC})/(1 - \theta_{BC})$. Consequently, $444 \times \theta_{AB}/(1 - \theta_{BC})$ of the $s_{BC} = 444$ nonrecombinants for *BC* are expected to fall into the upper cell and thus to contribute towards our number $\theta_{AB}n$ of gametes. The last type of observation to be considered here is the $k_{AC} = 453$ recombinants for *AC*, which are distributed over the diagonal of table 6.10, a proportion $\theta_{AB}/(\theta_{AB} + \theta_{BC})$ of which contributes towards our gametes in the upper right cell. The number of these recombinants to be counted as gametes recombinant for *AB* and nonrecombinant for *BC* is thus equal to $453 \times \theta_{AB}/(\theta_{AB} + \theta_{BC})$. Hence, the desired number of gametes recombinant for *AB* and nonrecombinant for *BC* amounts to $\theta_{AB}n = 4 + [444 \times \theta_{AB}/(1 - \theta_{BC})] + [453 \times \theta_{AB}/(\theta_{AB} + \theta_{BC})]$.

The number, $\theta_{BC}n$, of gametes recombinant for *BC* and nonrecombinant for *AB* can be determined in an analogous manner. That number certainly comprises all of the $k_{BC} = 11$ recombinants for *BC*. Next, the $s_{AB} = 275$ nonrecombinants for *AB* are distributed over the second row of table 6.10, $275 \times \theta_{BC}/(1 - \theta_{AB})$ of which fall into the left cell and are counted towards our number of gametes recombinant for *BC* and nonrecombinant for *AB*. Finally, the $k_{AC} = 453$ recombinants for *AC*, distributed over the diagonal of table 6.10, contribute towards our gametes with a number of $453 \times \theta_{BC}/(\theta_{AB} + \theta_{BC})$, the remainder having been counted as the other gamete type above.

A summary of gamete counts is shown in table 6.10. For information purposes, the number of nonrecombinant gametes is also given, which includes all of the $s_{AC} = 5,935$ nonrecombinants for *AC* (sum of upper left and lower right cells). The two proportions of gametes are now estimated by dividing their number (upper right and lower left cells of table 6.10 for θ_{AB}, lower left cell for θ_{BC}) by the total number of gametes ($n = 7122$),

$$\theta_{AB} = \frac{4 + 444\dfrac{\theta_{AB}}{1 - \theta_{BC}} + 453\dfrac{\theta_{AB}}{\theta_{AB} + \theta_{BC}}}{7122}, \tag{6.25a}$$

$$\theta_{BC} = \frac{11 + 275\dfrac{\theta_{BC}}{1 - \theta_{AB}} + 453\dfrac{\theta_{BC}}{\theta_{AB} + \theta_{BC}}}{7122}. \tag{6.25b}$$

Equations (6.25) are analogous to expressions for gene counting (Smith 1957) and contain the quantities to be estimated on both sides of the equations. The estimates are obtained iteratively by inserting initial values for the parameters in the right side, solving the equations, inserting the results as updated estimates on the right side, solving the equations again, etc. Suitable initial values for θ_{AB} and θ_{BC} are the pairwise estimates, $\hat{\theta}_{AB} = 0.014$ and $\hat{\theta}_{BC} = 0.024$, respectively, but the final results are independent of the initial values as long as $0 < (\theta_{AB}, \theta_{BC}) < \frac{1}{2}$. After a large enough number of iterations, the values converge to the multipoint estimates, $\hat{\theta}_{AB} = 0.0326$ and $\hat{\theta}_{BC} = 0.0367$. As one can see, they are quite different from the corresponding two-point estimates. The multipoint recombination estimate between the flanking loci is then $\hat{\theta}_{AB} + \hat{\theta}_{BC} = 0.0693$, which agrees fairly well with the two-point estimate, $\hat{\theta}_{AC} = 0.0709$, since this relation was based on a much larger number of observations than the other two pairwise recombination estimates.

Incidentally, gene counting equations other than (6.25) can be derived. The ones shown below are obtained on the basis of the log likelihood of the (two-point) observations, which is $[4 \times \log(\theta_{AB})] + [275 \times \log(1 - \theta_{AB})] + [11 \times \log(\theta_{BC})] + [444 \times \log(1 - \theta_{BC})] + [453 \times \log(\theta_{AB} + \theta_{BC})] + [5935 \times \log(1 - \theta_{AB} - \theta_{BC})]$. Taking partial derivatives with respect to θ_{AB} and θ_{BC}, setting these equal to zero, and solving the resulting equations as if they were obtained from multinomial data lead to the counting equations,

$$\theta_{AB} = \frac{e_1}{e_1 + 275 + \dfrac{5935(1 - \theta_{AB})}{1 - \theta_{AB} - \theta_{BC}}}, \tag{6.26a}$$

$$\theta_{BC} = \frac{e_2}{e_2 + 444 + \dfrac{5935(1 - \theta_{BC})}{1 - \theta_{AB} - \theta_{BC}}}, \qquad (6.26b)$$

where $e_1 = 4 + 453\theta_{AB}/(\theta_{AB} + \theta_{BC})$ and $e_2 = 11 + 453\theta_{BC}/(\theta_{AB} + \theta_{BC})$. Equations (6.26) differ from (6.25); depending on the starting values, one or the other pair of equations leads more rapidly to the results of a predetermined accuracy, but both lead to the same final estimates, $\hat{\theta}_{AB} = 0.0326$ and $\hat{\theta}_{BC} = 0.0367$.

This gene counting approach to estimating multipoint recombination rates is suitable for relatively uncomplicated situations and large numbers of offspring. For human family data, using one of the multipoint computer programs will generally be more practical.

6.8. Other Methodologic Issues

This last section of chapter 6 covers some of the problems commonly encountered in multipoint mapping. Although this chapter is primarily concerned with analysis by likelihood methods, a few other techniques will be mentioned below. At various places reference will be made to the excellent book chapter by Weeks (1991).

The first step in the ordering of a set of loci is to carry out a conventional two-point linkage analysis for each locus pair. For n loci, this will result in $\frac{1}{2}n(n - 1)$ estimates of θ with associated maximum lod score $Z_{\max}$. In principle, one may then proceed in one of two ways. A nucleus of about two or three loci with the highest $Z_{\max}$ values can be formed and, based on this starter map, new loci can be added in a stepwise fashion. At each step, each of the new loci can be tried, for example, using the LINKMAP program, and that locus with the highest location score can be added to the map.

The other way of proceeding works with all loci at the same time. Ideally, it would be best to evaluate the maximum log likelihood under each possible order and to rank locus orders by their associated maximum log likelihood. Since the total number, $n!/2$, of locus orders is usually much too high, often a preliminary ordering method is applied (Weeks and Lange 1987; for an overview of such methods, see Weeks 1991). One of the most reliable criteria seems to be the sum of adjacent recombination fraction estimates (MDMAP, "minimum distance map," Falk 1989; SARF, "sum of adjacent recombination fractions," Weeks 1988). This method is also one of the two recommended by Olson and Boehnke

(1990). For each order of loci, the sum of θ estimates in each interval is formed and locus orders are ranked by their sum of θ estimates, where the best order is the one with the smallest sum of θ estimates. For the best orders, a thorough multipoint analysis is then performed.

The SARF method is analogous to the well-known method of ordering loci such that the number of recombinations required to explain the data is as small as possible. To the untrained geneticist, these methods seem to suggest that recombination is something bad that ought not to happen. One should consider, however, that it is the occurrence of recombinations that allows us to order loci. Recombinations are thus essential for gene mapping and one should not try to explain away recombinations in one's data (this would, of course, bias the resulting estimates of recombination fractions and map distances; for a discussion of typing errors, see section 10.5).

To place a locus (a disease locus, say) on a map of known markers, one usually starts by carrying out two-point analyses between the disease and each of the marker loci. If a promising region of the map has been found, more elaborate multipoint analyses are undertaken. Often, not all of the loci can be accommodated in the linkage program used. A possible solution consists of defining a "window" of four marker loci and evaluating location scores at a number of map locations in the middle one of the three intervals. Then, the window is "moved" by one locus, for example, a marker is added on the right side of the previous map of four markers and the leftmost marker is left off, and location scores at various map positions of the disease locus are again evaluated in the middle interval. This process is repeated along the whole map of markers. Although this approach seems very appealing, in practice various problems occur, which cannot be discussed here in detail.

When a dense map of markers is available over the whole genome, it is no longer necessary to estimate x precisely. One may simply assume that the disease is located in the middle of one of the intervals and estimate the interval containing the disease locus. This is the basis of Lander and Botstein's (1986a) *interval mapping*, which these authors showed to be more powerful than using unmapped markers because, with a dense map of markers, the disease is always tightly linked with at least one marker.

With heterogeneous traits (several disease loci exist but only one segregates in each family), one usually estimates the proportion α of families in which the trait is located on a map of markers (with $1 - \alpha$ being the proportion of families in which the trait locus is elsewhere) and the map position x of the trait on the map. An extension of the interval-mapping approach to heterogeneous traits (*simultaneous search*, Lander and Botstein 1986a) consists of simultaneously finding the various disease loci on the gene map, which is more powerful than searching for one disease locus at a time. For up to four disease loci, one of the HOMOG programs may be used for this purpose (for an example, see Ott et al. 1990a).

Thus far in this section, it has been assumed that male and female map distances are the same. (General methods of investigating sex-specific map distances will be covered in section 9.1.) If, in addition to evaluating the maximum log likelihood under different locus orders, one also estimates the ratio R of female to male map distance, one may proceed in one of two ways. If under each locus order the ratio R is estimated separately, comparisons between the log likelihoods of different orders have approximately the same statistical interpretation as if R were fixed at some value such as $R = 1$. On the other hand, if R is estimated under the best order and if that value is retained in the evaluation of the maximum log likelihood under the next best order, the difference in log likelihood between these two orders will tend to be inflated unless one interprets these differences in log likelihood differently (they contain an extra degree of freedom).

Linkage analyses are being carried out by various methods, which sometimes yield different results. As an example, table 6.11 compares recently published map lengths of chromosomes and chromosome arms with the map lengths predicted by Morton et al. (1982) on the basis of chiasma counts. (With the exception of 16p-q, only those chromosome arms with good marker coverage over their entire length are listed in table 6.11.) The estimated map lengths are usually, but not always, somewhat

Table 6.11. Comparison of Male Map Lengths in centiMorgans as Determined by Marker Mapping (L_m) and Predicted from Chiasma Counts (L_c, see Table 1.2)

Chromosome	L_m	L_c	n[a]	Reference
1q	85	96	21	Buetow et al. 1990
7pter-qter	141	136	25	Lathrop et al. 1989
10pter-qter	131	127	32	Bowden et al. 1989
10pter-qter	214	127	57	White et al. 1990[b]
11qter-cen	88	60	31	Julier et al. 1990a
16p-q	164	108	40	Donis-Keller et al. 1987
16pter-qter	115	108	46	Keith et al. 1990
16pter-qter	187	108	24	Julier et al. 1990b
17p	46	48	18	Wright et al. 1990

[a] Number of markers.
[b] Consortium map.

larger than those predicted by the chiasma counts. They also vary strongly between different studies. Inasmuch as this variation is due to using different map functions, it is expected to become smaller as the gaps between markers decrease.

Before one embarks on finding a disease locus, it is essential to do a thorough search of the literature for previously published results on that locus. In many cases, genetic exclusions are known, which obviate the need for investigating markers in the excluded region of the genome. Similarly, deletions may be known, which exclude a locus from some section of the map. It has been debated whether one should try to combine results from physical mapping with those from genetic mapping. In principle, the two approaches are incompatible as they work with a different metric. In some respects, however, they are also complementary; for example, physical methods are good at ordering closely spaced loci, which is difficult by genetic mapping. Hence, it appears reasonable to accept in gene mapping a known locus order obtained by physical mapping methods. One must be aware, however, that physical methods are not error-free (either).

A technique based on the randomness of induced chromosome breaks rather than recombination is radiation hybrid mapping (Cox et al. 1990), which is an extension of the method of Goss and Harris (1975). For this technique, a particular human chromosome is irradiated by x-rays such that it breaks into several fragments. These are recovered in rodent cells, and the rodent-human hybrid cells are cloned. Several approximate methods for ordering loci based on radiation hybrids have been developed (for example, Cox et al. 1990; Falk 1991; Weeks, Lehner, and Ott 1991).

Problems

Problem 6.1. Show that the Kosambi map function is not multilocus-feasible, using the fact that $d\theta/dx = 1 - 4\theta^2$. To disprove multilocus feasibility, it suffices to show that (6.22) is violated for any value of x, where $x = 0$ is a convenient choice.

Problem 6.2. What steps would you have to carry out to determine the map length (independent of any mapping function) of a particular chromosome?

Problem 6.3. For three ordered loci *A-B-C*, assume recombination fractions in the two intervals of 0.05 and 0.08. What is the recombination fraction between loci A and C as predicted by the Haldane and Kosambi map functions?

Problem 6.4. For the recombination fractions of problem 6.3, what is the coefficient of interference predicted by the binomial map function with parameter $N = 2$?

7.

Penetrance

One of the problems that make linkage analysis complicated (and interesting) is that crossovers and recombinations take place on the genotypic level while observations occur on the phenotypic level, and phenotypes often do not fully exhibit the underlying genotypes. The concept of penetrance establishes the connection between genotypes and phenotypes and is thus of central importance in linkage analysis. This chapter introduces and discusses penetrance in a predominantly applied manner. In the first three sections, penetrance is assumed to have a fixed value, which helps develop the salient features of incomplete penetrance. The practically important situation of age-dependent penetrance will be discussed in section 7.4.

In this chapter, attention is focussed on incomplete penetrance for a particular phenotype, particularly for affliction with a disease. More general uses of the penetrance concept may be found in section 10.2.

7.1. Definitions of Penetrance

Penetrance in the *general sense* or *wide sense* is defined as the conditional probability $P(x|g)$ that an individual with a given genotype g expresses the phenotype x. For example, the zeros and ones in table 1.1 are penetrances—the probability is 1 that an individual with B/O genotype expresses the B phenotype, and the penetrance is 0 for such an individual to express the A or AB or O phenotype. Particularly for certain diseases, penetrances may be less than 1, in which case one speaks of incomplete or reduced penetrance. A given genotype may then lead to one of two or more phenotypes, where unspecified factors are responsible for determining which phenotype is expressed. For example, in insulin-dependent diabetes mellitus, penetrance of the disease has been estimated to be between 2 and 20 percent (Rotter 1981).

If phenotypes are mutually exclusive and exhaustive, the penetrances over all phenotypes for a given genotype sum to 1. In practice, one often works with phenotypes whose definitions "overlap" so that some of the phenotypes are not mutually exclusive. Table 2.4 shows such a case in which, depending on the antigen used for typing for the Lutheran blood group, various phenotypes are distinguished, some of which are not mutually exclusive, for example, the phenotypes $A + B -$ and $A +$. Another example occurs in RFLP marker typing with two alleles when one is unsure whether the *2* allele is present or not and one can only see the band corresponding to the *1* allele. In such cases, the penetrances for a given genotype do not sum to 1 over all phenotypes.

Most RFLPs show completely codominant inheritance so that the phenotypes reveal the underlying genotypes (1 : 1 correspondence between genotypes and phenotypes). Dominant inheritance and recessive inheritance are basically distinguished through the penetrance of heterozygotes (Mendel 1866)—that penetrance is 0 in the recessive case and 1 (with complete penetrance) in the dominant case. For example, consider a dominant disease with disease allele D and normal allele d and assume the penetrances $P(\text{affected}|\text{genotype } D/D) = P(\text{affected}|D/d) = f$ and $P(\text{affected}|d/d) = 0$. Hence, $P(\text{unaffected}|D/D) = P(\text{unaffected}|D/d) = 1 - f$ and $P(\text{unaffected}|d/d) = 1$. The phenotype "unknown" is the union of the phenotypes "affected" and "unaffected" so that it is characterized by a constant penetrance, $P(\text{unknown}|D/D) = P(\text{unknown}|D/d) = P(\text{unknown}|d/d) = 1$. When the penetrance for affecteds is small, $f \approx 0$, the penetrances for unaffecteds are almost all the same, $1 - f \approx 1$, which indicates that unaffected individuals contribute practically nothing to the linkage analysis. Occasionally, penetrances are purposely chosen to be small to carry out a so-called "affecteds-only" analysis, in which almost all information is derived from the affected individuals.

Penetrance is sometimes used in a *narrow sense* as the probability of being affected (with a disease) given a certain genotype. Thus, for a simple, fully penetrant recessive disease with disease allele d and normal allele D, the genotype d/d has penetrance 1, and genotypes D/D and D/d have penetrance 0 each. Penetrance in the wide sense coincides with penetrance in the narrow sense when the phenotype is fixed as $x = $ "affected." Narrow-sense penetrance refers only to diseases and is not used in any other context.

If only susceptible genotypes ever express the disease, an affected phenotype identifies an individual as a carrier of the disease allele (or alleles in the case of a recessive disease). In many diseases, however, *phenocopies* (also called *sporadic cases* or *false positives*) occur. These are individuals whose affection status is not the result of genetic predisposition but is due to some unspecified environmental factors, since genetic and nongenetic forms of disease are often undistinguishable. The presence of phenocopies is modeled by a nonzero penetrance for nonsusceptible genotypes. For example, consider a dominant disease with disease allele D and a normal allele d, with the disease allele having a population frequency of $p = P(D)$. The genotypes D/D, D/d, and d/d may have the respective associated penetrances $f_{DD} = 0.9$, $f_{Dd} = 0.9$, and $f_{dd} = 0.001$, where the genotypes D/D and D/d are susceptible and the genotype d/d is not susceptible to disease. The population frequency of genetically affected individuals is then equal to $A = p^2 f_{DD} + 2p(1 - p)f_{Dd}$, while the frequency of phenocopies is given by $C = (1 - p)^2 f_{dd}$. If the disease is rare, one has $A \approx 2pf_{Dd}$ and $C \approx (1 - 2p)f_{dd}$. The *phenocopy rate*, that is, the proportion of phenocopies among all affected individuals, is equal to $C/(A + C)$.

As will be seen in chapter 8, the LIPED computer program works with wide sense penetrance. In the LINKAGE programs, on the other hand, one uses penetrance in the narrow sense by defining a number of so-called liability classes (classes of phenotypes) and specifying in each class, for the different genotypes, the probability of being affected. It is easy to convert penetrances of one type into the other type; an example is provided in chapter 8.

7.2. The Cost of Incomplete Penetrance

Incomplete penetrance clouds our view of the genotypes—phenotypes no longer unambiguously exhibit underlying genotypes. The consequence of this ambiguity is a loss of information which, for simple situations, may be assessed by computing expected lod scores. The reader interested only in results may turn directly to the discussion of table 7.2 at the end of this section.

Assume a dominant trait with disease allele D and normal allele d and a codominant marker locus with alleles *1* and *2*. The penetrance $f = P(\text{affected}|\text{genotype } D/d)$ at the disease locus is taken to be known, and phenocopies are assumed absent. For full penetrance, $f = 1$. Consider a phase-known double backcross mating, $D1/d2 \times d1/d1$. Table 7.1 shows the four possible offspring genotypes, g, and their probabilities $P(g; r)$ of occurrence, where r is the true recombination fraction between the disease and marker loci. The recessive genotypes, $d2/d1$ and $d1/d1$, produce only the respective recessive phenotypes, d21 and d11. Owing to incomplete penetrance, however, the $D1/d1$ genotype expresses the D11 phenotype

Table 7.1. Offspring Phenotype Probabilities in Phase-known Double Backcross Families with Incomplete Penetrance at the Disease Locus

Genotype g	$P(g; r)$	Phenotype x			
		D11	d21	D21	d11
$D1/d1$	$\frac{1}{2}(1-r)$	f	0	0	$1-f$
$d2/d1$	$\frac{1}{2}(1-r)$	0	1	0	0
$D2/d1$	$\frac{1}{2}r$	0	$1-f$	f	0
$d1/d1$	$\frac{1}{2}r$	0	0	0	1
	$P(x)$	$\frac{1}{2}(1-r)f$	$\frac{1}{2}(1-rf)$	$\frac{1}{2}rf$	$\frac{1}{2}(1-f+rf)$
	$L(\theta)/L(\frac{1}{2})$	$2(1-\theta)$	$\dfrac{1-\theta f}{1-\frac{1}{2}f}$	2θ	$\dfrac{1-f+\theta f}{1-\frac{1}{2}f}$

with probability f and the d11 phenotype with probability $1 - f$. Similarly, $D2/d1$ expresses D21 and d21 with the respective probabilities f and $1 - f$. The unconditional probabilities of occurrence of the offspring phenotypes are computed as $P(x; r) = \Sigma_g P(x|g)P(g; r)$, with $P(x|g) = f$, and are given in table 7.1.

The lod score corresponding to a particular phenotype x is given by $Z_x(\theta) = \log[L(\theta)/L(\frac{1}{2})]$, where $L(\theta) = P(x; \theta)$. The likelihood ratios given in table 7.1 show that, for the dominant phenotypes, which unequivocally exhibit underlying genotypes, the lod scores do not involve the penetrance (this is the basis for the affecteds-only analysis mentioned above). The expected lod score is calculated as the weighted average of the lod scores, $\Sigma_x P(x; r)Z_x(\theta)$. Of interest here is only its maximum (the ELOD), which is attained at $\theta = r$ and is denoted as $E[Z(r; f)]$. The ratio, $R = E[Z(r; f)]/E[Z(r; 1)]$, of the expected lod score with incomplete penetrance over that with full penetrance yields the relative informativeness for detecting linkage when the penetrance is f. For values of r close to ½, the relative ELOD, R, is numerically almost the same as the ratio of the corresponding expected informations (the relative efficiency, Elandt-Johnson 1971).

For the mating type discussed above, table 7.2 shows relative ELODs, R, associated with various values of penetrance, f, and recombination fraction, r. They strongly depend on the penetrance but not very much on the recombination fraction. For example, with a penetrance of 50 percent, the ratio of ELODs is approximately ⅓ only. Consequently, one needs three times as many observations to obtain the same ELOD as with full penetrance. Generally, $1/R$ is the factor by which one has to multiply the number of observations when the relative ELOD is R. As another ex-

Table 7.2. Ratio of Expected Lod Scores at True Recombination Fraction, r, under Incomplete Penetrance, f, versus Full Penetrance

f	Recombination Fraction, r					
	0^a	0.01	0.05	0.10	0.20	0.50^a
1	1	1	1	1	1	1
0.95	0.855	0.867	0.883	0.891	0.899	0.905
0.90	0.758	0.769	0.787	0.798	0.809	0.818
0.80	0.610	0.618	0.634	0.644	0.656	0.667
0.50	0.311	0.314	0.319	0.323	0.328	0.333
0.20	0.108	0.108	0.109	0.110	0.110	0.111

^{a}Limiting values.

ample, at $f = 0.20$, table 7.2 shows $R \approx 0.1$, so that $1/R = 10$ times the number of observations are required for the same ELOD as under full penetrance.

The figures presented in table 7.2 are calculated under the assumption of known penetrance. When f is unknown and must be estimated from the data (which situation is briefly discussed in section 7.3), informativeness presumably is even smaller because some of the information in the data is required to estimate f. When penetrance is incomplete yet full penetrance is assumed in the analysis, the estimate of the recombination fraction is biased upward. This will be discussed in chapter 10.

In principle, there is no lower bound on the penetrance below which linkage analysis could not be carried out. With very low penetrance, one simply needs a much larger set of data. As an example, which was pointed out to me by Dr. David Pauls, the gene for dystonia was successfully mapped to the long arm of chromosome 9, although penetrance is only about 31 percent (Ozelius et al. 1989; in the analysis, a maximum penetrance of 75 percent at high age was assumed).

7.3. Estimating Penetrance and Recombination

For diseases, penetrance is the probability that a susceptible individual is affected. In principle, therefore, the penetrance f is estimated as the proportion of affecteds among susceptible individuals. The problem is that it is not always easy to find a collection of susceptible individuals and to unbiasedly estimate the proportion of affecteds. While a detailed coverage of penetrance estimation is beyond the scope of this book (such a topic falls in the realm of segregation analysis), a few simple approaches are given below.

When a rare dominant disease segregates in a sibship, only one of the parents is expected to carry the disease allele, and that parent may or may not be affected. On average, half of the offspring will receive the disease allele and, of those, a proportion f will develop the disease. The proportion of affected offspring is thus $p_A = \frac{1}{2}f$ so that an estimate of f is given by $2p_A$. The relevant procedure for estimating f would then be to find affected individuals and count affected and unaffected individuals among their offspring, including sibships without affecteds.

In practice, it is easier to collect sibships through an affected sibling, the proband. That way, however, one misses sibships not containing any affected individuals, which would lead to an *ascertainment bias*, if estimation of f is carried out as described in the previous paragraph. Properly correcting for ascertainment biases is difficult (Greenberg 1986; see also section 3.3.4 and appendix 3 in Vogel and Motulsky 1986 and chapter 17 in Elandt-Johnson 1971). The easiest ascertainment correction is to leave off the proband from all calculations, which is known as Weinberg's (1912) proband method. If k_i is the number of affecteds in the ith sibship of size n_i, the corrected estimate for the proportion of affecteds is given by

$$\hat{p}_A = \sum_i \frac{k_i - 1}{n_i - 1}. \tag{7.1}$$

The penetrance estimate is simply double the estimate of p_A. If the estimate of f exceeds 1, then 1 is assumed as the penetrance estimate. In large pedigrees segregating a dominant disease, when the pedigrees are collected on the basis of one or a few probands (and not because they contain a large number of affecteds), effects of ascertainment are probably small (Elston 1973). Thus, one may estimate the penetrance numerically using one of the programs for linkage analysis by repeatedly calculating the likelihood with respect to f until an approximate maximum likelihood estimate of f is found.

For rare recessive diseases, the situation is somewhat more complicated as one cannot ascertain sibships through parents—both parents are usually unaffected carriers of the disease allele. In other respects, the situation is similar to the one discussed above for dominant diseases. When the two parents are heterozygous, the probability for an offspring to be susceptible (homozygous for disease allele) is $\frac{1}{4}$. Hence, the proportion of affecteds is expected to be $p_A = \frac{1}{4}f$, so that an estimate of the penetrance is obtained as $4p_A$ (as opposed to $2p_A$ in the dominant case). Corrected estimates of p_A may again be calculated using equation (7.1).

Thus far, our discussion of penetrance estimation has focused on one locus only (the one with possibly incomplete penetrance). However, it is often useful also to incorporate information from phenotypes at a closely linked locus in these estimates, usually a genetic marker locus. This may be beneficial, for example, when in a large pedigree some parents are unaffected so that it is unclear with what probability offspring are susceptible. Marker information may then be able to help identify the carrier status of unaffected individuals.

In a collection of large pedigrees, or generally when ascertainment biases can be ignored, the joint estimation of penetrance f and recombination fraction θ is carried out best by calculating the likelihood, $L(f, \theta)$, for various pairs (f, θ). $L(f, \theta)$ may then be pictured as the height above a plane with coordinates f and θ, and the estimates of f and θ are determined by the maximum of $L(f, \theta)$. An example of such an estimation may be found in Rossen at al. (1980). Notice that it is the likelihood (or log likelihood) that has to be maximized, not the lod score (but see chapter 11 for more discussion on this).

When a test for linkage is carried out, one generally compares the maximum of the likelihood $L(\theta)$ under linkage with the likelihood $L(\frac{1}{2})$ under absence of linkage, the relevant test statistic being the maximum lod score, $Z_{max} = \log[L(\hat{\theta})/L(\frac{1}{2})]$. If penetrance is reduced, an analogous test statistic is

$$Z_{max} = \log[L(f, \hat{\theta})/L(f, \frac{1}{2})]. \tag{7.2}$$

In regular cases, $4.6 \times Z_{max}$ then corresponds to a chi-square variable with 1 df. This involves no particular problem when the penetrance is known and is independent of the recombination fraction. In practice, however, penetrance is often estimated and the estimates are positively correlated (see below). Then, equation (7.2) must be modified to allow for these dependencies.

When penetrance f and recombination fraction θ are estimated simultaneously such that $L(\hat{f}, \hat{\theta})$ is the maximum likelihood under the hypothesis H_1 of linkage, there are two ways of comparing this with the likelihood under the hypothesis H_0 of absence of linkage. Either the penetrance is kept at its estimated value $\hat{f}$ obtained under linkage and one computes the maximum lod score,

$$Z_2 = \log[L(\hat{f}, \hat{\theta})/L(\hat{f}, \frac{1}{2})], \tag{7.3}$$

or one obtains a separate estimate $\hat{f}_1$ under absence of linkage and computes the maximum lod score,

$$Z_1 = \log[L(\hat{f}, \hat{\theta})/L(\hat{f}_1, \frac{1}{2})]. \tag{7.4}$$

It should be noted that Z_1 is associated with 1 df, for one restriction ($\theta = \frac{1}{2}$) leads from H_1 to H_0, but Z_2 is associated with 2 df corresponding to the two restrictions ($\theta = \frac{1}{2}$, $f = \hat{f}$) characterizing H_0. Therefore, it is easier to obtain Z_2 than Z_1; in other words, the same maximum lod score obtained by (7.3) is not as strong an indication of linkage as when it is obtained from (7.4).

These considerations have consequences for the determination of support intervals for θ, for example, by including in the support interval all points θ with associated lod score $Z(\theta) \geq Z_{max} - 1$. When the lod scores $Z(\theta)$ are based on (7.3) (i.e., are computed with a fixed penetrance estimate), then the support interval will generally be too small. The proper way of calculating lod scores $Z(\theta)$ associated with 1 df would be to calculate, at each point of θ, a likelihood $L(\hat{f}_\theta, \theta)$, where L is maximized over f at each θ, so that one obtains $Z(\theta) = \log[L(\hat{f}_\theta, \theta)/L(\hat{f}_{1/2}, \frac{1}{2})]$. These lod scores will furnish a support interval of the proper length (associated with 1 df). Alternatively, a bivariate support region for f and θ may be constructed (see chapter 8).

The remainder of this section is devoted to two more theoretical aspects of the joint estimation of penetrance f and recombination fraction r. The first point of discussion is that generally these estimates are correlated. For a particular simple mating type such as the phase-known double backcross considered in the previous section, it is straightforward to calculate the expected asymptotic correlation $\rho(\hat{f}, \hat{\theta})$ via the inverse of the information matrix (equation [5.9]). One obtains

$$\rho(\hat{f}, \hat{\theta}) = \frac{f(1 - 2r)\sqrt{r - r^2}}{\sqrt{1 - f + 2f^2r(1 - r)(1 - 2r + 2r^2)}}, \quad (7.5)$$

where f and r refer to true parameter values. The correlation is positive for $r < \frac{1}{2}$ and equal to 0 for $r = \frac{1}{2}$. Selected values of ρ (equation [7.5]) are given in table 7.3. For example, with a penetrance of $f = 0.70$ and a recombination fraction of $r = 0.05$, the corresponding estimates are correlated with $\rho(\hat{f}, \hat{\theta}) = 0.23$.

Analogous calculations can be carried out for larger families. For example, assume a family composed of a phase known double backcross mating $D1/d2 \times d2/d2$, with a daughter of this mating married to a $d2/d2$ man, and their son. When the correlation between $\hat{f}$ and $\hat{\theta}$ is calculated from the joint phenotype distribution of the daughter and her son, that correlation turns out to be negative, but it is never larger than 0.32 in absolute value in the range $0 < f \leq 1$, $0 < r \leq \frac{1}{2}$. In practice, the correlation between estimates of f and r obtained from pedigree data may

Table 7.3. Asymptotic Correlation $\rho(\hat{f},\ \hat{\theta})$ between Estimates of Penetrance f and Recombination Fraction r in Phase-known Double Backcross Families

f	Recombination Fraction, r				
	0.01	0.05	0.10	0.20	0.30
1	0.70	0.67	0.62	0.51	0.37
0.9	0.26	0.43	0.46	0.41	0.30
0.7	0.12	0.23	0.28	0.26	0.20
0.5	0.07	0.14	0.16	0.16	0.12
0.3	0.03	0.07	0.09	0.08	0.06

be approximated by the methods introduced in chapter 8 (VARCO6 program).

Another statistically interesting aspect of jointly estimating f and r is that, in simple situations, $\hat{f}$ and $\hat{\theta}$ can be obtained directly as transformations of multinomial proportions. For example, for the phase-known double backcross mating $D1/d2 \times d1/d1$ considered previously in this section and the previous section, there are four types of offspring, $D2$, $d2$, $D2$, $d1$ (table 7.1), with respective probabilities of occurrence $p_1 = \frac{1}{2}(1 - r)f$, $p_2 = \frac{1}{2}(1 - rf)$, $p_3 = \frac{1}{2}rf$, and $p_4 = \frac{1}{2}(1 - f + rf)$. Because of two linear constraints, $p_4 = 1 - p_1 - p_2 - p_3$ and $p_2 + p_3 = \frac{1}{2}$, these four probabilities are completely specified by the two parameters f and r. Their estimates, therefore, can be obtained directly as

$$\hat{f} = 2(\hat{p}_1 + \hat{p}_3), \quad \hat{\theta} = \frac{\hat{p}_3}{\hat{p}_1 + \hat{p}_3}, \tag{7.6}$$

where $\hat{p}_1$ and $\hat{p}_3$ are the MLEs of the trinomial proportions p_1 and p_3. For example, p_3 is the proportion of $D2$ phenotypes. Equation (7.6) provides a striking example of biased MLEs in human genetics. The existence of the bias can be seen as follows: The $\hat{p}_i$ are known to be unbiased estimates of p_i and will assume values ranging from 0 through 1. However, the limited ranges of f and r in (7.6) impose severe restrictions on the ranges of p_1 and p_3, which induces bias. First, the requirement, $0 \le f \le 1$, imposes the restriction, $p_1 \le \frac{1}{2} - p_3$. The region in the parameter space of p_1 and p_3 corresponding to this inequality is identified in figure 7.1 as area 1. In addition, the requirement that $0 \le \hat{\theta} \le \frac{1}{2}$ imposes the restriction $p_3 \le p_1$ with associated parameter region 2 in figure 7.1. The intersection of areas 1 and 2 identifies a small triangle (black area in fig. 7.1) as the only admissible set of parameter values, p_1 and p_3, in the joint estimation of f and r from the offspring of phase-known double backcross families. In other mating types, the situation presumably is very similar so that, in

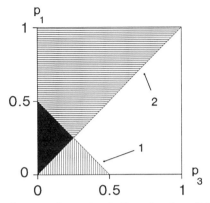

Figure 7.1. Restricted ranges of p_1 and p_3 in the estimation of f and θ.

general, joint estimates of f and r must be strongly biased, since often these parameters will be estimated at their boundary values. For example, $\hat{f} = 1$ whenever $\hat{p}_3 \geq \frac{1}{2} - \hat{p}_1$ ($f > 1$ for $p_3 > \frac{1}{2} - p_1$ in equation [7.6]). For large sets of observations, the bias is expected to vanish because MLEs are consistent.

7.4. Age-dependent Penetrance

Several genetic traits, for example, Huntington's disease (Folstein 1989), are not expressed at birth and develop only later in life, that is, the penetrance is age dependent. In this section, age-dependent penetrance is first introduced for simple situations with complete penetrance at high age and no phenocopies. This will provide the necessary knowledge for handling many common situations. In the second half of this section, a more thorough treatment of age of onset follows, which will enable linkage analysts to tackle more complicated cases.

The conceptually easiest approach to age-dependent penetrance is to group the individuals in a pedigree into age classes, where the kth age class comprises individuals between the ages of x_{k-1} and x_k. If one could identify susceptible individuals at birth, the proportion of susceptible unaffected individuals entering age class k who develop the disease between the ages of x_{k-1} and x_k would be an estimate of the penetrance for the kth age class. In practice, one usually approaches this problem in a retrospective rather than prospective way by focusing on a collection of affecteds whose ages at disease onset are recorded. The cumulative distribution of these onset ages are then used as "age-of-onset curves," as outlined below. As pointed out by Heimbuch, Matthysse, and Kidd (1980), this method suffers from serious drawbacks. These authors presented an analysis method that takes the population age structure into account. Practice shows that a rough approximation to age-of-onset distributions is sufficient in linkage analysis so that the simple procedures given in this section for determining age-of-onset curves should be adequate.

The approximate method of recording ages at disease onset of affecteds works as shown below. Let x_k be the upper boundary of the kth age class. The proportion of affecteds falling into the kth age class is then taken as an estimate for the probability that a susceptible individual will develop the disease between the ages of x_{k-1} and x_k. Since the penetrance at age x_k is the probability of becoming affected (i.e., of developing the disease by age x_k), it is given by the sum of the proportion of all affecteds from the first to the kth age class. Let $F(x_k)$ denote the proportion of all affecteds who developed the disease by age x_k. The graph of $F(x_k)$ will usually take a sigmoid shape. As a simple example, consider the four age categories taken from table 3 in Bird and Kraft (1978), which presents age at onset of Charcot-Marie-Tooth disease (the example is for illustration purposes only; see chapter 9 for genetic heterogeneity in this disease). Among the fifty-three affected individuals, eighteen had onset by age 10, so that $F(10) = 18/53 = 0.34$; $18 + 21 = 39$ had onset by age 15 so that $F(15) = 39/53 = 0.74$; $18 + 21 + 9 = 48$ had onset by age 20 so that $F(20) = 0.90$; and the remaining five individuals developed the disease at a later age (say, by age 30) so that $F(30) = 1$. The age-of-onset curve for these data is shown in figure 7.2.

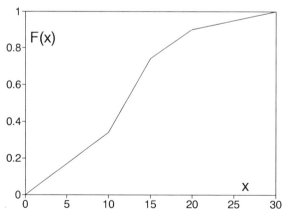

Figure 7.2. Age-of-onset curve $F(x)$ from small sample of affecteds with Charcot-Marie-Tooth disease (x = age of onset).

In a computer program for linkage analysis, the penetrance for each class is required. It may be obtained from the graph of $F(x)$ as the average height of the curve in the kth age class. The penetrance for the kth age class is thus approximately given by

$$h(x_k) \approx \frac{1}{2}[F(x_{k-1}) + F(x_k)]. \tag{7.7}$$

For the given example, one computes $h(x_1) = \frac{1}{2}(0 + 0.34) = 0.17$ (for age class 1), $h(x_2) = \frac{1}{2}(0.34 + 0.74) = 0.54$, $h(x_3) = 0.82$, and $h(x_4) = 0.95$. These values are examples of (narrow sense) penetrances as they would be used in one of the LINKAGE programs. In the LIPED program, which uses penetrances in the general sense, the values $h(x_k)$ are the penetrances for affecteds; the corresponding penetrances for unaffecteds are given by $1 - h(x_k)$. Notice that affecteds are known to carry the disease allele (since phenocopies are assumed to be absent), whatever their age. Hence, in a table of penetrances with rows referring to genotypes and columns referring to phenotypes by age categories, only one column for affecteds (penetrance class) is needed, provided that heterozygotes and homozygotes for the disease allele have the same penetrances. For the disease example discussed here, the relevant wide-sense penetrances are shown in table 7.4. Generally, whenever the penetrances for one phenotype can be obtained from those for another by multiplying the penetrances by a constant factor, these two phenotypes require only one penetrance class (multiplication by a constant does change the likelihood of the data but leaves the lod score unchanged). For example, for genotypes D/D, D/d, and d/d, the penetrance array $(0.17, 0.17, 0)$ for affecteds in age class 1 can be translated into the penetrance array $(0.54, 0.54, 0)$ for affecteds in age class 2 by multiplying each penetrance by 54/17, while no such translation of penetrances for unaffecteds is possible. This applies to affecteds in all age classes so that, as shown in table 7.4, only one

Table 7.4. Age-dependent Penetrances in the Wide Sense, $P(\text{phenotype}|\text{geno-type})$, Calculated for Example Data (D = Disease Allele, d = Normal Allele)

| | | Phenotype | | | |
| | | Unaffected at Age: | | | |
Genotype	Affected	0–10	11–15	16–20	>20
D/D	1	0.83	0.46	0.18	0.05
D/d	1	0.83	0.46	0.18	0.05
d/d	0	1	1	1	1

general class for affecteds is required. Of course, the values shown in table 7.4 are based on a very small sample and are given here for illustration purposes only.

Instead of estimating penetrances in different age classes, one may determine the functional form of an age-of-onset curve $F(x)$, for example, the cumulative normal or lognormal distribution function. Age is then treated as a continuous variable so that penetrance at age x is given by $F(x)$. A particularly suitable curve is the logistic distribution,

$$F(x) = \frac{1}{1 + \exp(-1.8138 z_i)}, \tag{7.8}$$

where $z_i = (x_i - \mu)/\sigma$, μ and σ being mean and standard deviation of age at onset. For example, in Bird and Kraft (1978), mean and standard deviation for age at onset are given as $\mu = 12.2$ and $\sigma = 7.3$ years. With this, equation (7.8) yields for a susceptible individual at age 5 a disease penetrance of $F(5) = 0.143$. One of the advantages of the logistic distribution (7.8) is that it has a closed form inverse,

$$x = \mu - (\sigma/1.8138) \ln[(1 - F)/F], \tag{7.9}$$

which yields the age at onset for a given penetrance. For example, with $\mu = 12.2$ and $\sigma = 7.3$, a penetrance of $F = 0.99$ leads to $x = 30.7$, that is, it is expected that, by age 31, 99 percent of all *susceptible* individuals will have expressed the disease.

Other functional forms for the age-of-onset distribution have been used. These curves are generally characterized by a small number of parameters which may be estimated numerically from pedigree data using one of the linkage programs. Estimating these parameters from pedigree data is a better way of determining age-of-onset curves than recording age at onset of affected individuals because information from unaffecteds is used as well. Notice, however, that such estimates do not incorporate any ascertainment corrections.

A cruder but generally satisfactory approach is to work with an age-of-onset curve composed of straight lines: $F(x)$ is zero up to age x_1, then rises linearly until it reaches 1 at age x_2:

$$F(x) = \begin{cases} 0 & \text{if } x \leq x_1 \\ (x - x_1)/(x_2 - x_1) & \text{if } x_1 < x < x_2 \\ 1 & \text{if } x \geq x_2. \end{cases} \tag{7.10}$$

The two parameters of this curve may be approximately determined as the earliest and latest ages, x_1 and x_2, respectively, at which anyone ever expressed the disease. If age at onset is taken as a random variable with distribution (7.10), its density is uniform, $f(x) = 1/(x_2 - x_1)$ for $x_1 < x < x_2$ and $f(x) = 0$ otherwise, with mean $\mu = \frac{1}{2}(x_2 - x_1)$ and standard deviation $\sigma = (x_2 - x_1)/\sqrt{12} = (x_2 - x_1)/3.464$.

We now turn to more complex situations allowing for the presence of phenocopies. A relatively easy approach to these situations is to take *age at onset* as the (quantitative) phenotype rather than affection status. The latter will be seen to be special cases of the distribution of age at onset when onset age is unavailable (either not recorded for affecteds or not observed for unaffecteds). Age at onset, x, generally has a bell-shaped density, $f(x)$, whose corresponding distribution function, $F(x)$, is the "age-of-onset curve" discussed above. Since the phenotype x is now quantitative rather than qualitative, as outlined in section 7.6, the penetrance in the likelihood (4.17) is replaced by the density, $f(x)$. Several different situations have to be distinguished (Elston 1973), as shown below.

For an affected individual with known age at disease onset, x, the age at onset is the phenotype and the corresponding conditional likelihood, given a susceptible genotype, is $f(x)$. In computer programs, one usually groups individuals into age classes and, in each class, uses the average of $f(x)$ as the density representative for each individual in that class. In the LINKAGE programs, the values of $f(x)$ associated with the different age classes ("liability classes") are still called penetrances. However, the values of $f(x)$, being densities, may assume values larger than 1 and cannot be interpreted in the same way as true penetrances.

If age at onset for an affected individual is unavailable, then at the current age (or age last seen), a, affection status is a binomial variable, that is, an individual is affected with probability $F(a)$ and unaffected with probability $1 - F(a)$, given a susceptible genotype, where F is the distribution function of $f(x)$ evaluated at the current age, a. Therefore, in a computer program, the penetrance to be assigned to an affected individual with unknown age at onset is $F(a)$, and the penetrance for an unaffected individual should be $1 - F(a)$.

Nonsusceptible genotypes (potentially leading to phenocopies) are sometimes taken to have a fixed small penetrance (e.g., 0.001) independent of age. For most diseases, however, when penetrance for susceptible genotypes is age dependent, the penetrance for nonsusceptible genotypes should also be age dependent.

Penetrance at high age may never reach 100 percent but may stay at some lower level, t, beyond a certain age. Then, the age at onset distribution may be defined as $G(x) = F(x)$ with probability t, and $G(x) = 0$ with probability $1 - t$, where, for example, $F(x)$ is the straight-line age-at-onset distribution (7.10). This leads to the following straight-line age-of-onset distribution with incomplete penetrance, t, at high age:

$$G(x) = \begin{cases} 0 & \text{if } x \le x_1 \\ t(x - x_1)/(x_2 - x_1) & \text{if } x_1 < x < x_2 \\ t & \text{if } x \ge x_2. \end{cases} \quad (7.11)$$

When the age x at disease onset is known, the density corresponding to (7.11) is then given by $g(x) = t/(x_2 - x_1)$ if $x_1 < x < x_2$ and $g(x) = 0$ otherwise.

These parametrizations have been implemented in the PC-LIPED program. When age-of-onset curves are to be used with other programs, one must make certain that the phenotype of each individual is associated with the corresponding correct penetrance. Actual age at disease onset is relevant only when disease can occur under different genotypes with different nonproportional penetrances. If this is not so (in many cases it is not), then present age may be used for all affecteds, that is, one may use $G(a)$ for all individuals and disregard the actual age at disease onset (this is how age-of-onset curves are usually handled). This is incorrect, however, in the presence of phenocopies unless at any age the penetrances for nonsusceptible genotypes are constant multiples of those for susceptible genotypes. Of course, if the age-at-onset distribution is to be estimated from family data, then age at disease onset (not current age) should be used when it is known.

As an example, consider an analysis of familial osteoarthrosis (Palotie et al. 1989), in which equation (7.10) was used as the age-at-onset distribution for individuals with genetic predisposition ($x_1 = 0$ and $x_2 = 60$ years of age). In addition, for nongenetic cases (phenocopies), onset was also assumed to be age dependent (equation [7.11]) with $t = 0.8$, $x_1 = 40$, and $x_2 = 100$ years of age because, at high age, close to 80 percent of individuals in the Finnish population suffer from osteoarthrosis. The curves of $f(x)$ and $F(x)$ assumed in this example are shown in figure 7.3. A few sample penetrances are as follows: An affected individual with age at onset $x = 20$ years has "penetrance" $f(20) = 1/60 = 0.017$ (all affecteds with known age at onset have the same penetrance). An affected individual with unknown age at onset and current age $a = 40$ years has penetrance $F(40) = 40/60 = 0.67$, and an unaffected individual with current age $a = 40$ years has penetrance $1 - F(40) = 0.33$. Discrimination between genetic and nongenetic cases is modeled primarily through the different ages of onset and to a lesser degree also through incomplete penetrance in nongenetic cases. The densities of age at onset for genetic and nongenetic cases overlap only for ages 40 through 60. Any onset at

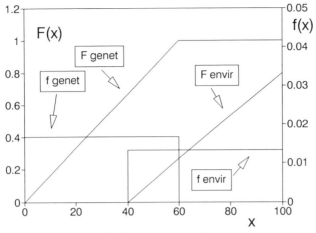

Figure 7.3. Density $f(x)$ and distribution function $F(x)$ for age at onset assumed for familial osteoarthrosis (Palotie et al. 1989).

age below 40 must be a genetic case, and any onset above age 60 must be a nongenetic case. The results of this study were confirmed by the detection of a base-pair substitution in the type 2 procollagen gene, which was present in all affected members of a large family and absent in the unaffected members and in fifty-seven unrelated individuals (Ala-Kokko et al. 1990).

7.5. The Factors Influencing Penetrance

Penetrance (the conditional probability of being affected) can depend on a number of covariates (e.g., age or sex), but other variables may also influence penetrance. In a linkage analysis, the effect of such covariates is generally taken into account by forming covariate classes and, for each such class, defining the appropriate set of penetrances. The example of age classes was covered in the previous section. To take sex difference in penetrance into account, one may distinguish two sets of age classes, one for males and one for females. Another example is the presence or absence of cytologic abnormalities in the fragile X syndrome (see section 11.3).

Incomplete penetrance for a disease, say, implies a certain randomness in the occurrence of the disease. It is usually assumed that unspecified environmental factors determine the probability with which a susceptible genotype expresses the disease. Alternatively, other genes might epistatically interact with the disease gene, such that genetic factors are responsible for incomplete penetrance at the disease locus. Computer simulation experiments have shown (Greenberg and Hodge 1989) that the source of the reduction in penetrance has little influence on the outcome of linkage analyses.

7.6. Quantitative Phenotypes

In section 7.5 on penetrance, a particular quantitative phenotype, the age at disease onset, was discussed at length. Generally, quantitative phenotypes at a monogenic gene locus, such as the level of blood cholesterol, are not usually thought of in terms of penetrance. There is a strong analogy, however, and it will be convenient to discuss quantitative phenotypes in the context of penetrance, first in general terms and then in a more theoretical framework.

Several methods for using quantitative phenotypes in linkage analyses have been proposed, for example, by Haseman and Elston (1972), Hill (1975), Smith (1975), and Cockerham and Weir (1983). To elucidate the properties of the lod score method for quantitative traits, Lange, Spence, and Frank (1976) carried out a simulation study, in which susceptible and nonsusceptible genotypes were associated with two normal distributions separated by a certain difference in their mean values. They found that the peak lod score dropped from 4.5 for practically complete separation of the phenotype distributions to a value of about 1.7 when the difference between the means was 2 units of standard deviation. Although a drop of 2.8 units of lod score seems like a huge loss in information, one must remember that the sum of two normal distributions with a standardized mean difference of 2 or less is no longer bimodal. It is thus encouraging that, even with strongly overlapping distributions, one can still expect positive lod scores.

In linkage analyses involving quantitative traits, the lod score method is applied as shown below. Assume a monogenic trait (e.g., an autosomal dominant disease) where the phenotype is a measurement such as the blood cholesterol level, which is elevated in individuals carrying one or two disease alleles. For normal individuals the phenotype randomly fluctuates around the mean μ_1; for individuals with one or two disease genes, however, the phenotype mean is $\mu_2 > \mu_1$. With given means and standard deviations, the likelihood can be computed simply by replacing the penetrance, $P(x|g)$, in equation (4.17) by the density, $f(x_i; \mu_g, \sigma_g)$, where x_i is the ith individual's phenotype and the parameters μ_g and σ_g are means and standard deviations depending on the genotype g. In some linkage programs such as ILINK, these parameters can be estimated from family data, or they may be estimated from sets of normal individuals and obligate carriers of the disease gene.

In practice, few quantitative phenotypes are analyzed as continuous variables (e.g., the creatine kinase level in Duchenne muscular dystrophy, which is elevated in female carriers of the disease allele). Usually, a cutoff point separating abnormal (high) from normal (low) phenotypes is defined, thus defining a qualitative phenotype with two classes, affecteds and unaffecteds. In principle, removing the overlap by creating two distinct classes leads to an increase in misclassifications and to a bias in parameter estimates; mixed observations should be analyzed under a model of a mixture of distributions whenever possible. On the other hand, forming distinct classes obviates the need for estimating means and standard deviations.

An overlap of quantitative phenotypes gives rise to misclassification, even when they are analyzed taking the overlap into account, and hence leads to a reduction in the amount of information in the data on the recombination fraction r. To quantify this loss of information, assume a normally distributed phenotype with standard deviation 1, divided into a large number, c, of classes. The density $f(x_i; \mu_g)$ is then replaced by a histogram, with one bell-shaped histogram for each of the two means, separated by $\Delta\mu = \mu_2 - \mu_1$, where the probability of occurrence of the phenotype x_i is its penetrance.

In addition to the main locus, assume a dominant marker locus with two alleles and two phenotypes, B and b. Consider a phase-known double backcross mating $AB/ab \times ab/ab$. For the ith phenotype at the main locus, let the penetrance be q_i when a given genotype contains the A allele and p_i otherwise. When $\Delta\mu = 0$, one has $p_i = q_i$. The phenotypes, considered jointly at the two loci, occur with probabilities

$$P(x_i, B) = \tfrac{1}{2}[rp_i + (1 - r)q_i] \tag{7.12}$$

$$P(x_i, b) = \tfrac{1}{2}[(1 - r)p_i + rq_i]$$

where $i = 1 \ldots c$, and r is the true recombination fraction. From this, with a given difference $\Delta\mu$ of the means, Fisher's expected information per offspring can be calculated as

$$i(r) = \tfrac{1}{4} \sum_{i=1}^{c} (p_i - q_i)^2 [1/P(x_i, B) + 1/P(x_i, b)]. \tag{7.13}$$

For complete separation of the two distributions ($\Delta\mu = \infty$), $i(r)$ (7.13) becomes $1/[r(1 - r)]$, as it should. Sample values of the relative effi-

Table 7.5. Relative Efficiency of the Recombination Fraction Estimate with Two Overlapping Distributions of the Phenotype at the Main Trait

	Recombination Fraction, r				
$\Delta\mu$	0.01	0.05	0.10	0.20	0.50
∞	1	1	1	1	1
5	0.92	0.96	0.97	0.97	0.97
4	0.77	0.85	0.88	0.90	0.92
3	0.47	0.62	0.69	0.74	0.78
2	0.15	0.30	0.39	0.46	0.52
1	0.02	0.06	0.10	0.14	0.19

ciency, $i(r; \Delta\mu)/i(r; \Delta\mu = \infty)$, are given in table 7.5. As one can see, as long as $\Delta\mu \geq 3$, the relative efficiency is no less than 50 percent, that is, the loss of information due to such an overlap can be compensated for by doubling the number of observations. The values in table 7.5 were obtained under the assumption of known means and variances. When these have to be estimated, efficiency is expected to be reduced further.

Problems

Problem 7.1. For the example shown in figure 7.3, what is the appropriate penetrance for an affected individual with age at onset $x = 15$ years and current age $a = 65$ years?

Problem 7.2. For some disease with age-dependent penetrance, assume a straight-line age-of-onset curve, starting with $F(x_1) = 0$ at age $x_1 = 5$ years and ending with $F(x_2) = 1$ at age $x_2 = 40$ years. At what age are 80 percent of all susceptible individuals expected to have expressed the disease?

8.

Numerical and Computerized Methods

Human linkage analysis applies statistical procedures to observations of family members. As in many applications of classical statistical methods such as analysis of variance, linkage analysis may involve extensive calculations. This aspect of linkage analysis will be covered in this chapter. It would be a mistake, however, to assume that carrying out a linkage analysis is basically a matter of using a computer program.

In some simple situations, it is possible to obtain the solution to a linkage problem by analytical means (section 8.1). In more complicated cases, analytical solutions may still be possible but are simply too tedious to carry out. One may then write a computer program or use one of the commercially available spreadsheet programs to find the desired solution. An example is provided in the second half of section 8.1. Often, however, analytical solutions are not feasible, in which case so-called numerical methods may be applied, which generally result in any desired accuracy. Examples may be found in section 8.4. Finally, some problems are so complex or time-consuming to carry out that even numerical solutions are inappropriate, in which case one may resort to computer simulation (section 8.7).

8.1. Calculating Lod Scores Analytically

In chapter 4, some simple lod scores were calculated, for example, in equation (4.7). For a few families (Ott and Frater-Schröder 1981), it is demonstrated below how to derive two-point lod scores analytically (instructive examples can also be found in Morton 1956). Four two-generation families have been selected for this purpose (table 8.1). One of the loci used is that coding for transcobalamin II (TCN2, now known to be on chromosome 22), a vitamin B_{12}-binding protein, whose alleles are num-

165

Table 8.1. Four Families from a Linkage Investigation of TCN2

Family	Individual[a]	Phenotype	Possible Genotypes
Bu	F	1/3; a/b	(I) *1a/3b* or (II) *1b/3a*
	M	3/3; c/d	*3c/3d*
	S	3/3; a/c	*3a/3c*
	D	3/3; b/c	*3b/3c*
De	F	—	(I) *1a/3b* or (II) *1b/3a*
	M	3/3; c/d	*3c/3d*
	S	1/3; a/c	*1a/3c*
	D	1/3; b/c	*1b/3c*
	D	3/3; a/d	*3a/3d*
A47	F	1/3; O	*1o/3o*
	M	1/3; A	(I) *1a/3o* or (II) *1o/3a*
	S	1/3; O	*1o/3o*
	S	1/1; O	*1o/1o*
	S	3/3; A	*3a/3o*
B5	F	—	(p^2) *3a/3o* or ($2p(1 - p)$) [*3a/xo* or *3o/xa*]
	M	1/1; O	*1o/1o*
	D	1/3; O	*3o/1o*
	S	1/3; A	*3a/1o*
	S	1/3; O	*3o/1o*

Source: Ott and Frater-Schröder 1981.
[a] M = mother, F = father, D = daughter, S = son.

bered *1*, *2*, and *3*. The marker locus is either *HLA*, whose haplotypes are designated by *a*, *b*, *c*, and *d*, or the *ABO* locus with alleles *a*, *b*, and *o* and phenotypes (blood types) A, B, AB, and O. Phases are distinguished by roman numerals, I, II, etc.

Family Bu. Of the four individuals in family Bu, three unequivocally exhibit their genotypes through the phenotypes. In the father, however, a double heterozygote, two phases can be distinguished. Under phase I, the son is a recombinant and the daughter is a nonrecombinant, while the reverse is true under phase II. The phases are assumed to occur with equal frequencies in the population so that the likelihood is proportional to

$$L(\theta) = \tfrac{1}{2}\theta(1 - \theta) + \tfrac{1}{2}(1 - \theta)\theta = \theta(1 - \theta).$$

With θ set equal to $\tfrac{1}{2}$, this leads to $L(\tfrac{1}{2}) = \tfrac{1}{4}$, so that the lod score is obtained as

$$Z(\theta) = \log[4\theta(1 - \theta)].$$

This is the same lod score as the one for a phase-known double backcross family with one recombinant and one nonrecombinant offspring. In family Bu there is one known recombinant but, since the phase of the father is unknown, one cannot tell which of the children is the recombinant. The maximum of Z occurs at $\theta = \frac{1}{2}$, that is, all other lods in this family are negative.

Family De. Although the phenotype of the father is unknown, his single-locus genotypes can be inferred from those of the other family members. The mating type in this family turns out to be the same as that in the previous family. In phase I, there are one nonrecombinant and two recombinants, and the reverse is true in phase II. The likelihood is thus proportional to

$$L(\theta) = \frac{1}{2}(1 - \theta)\theta^2 + \frac{1}{2}\theta(1 - \theta)^2 = \frac{1}{2}\theta(1 - \theta).$$

It differs from the likelihood for family Bu by a constant that cancels in the likelihood ratio, so that the lod score for family De is identical to that for family Bu. The three children in family De are as informative for linkage as the two children in family Bu.

Family A47. Both parents are heterozygous at the TCN2 locus. As one can infer from the occurrence of children with blood type O, the mother is also heterozygous at the *ABO* locus. Under phase I, the first son is a recombinant if the *Io* haplotype was received from the mother and a nonrecombinant if that haplotype was received from the father; the reverse is true under phase II. Given either of the two phases, the first son's phenotype occurs with probability $\frac{1}{2}[\frac{1}{2}\theta + \frac{1}{2}(1 - \theta)] = \frac{1}{4}$, that is, all he contributes to the likelihood is a constant factor, which will cancel in the likelihood ratio. In this family, therefore, such a phenotype is not informative for linkage (there were two such children in this family, but only one is listed in table 8.1). Under phase I, sons 2 and 3 are both recombinants; under phase II, however, they are both nonrecombinants. The likelihood is thus proportional to

$$L(\theta) = \theta^2 + (1 - \theta)^2. \tag{8.1}$$

Family B5. As in family De, the father's phenotype is unknown. From the other family members it can be concluded that his *ABO* genotype must be *a/o*. The first son is a double heterozygote; the phase of his genotype is known, since the mother is doubly homozygous. At the TCN2 locus, the father may have one of several genotypes whose probabilities depend on the population allele frequencies. As will be seen, one may simply consider the *3* allele and lump the other alleles together into an unspecified allele, *x*. The gene frequencies at the *ABO* locus are not relevant, since the *ABO* genotypes are known in both parents.

Let *p* denote the gene frequency of the *3* allele at the TCN2 locus. For the father, the following three genotypes at the TCN2 locus must then be distinguished: (1) If he has genotype *3/3*, each of the children's genotypes occurs with probability ½, that is, the conditional likelihood is equal to ⅛. In this case, the family is uninformative for linkage, but this possibility must still be taken into account. It occurs with probability p^2. (2) If the father has one *3* allele (the other TCN2 allele is denoted by *x*), then in phase I the daughter, son 1, and son 2 are a recombinant, a nonrecombinant, and a recombinant, respectively, and the reverse holds in phase II. Hence, under phase I, the likelihood is equal to $\frac{1}{8}\theta^2(1 - \theta)$, and under phase II it is equal to $\frac{1}{8}\theta(1 - \theta)^2$. Since each phase occurs with probability ½, the conditional likelihood for case 2 turns out to be equal to $\theta(1 - \theta)/16$, and this case occurs with probability $2p(1 - p)$. (3) The father must have at least one *3* allele so that the genotype *x/x* need not be considered. The total likelihood is then the weighted average of the two conditional likelihoods,

$$L(\theta, p) = \tfrac{1}{8}p^2 + \tfrac{1}{8}p(1 - p)\theta(1 - \theta), \tag{8.2}$$

so that the lod score is given by

$$Z(\theta; p) = \log\left\{\frac{4[\theta(1 - \theta)(1 - p) + p]}{1 + 3p}\right\}. \tag{8.3}$$

The maximum of *Z* occurs at $\theta = $ ½ so that all other lod scores are negative. For instance, with $p = 0.52$ and $\theta = 0.10$, $Z(0.10) = -0.055$. Equation (8.3) is an example of a lod score whose value depends on parameters other than θ alone. In a large pedigree the gene frequencies influence genotype probabilities of the founder members only and will not usually have much effect on the lod score; in this small family, however, varying *p* greatly affects the lod score. For example, at $\theta = 0$ the lod score (8.3) is given by $Z(\theta = 0; p) = \log[4p/(1 + 3p)]$, which is equal to -0.09 for $p = 0.52$ and equal to -3.08 for $p = 0.10$. The reason for this dependency on *p* can be seen as follows: Since only the ratio between $2p(1 - p)$ and p^2 matters, the relative probability of the father's being a double heterozygote—and thus being informative for linkage—is given by $2p(1 - p)/[2p(1 - p) + p^2] = 2(1 - p)/(2 - p)$, and this is largest as $p \rightarrow 0$.

8.2. The Elston-Stewart Algorithm

As mentioned in section 4.1, calculating lod scores in large families by hand is extremely tedious and becomes prohibitive in the multilocus case. Early on, therefore, attempts were made to have computers carry out this task (see section 8.3), but with only limited success. A particular representation of the likelihood, published by Elston and Stewart (1971), made it possible to calculate likelihoods for large families in a recursive (or telescopic) manner. The resulting method for rapidly calculating pedigree likelihoods is called the Elston-Stewart algorithm and is the subject of this section, which is necessarily somewhat technical (a special issue of *Human Heredity* in 1991 was devoted to the celebration of the twentieth anniversary of the publication of this algorithm).

Consider a human pedigree of size m. Let x_i denote the phenotype and g_i a particular genotype of the ith pedigree member, where phenotype and genotype may refer to several loci simultaneously. The pedigree likelihood is then expressed as given by equation (4.17), with $P(x|g) = \Pi \, P(x_i|g_i)$, where $P(x_i|g_i)$ refers to an array of multilocus penetrances of the ith family member. Assuming absence of phenotypic interactions at different loci, each $P(x_i|g_i)$ factors into the corresponding single-locus terms.

To evaluate the likelihood (4.17), one would have to take a multiple sum over all possible combinations of genotypes, which can be very complex (Bailey 1961) and too time-consuming for even a modern computer. The Elston-Stewart (1971) algorithm provides a means of evaluating the multiple sum (4.17) in a streamlined fashion, which is particularly suitable for implementation in computers if the pedigrees are of the so-called simple type, as follows: Consider the commonly used graphical representation of pedigrees as shown, for example, in figure 6.1, with lines connecting related and/or married individuals. A path is said to exist between two individuals (e.g., two unrelated mates) when they are connected by an uninterrupted sequence of lines. A *loop* is said to exist in a pedigree when a path consists of a complete circle, leaving an individual by one line and returning to that individual by a different line. One loosely distinguishes two types of loops: a *consanguinity loop* contains at least two mates who are blood related; in a *marriage loop*, however, no mating of related individuals exists. A commonly encountered marriage loop occurs when, in two pairs of siblings, each sib of one pair is married to one sib in the other pair (an example is shown in fig. 1 of Sandkuyl and Ott 1989). Genetically, two individuals (whether married or not) form a mating only when they have offspring, not all of which have phenotypes completely unknown. With these terms, a *simple pedigree* is defined as any family in which no loops occur and in which, for any mating, at most one of the mates has his or her parents in the pedigree. A pedigree not falling in this category is termed a *complex pedigree*.

In a simple pedigree, consider the individuals ordered such that parents precede their children. The pedigree likelihood (4.17) can then be represented as the telescopic sum

$$L(\theta) = \sum P(x_1|g_1)P(g_1|\cdot) \ldots$$
$$\sum P(x_{m-1}|g_{m-1})P(g_{m-1}|\cdot) \sum P(x_m|g_m)P(g_m|\cdot) \qquad (8.4)$$

(Elston and Stewart 1971), where $P(g_i|\cdot)$ represents either the ith child's genotype given the parental genotypes, in which case it may involve the recombination fraction, or the probability that a founder individual (no parents in pedigree) has genotype g_i. Calculating a pedigree likelihood (8.4) by the Elston-Stewart algorithm starts with the innermost (rightmost) sum, which is evaluated for each genotype in the next outer sum, and each summation result is "tagged on" to the appropriate term corresponding to that genotype in the outer sum. Once the summations have been carried out for all genotypes in the outer loop, the rightmost sum is no longer required (for a detailed description, see Ott 1974a). This recursive procedure can be seen to "clip off" branches (sibships) of the pedigree, one after the other, starting at the bottom and finishing at the top of the pedigree. One such round of calculations yields the pedigree likelihood for a given value of the recombination fraction. To evaluate $L(\theta)$ at other θ values, the procedure must be repeated.

The Elston-Stewart algorithm has proved to be very effective in practical applications (see subsequent section). It was extended by me (1974) to nonloop complex pedigrees and by Lange and Elston (1975) to general complex pedigrees. The latter extension is based on the principle demonstrated below. For example, consider an individual who is both an offspring and a mate. If his or her genotype (including phase) is known or can be deduced for certain, for calculation purposes one may represent that individual as two separate individuals, one being an offspring and one being a mate, and treat these two individuals as if they were independent. This "doubling" of individuals results in at most a multiplication of the likelihood by a constant factor, which may involve gene frequencies but no recombination fractions, and this factor can be accounted for in a computer program. Consider now the representation of the likelihood,

$$L(\theta) = P(x) = \sum_{g_i} P(x, g_i), \qquad (8.5)$$

where each term in the sum is conditioned on one (multilocus) genotype of the ith individual and the sum is evaluated over all genotypes of that individual. In each evaluation, the exact genotype of the ith individual is known; therefore, that individual can be "doubled" or "tripled" as described above. The original form of this technique has been implemented in the LIPED program (see below) to allow the processing of complex pedigrees by the Elston-Stewart algorithm. Clearly, this extension is purchased at a price—the likelihood must be evaluated a number of times, this number being equal to the number of possible genotypes of the ith individual. It is thus beneficial, for example, to break a loop at an individual whose phenotype or pedigree relationships exhibit as much as possible of the underlying genotype, so that the sum in (8.5) has to calculated over as small a number of terms as possible.

Other recursive algorithms, allowing pedigree traversal in any direction, have since been proposed (for example, by Cannings, Thompson, and Skolnick 1978). In the MENDEL program (see below), a particular "clipping" or "peeling" algorithm has been implemented, which corresponds to moving the summation signs in equation (8.4) inward (to the right) as much as possible. This way, loops are handled in the framework given by equation (8.4) and not by conditioning on the genotypes of a specific individual. An intermediate implementation of the Elston-Stewart algorithm has been accomplished in the LINKAGE programs (see below): free-ending branches of a pedigree (not involved in a loop) are "peeled" upward (by a partial application of equation [8.4]) or downward (by a modification of [8.4]) as needed, and loops are handled by conditioning on an individual's genotypes (equation [8.5]).

Calculating genetic risks is not directly related to the Elston-Stewart algorithm but is more generally related to the pedigree likelihood (Elston and Stewart 1971): the risk that the ith individual has a particular genotype g_i is given by the conditional probability, $P(g_i|x) = P(x, g_i)/P(x)$, which may be evaluated as shown below. For example, consider equation (8.5) and assume that the summation is taken over the three genotypes of the ith individual at a particular recessive disease locus, $g_i^{(1)} = d/d$, $g_i^{(2)} = d/D$, and $g_i^{(3)} = D/D$, d being the disease allele and D being the normal allele. Each of these genotypes is associated with a particular penetrance, $P(x^{(j)}|g^{(j)})$. The jth term in (8.5) is then obtained as that pedigree likelihood, L_j, in which penetrance for the jth genotype of the ith individual is equal to $P(x^{(j)}|g^{(j)})$, and the other two single-locus penetrances are set equal to zero. The total likelihood is simply the sum, $L = \Sigma_j L_j$, and the risk of having the jth genotype is given by L_j/L. Genetic risks may be calculated in exactly this manner by carrying out two likelihood calculations using the LIPED program (see below). In other computer programs, however, particular procedures are implemented for directly calculating genetic risks. In the MLINK program of the LINKAGE package, for example, the pedigree likelihood is "peeled" onto the proband (the individual for whom a risk is to be calculated), such that the proband is the last individual in the recursive likelihood calculations.

8.3. Computer Programs for Linkage Analysis

After a slow start some dozen years ago, quite a few linkage programs are available now and are still being developed. I am familiar with some but not all of them, so the programs discussed in this section necessarily represent a subset of the existing programs. For a list of programs available from me, please write: Columbia University, Box 58, 722 West 168th Street, New York, New York 10032. I also distribute a *Linkage Newsletter* approximately three times a year. It contains information on software, discussions of special topics in linkage analysis, contributions from readers, etc.

Most linkage programs in current use compute lod scores by calculating pedigree likelihoods numerically for each set of parameter values, whereas early approaches consisted of calculating by hand some lod scores for certain well-defined family types and simply storing them on a computer. The first lod scores for nuclear families were tabulated on a vacuum-tube predecessor of the IBM 650 computer (Morton 1955). A remarkable program was developed by Renwick (Renwick and Schulze 1961; Renwick and Bolling 1967). It ran on an IBM 7094 in Baltimore and calculated lod scores for large pedigrees. Being written in machine language, it was unfortunately not transportable. Later approaches included storage of Morton's lod scores on computers for small families (MOSM program; Gedde-Dahl et al. 1972) and numerical calculation of lod scores for linkage analysis in three-generation families (Falk and Edwards 1970; Edwards 1972). In the PEDIG program (Heuch and Li 1972), genetic risks were calculated via pedigree likelihoods.

The first generally available program to compute likelihoods numerically in large pedigrees was LIPED (for LIkelihood in PEDigrees) (Ott 1974, 1976). It is based on the Elston-Stewart algorithm (Elston and Stewart 1971) and extensions of it (Lange and Elston 1975) and allows calculation of two-point lod scores. As the source code is freely available—it is written in FORTRAN—several groups have made modifications to the original version. The only version currently supported by me is PC-LIPED for IBM type microcomputers, which is available from me. I have generalized it to allow for allelic association and age-dependent penetrance (onset age known or unknown). Its first application was in a large kindred of over ninety individuals, where the linkage relationships between familial hypercholesterolemia (LDLR) and sixteen genetic markers were estimated (Ott et al. 1974). The results showed a weak suggestion of linkage between LDLR and complement C3, which was later confirmed by other groups (Berg and Heiberg 1976; Elston, Namboodiri, et al. 1976; Berg and Heiberg 1978).

The LIPED program is still used by many researchers because it has been error-free for more than ten years and because it is able to detect a large percentage of errors in the input data by carrying out many checks for data consistency. LIPED works with penetrances in the wide sense; the user must furnish at each locus a table of penetrances such as the one given in table 1.1. The program produces lod scores at predetermined values of θ or (θ_m, θ_f) (male and female fractions jointly), but it does not iteratively find maximum likelihood estimates.

The LIPED program (as well as most other linkage programs) makes very restrictive assumptions on the genetic models for the phenotypes. While these are allowed to be qualitative or quantitative, they are assumed to be made up of two components only—a genetic component due to a mendelian gene and a random environmental deviation. Many traits may be influenced also by polygenic effects and nonrandom or common environmental factors contributing to the similarity among relatives. A computer program approximately taking such effects into account was developed by Hasstedt (1982).

The PAP program extends linkage analysis to several (currently four) loci jointly. It is being used by many researchers. For details, the reader is referred to its original description (Hasstedt and Cartwright 1981).

The original purpose of developing the LINKAGE programs (Lathrop et al. 1984) was for gene mapping. Presently, they exist in two versions, a set of programs for general pedigrees and a specialized version for the analysis of codominant markers in the CEPH panel of reference families (Dausset et al. 1990). As pointed out in the previous section, the LINKAGE programs basically use the Elston-Stewart algorithm but can peel upward or downward in a pedigree. The specialized LINKAGE version for CEPH families employs a technique of factorizing the multilocus likelihood (Lathrop, Lalouel, and White 1986), which, in comparison with the version for general pedigrees, allows more rapid analysis and joint processing of a greatly increased number of loci. The description below focuses on the version for general pedigrees.

The LINKAGE package consists of three analysis programs, each of which calculates two-point or multipoint likelihoods in human pedigrees. MLINK calculates likelihoods by stepwise variation of the recombination fraction in one of the interlocus intervals. It also computes genetic risks. The LINKMAP program assumes a fixed map of markers and calculates likelihoods for a new locus at various points in each interval along the known map. The third program, ILINK, iteratively estimates recombination fractions and other model parameters. Except for three-locus analysis, these programs (like most other linkage programs) assume absence of interference in the calculation of gamete probabilities given parental genotypes (see discussion in chapter 6). Work is in progress to implement some form of interference. Recently, the three analysis programs have been extended to allow for a two-locus mode of inheritance of a qualitative phenotype, which is of particular interest for linkage analysis of disease loci (Lathrop and Ott 1990).

The LINKAGE programs are written in PASCAL and are available from Dr. Mark Lathrop in Paris or from me. The number of loci that can be analyzed jointly is limited only by the available memory. The version for microcomputers (available from me) presently allows for no more than six two-allele loci (less for multiallelic systems) at any one time when run under the MS-DOS operating system. A version for the OS/2 operating system is in preparation and should be more flexible than the DOS version. One must be aware, however, that the calculation of multipoint likelihoods is very computer intensive and may require long execution times.

A major difference between LIPED and the LINKAGE programs consists in the definition of penetrance (see section 7.1). While LIPED uses penetrance in the general (wide) sense, penetrance in the LINKAGE programs is the probability of being affected given a genotype. A table of penetrances such as table 1.1 is suitable for direct input to LIPED. To use such penetrances in the LINKAGE programs, it is easiest to treat such a locus as an "affection status locus," to call each individual affected at this locus and to consider each phenotype (column in table 1.1) as representing a so-called liability or penetrance class (examples and more detailed explanations are provided in the manual accompanying the LINKAGE programs).

Another difference between the two program sets is in the way they handle male (θ_m) and female (θ_f) recombination fractions. While LIPED directly uses these two parameters and the LINKAGE programs output both θ_m and θ_f, for input the LINKAGE programs work with the two parameters θ_m and the ratio, $R = x_f/x_m$, of female-to-male map distances. Using the Haldane mapping function (absence of interference), conversions between θ_f and R (with given θ_m) can be accomplished by the following two formulas:

$$R = \frac{\ln(1 - 2\theta_f)}{\ln(1 - 2\theta_m)}, \tag{8.6}$$

$$\theta_f = \frac{1}{2}[1 - (1 - 2\theta_m)^R], \tag{8.7}$$

where ln denotes the natural logarithm (base e). These conversions may also be carried out by the SEXDIF utility program.

The FAP (Family Analysis Package; Neugebauer and Baur 1991) was originally developed to estimate allele and haplotype frequencies at the *HLA* locus. It has been extended to carry out many other tasks including linkage analysis.

MAPMAKER (Lander et al. 1987) is a user-friendly linkage program specializing in analyzing codominant loci in CEPH-type families. Using the EM algorithm (for a review, see Weir 1990), it maximizes the likelihood recursively over loci rather than over individuals in a pedigree, which allows analysis of a large number of loci jointly but limits the size of the pedigrees it can handle. For families with unambiguous genotypes, MAPMAKER evaluates likelihood at an impressive speed, but it can be slow for phase-unknown matings. Also, it does not seem to make full use of all of the data (White et al. 1990).

CRI-MAP was developed by Dr. Phil Green to analyze codominant marker systems in small families. It has been extended to more general pedigrees and to simple dominant systems (Goldgar et al. 1989). Single-locus genotypes must be known (through phenotypes or inference) or else some information will be lost in the analysis.

The MENDEL program (Lange, Weeks, and Boehnke 1988) is comparable in its capabilities to the general version of the LINKAGE programs. It is written in FORTRAN and provides routines for special tasks such as risk calculation and estimating parameters for homogeneity tests. Loops in pedigrees are handled by basically condensing pedigree information onto individuals in the loops and analyzing with the loops unbroken. This method of handling loops appears to be more efficient and leads to shorter analysis times than the method implemented in LIPED and LINKAGE, for example. On the other hand, for analyzing the same problem, MENDEL tends to require more memory than the LINKAGE program, which is particularly problematic on microcomputers.

MAP (Morton and Andrews 1989) is an updated version of an older program based on the method of Rao et al. (1979) for combining two-point lod scores into a multipoint framework. The MAP program uses the Rao mapping function (section 1.5). As it treats pairs of loci in the same linkage group as if they were independent, the resulting multipoint likelihood is approximate only.

In linkage analysis, the likelihood is maximized over θ values and perhaps other parameters. Some programs such as LIPED do this by simply evaluating the likelihood at a predefined set of parameter values, while other programs use various iterative numerical maximization techniques. For example, in ILINK, the GEMINI routine (Lalouel 1979) for numerical maximization of the likelihood is implemented. The MAPMAKER program makes use of the EM algorithm (Dempster, Laird, and Rubin 1977), which is known to be very stable and to converge quickly when parameter values are far away from their estimates, but it tends to be slow close to the maximum of the likelihood. In MENDEL, a hybrid technique is implemented in that the EM algorithm is used first, which is later switched to a quasi-Newton algorithm (Lange and Weeks 1989). Most of these techniques always lead "uphill" to parameter values of higher likelihood so that maximization may be trapped at a local maximum, particularly in multipoint analysis where the likelihood often is multimodal. Choosing good starting values for iterations is thus important. It is also advisable to try several different starting values for the same problem. One maximization technique, simulated annealing, is known to tend to find global maxima, but a discussion of it is beyond the scope of this book (see reviews in Weeks and Lange 1987; Weeks 1991). It does not seem to have been incorporated in any linkage programs.

As already pointed out, multipoint linkage analysis requires many calculations and can take considerable time even on a fast computer. This problem is exacerbated in the presence of loops, particularly when they contain untyped individuals (i.e., with unknown phenotype). When an entire family is untyped at one locus, a simple remedy is to make every individual homozygous at that locus. In other cases, one must be careful to point out to the program that the loop should be broken at an individual with as little ambiguity on the genotype as possible. This means that one should choose an individual with known phenotype and unambiguous genotype at as many loci as possible. When two individuals are both typed at each locus, choose the one who is more often homozygous than the other. In still other cases, one may have to reduce the number of loci analyzed jointly, or one may even have to disregard a loop, which will generally have little effect when the loop is relatively wide.

8.4. Special Applications of Linkage Programs

Linkage programs are generally designed to estimate recombination fractions. Because they calculate pedigree likelihoods for various genetic parameters, they also lend themselves to the maximum likelihood estimation of these parameters. For example, the ILINK program numerically estimates gene frequencies, haplotype frequencies, penetrances, the ratio of female-to-male map distance, etc. Notice, however, that such estimates are obtained without ascertainment corrections, which may represent serious problems. For example, for linkage analyses involving a disease locus, families are often collected to contain as many affected individuals as possible. In those cases, uncorrected estimates of penetrance based on the collected families will yield inflated values.

The purpose of this section, however, is not to discuss parameter estimation but to point out some less well known applications of linkage programs, which can be of considerable value to linkage analysts. The first examples outlined below involve tricking a program into carrying out analyses for which it was not directly designed. Later examples will show how to obtain numerically some probability distributions, whose calculation would be very tedious to carry out in any other way.

Linkage programs perform analyses between autosomal loci or between X-linked loci, but there is generally no provision for an analysis between an X-linked and a pseudoautosomal locus, between an X-linked and a Y-linked locus, or between two Y-linked loci. No new programs are required, however. Linkage investigations involving pseudoautosomal loci can be handled with an appropriate use of penetrances (Ott 1986a). The principle applied here is to emulate X-linked and Y-linked inheritance as special forms of autosomal inheritance. For the pseudoautosomal region, recombination in females occurs when two X chromosomes pair up, whereas recombination in males takes place when the X and Y chromosomes unite. The cases described below have to be distinguished.

Loci located in the pseudoautosomal region (section 1.4) behave in their inheritance pattern exactly like autosomal loci. Hence, linkage analyses among pseudoautosomal loci may be carried out as if the loci followed an autosomal mode of inheritance except that a low female-to-male map distance ratio of approximately 0.066 should be applied (section 1.6). With genetic marker loci, it may often be possible to count recombinations and nonrecombinations so that a linkage analysis need not be carried out with a computer program. For example, Gough et al. (1990) analyzed families for linkage between the granulocyte-macrophage

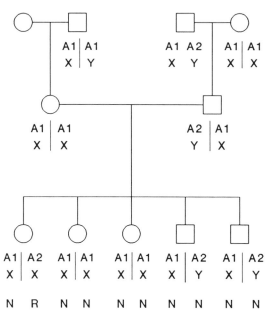

Figure 8.1. A family showing linkage between the GM-CSF receptor gene and gender (adapted from Gough et al. 1990).

colony-stimulating factor (GM-CSF) receptor gene in the pseudoautosomal region and the gender phenotype (male/female), which is thought to be the expression of a sex-determining locus. One of their families is depicted in figure 8.1, where X and Y refer to the pseudoautosomal portions of the X and Y chromosomes, respectively. This family provides a good object for studying the inheritance of pseudoautosomal loci.

To assess linkage relationships involving pseudoautosomal as well as X-linked and Y-linked loci, it is easiest to model X linkage and Y linkage in the framework of autosomal inheritance by adding a dummy allele to each locus (x in Y-linked loci and y in X-linked loci) and setting the penetrances such that, for instance, no male can ever have a genotype x/x or y/y. As an example, assume a codominant X-linked locus with alleles A, a, and y, the corresponding gene frequencies being taken as p_A, p_a, and ½ (the gene frequencies then sum to 1.5). Similarly, assume a Y-linked locus with alleles D, d, and x. Tables 8.2 and 8.3 show the penetrances required in this situation. Pairwise analyses between an X-linked and a pseudoautosomal locus or between a Y-linked and a pseudoautosomal locus will yield correct lod scores under this scheme (the likelihoods will be incorrect by a constant factor). For multipoint analyses, haplotypes

Table 8.2. Penetrances at an X-linked Locus with an Emulated Autosomal Inheritance Pattern

Genotype	Female Phenotypes				Male Phenotypes		
	A	Aa	a	Unknown	A	a	Unknown
A/A	1	0	0	1	0	0	0
A/a	0	1	0	1	0	0	0
A/y	0	0	0	0	1	0	1
a/a	0	0	1	1	0	0	0
a/y	0	0	0	0	0	1	1
y/y	0	0	0	0	0	0	0

Table 8.3. Penetrances at a Y-linked Locus with an Emulated Autosomal Inheritance Pattern

Genotype	Any Female Phenotype	Male Phenotypes		
		D	d	Unknown
D/D	0	0	0	0
D/d	0	0	0	0
d/d	0	0	0	0
D/x	0	1	0	1
d/x	0	0	1	1
x/x	1	0	0	0

instead of alleles must be defined (Ott 1986a), but this can be tricky. The methods outlined above are easiest to use in two-point linkage.

As an example for a linkage investigation between an X-linked and a pseudoautosomal locus, consider the artificial pedigree shown in figure 8.2. Phenotypes are made up to allow counting recombinants and nonrecombinants. Shown in figure 8.2 are the genotypes including phase where known. The estimated male recombination fraction is $\hat{\theta}_m = \frac{1}{6}$, and the female recombination fraction is $\hat{\theta}_f = \frac{2}{6}$ (as pointed out above, θ_m is expected to be much larger than θ_f because at least one crossover occurs in the pseudoautosomal region). One may verify the correct operation of this coding scheme by running the example pedigree with one of the usual linkage programs. Needless to say, one must be extremely careful when applying such a scheme. Linkage programs have no way of detecting an error in coding (e.g., when a male phenotype is used in a woman or vice versa), but such errors easily lead to completely wrong results.

To calculate the expected lod score (section 5.2) or the risk distribution (section 11.8) in a given family, one must evaluate all possible values

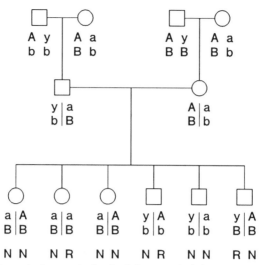

Figure 8.2. Theoretical example for the linkage analysis between a pseudoautosomal locus (alleles *A*, *a*) and an X-linked locus (alleles *B*, *b*). *R* and *N* indicate recombinant and nonrecombinant haplotypes.

of the lod score or the genetic risk and calculate the probability of occurrence of each value. Even when the number of values is not too large, evaluating their probabilities is often impossible by analytic means. As these probabilities are proportional to the pedigree likelihood, linkage programs may conveniently be used to obtain the required outcome probabilities. The subsequent example was pointed out to me by Drs. Leena Peltonen and Irma Järvelä.

Infantile neuronal ceroid lipofuscinosis (CNL1; Santavuori disease, MIM no. 25673) is a recessive disorder that leads to blindness by the age of two years and to brain death by three years and that is fatal by ten years of age. CNL1 has been mapped to the short arm of chromosome 1 (Järvelä et al. 1990). Two parents with an affected child wanted to know with what precision geneticists could predict the risk to a future child. Blood was drawn from the parents (who are obligate carriers of the disease gene) and from their affected child, and genotypes were determined for the two genetic markers nearest the disease, the locus order being *CNL1-D1S62-D1S57* with interval recombination rates of 0.02 and 0.082. Father, mother, and affected child turned out to have the following respective marker phenotypes: 2/2, 1/2, and 2/2 at *D1S62* and 1/2 each at *D1S57*.

To evaluate the range of risks to a future child, one compiles a list of all possible marker phenotypes for that child. At *D1S62*, an offspring can be either 1/2 or 2/2, and at *D1S57*, it can be 1/1, 1/2, or 2/2. Hence, there are a total of six possible phenotypic outcomes at the two marker loci. At each of these outcomes, a risk can be calculated, and each occurs with a certain conditional probability given the known phenotypes of parents and affected child. Using the MLINK program, assuming linkage equilibrium and equal male and female recombination fractions, the pedigree likelihood (the antilog of the log likelihood) and a risk of being affected are then computed. Also, a likelihood must be obtained under the assumption that the future child has unknown phenotype at each of the two markers—that likelihood should be the sum of the likelihoods over all six outcomes, which serves as a check that the outcomes are mutually exclusive and exhaustive. The likelihoods are then divided by their sum, which yields the probabilities of the various outcomes.

Table 8.4 displays the various risks that may be given to a future child, as determined by the marker phenotypes it can have. The probabilities of the different outcomes appear simple, but it is in general difficult to compute these by hand. The weighted average of the risks is ¼, which is the risk without marker information. The following answers may now be given to the parents: The risk to a future child is generally low (i.e., ¼). When marker information is available on a new fetus, there is a 50 percent chance that the test will result in a much lower risk of 1–3 percent. Otherwise, there is an equal chance that the test is uninformative (no change to the expectation of a risk of ¼) or that it increases the risk to 70 percent. The test will never result in a risk higher than 70 percent, but that does not, of course, mean that a future child could not be affected. Obviously, such probabilistic details are not generally useful for counselees, but they can be very valuable for counselors.

In larger families, generally many different risks to a proband can occur. In these cases, risk distributions can be approximated using com-

Table 8.4. Example of Determining the Distribution of Risks, R, to a Future Child in a Specific Family (See Text)

D1S57	D1S62	Risk	L^a	Probability $L/\Sigma L$
1/1	1/2	0.028	1.4324	0.125
1/1	2/2	0.264	1.4324	0.125
1/2	1/2	0.011	2.8648	0.250
1/2	2/2	0.697	2.8648	0.250
2/2	1/2	0.028	1.4324	0.125
2/2	2/2	0.264	1.4324	0.125
	Total		11.4592	1

^aL = likelihood, multiplied by 10^9.

puter simulation (see section 8.7). Techniques analogous to the one described above can be used to find the distribution of lod scores, their average, and the probability that they exceed a certain threshold but, as mentioned before, this is feasible only when the number of possible outcomes is not too large. For these problems, too, one would in general use computer simulation. Section 11.2 quotes an example in which all possible outcomes for a small family type are evaluated with the aid of a computer program written for that purpose.

8.5. Linkage Utility Programs

In linkage analysis, calculations are sometimes required that would be somewhat tedious to carry out on a calculator. A set of small computer programs called Linkage Utility programs is available from me; these have proven useful in a linkage analyst's daily routine. Some of them are discussed elsewhere, for example, the ASSOCIATE program is mentioned in section 11.4. This section briefly describes a selection of these programs. Details are given in the manual that comes with the programs in the form of a disk file. The programs for analyzing genetic heterogeneity are discussed in chapter 9.

The BINOM program computes binomial class frequencies and exact confidence intervals (not support intervals) for binomial proportions for values of n up to 8,000. A typical application is shown below. In $n = 20$ recombination events, $k = 3$ recombinations have occurred. The corresponding recombination fraction estimate is $\frac{3}{20} = 0.15$ with a maximum lod score of $Z_{max} = 2.35$. The empirical significance level associated with this Z_{max}, that is, the probability under $\theta = \frac{1}{2}$ of obtaining three or fewer recombinants, is obtained from the BINOM program as $p = 0.0013$.

In the 2BY2 program, Fisher's exact test (Armitage and Berry 1987, 129) is carried out for a comparison between two binomial proportions (total number of observations at most 8,000), to compare, for example, two recombination rates obtained from different meiosis counts.

The CHIPROB program computes p-values for given values of chi-square and number of degrees of freedom. For the normal distribution, NORPROB computes the p-values associated with a given normal deviate, while NORINV finds the normal deviate associated with a given p-value. The following is a useful application of the CHIPROB program: When p-values from n independent investigations should be combined into one p-value, Fisher's (1970) method specifies that one should transform each value of p into $c = -2 \times \ln(p)$. The resulting n c-values are added together. Their sum, Σc, represents a chi-squared variable with $2n$ df. So, if Σc is entered in the CHIPROB program with $2n$ df, the p-value returned is the overall observed level of significance. For example, assume that three independent tests (not necessarily chi-square tests) have furnished the respective p-values 0.011, 0.047, and 0.35. The corresponding c-values are 9.02, 6.12, and 2.10. Their sum, 17.24, with 6 df, yields a combined p-value of 0.008.

EQUIV computes equivalent observations (section 4.5), either from Z_{max} and $\hat{\theta}$ or from a pair of lod scores, Z_1 and Z_2 at θ_1 and θ_2. It also computes lod scores for given numbers of recombinants and fully informative meioses.

The MAPFUN program converts recombination fractions into map distances and vice versa using seven different map functions, while SEXDIF converts (θ_m, θ_f) into (θ_m, R) and vice versa (using Haldane or Kosambi map functions), where $R = x_f/x_m$ is the female-to-male map distance ratio.

NOCOM (on a separate disk in the list of programs) analyses a mixture of distributions by estimating means, variances, and proportions of the single components (Ott 1979b). The distributions are taken to be normal with optional power transformation of the observations, which accommodates the lognormal and a range of other distributions.

PIC furnishes the PIC value and the heterozygosity for given allele frequencies.

Lod scores are usually computed at each of a set of θ values. One may then want to carry out interpolation and approximately find the maximum lod score and its curvature, the latter being used to compute a standard error for $\hat{\theta}$. The VARCO programs (for variance components) perform these tasks for univariate (VARCO3—three θ points) or bivariate (VARCO6—six points) lod scores. In the univariate case, the observed likelihood is taken to represent approximately a normal density with mean at $\hat{\theta}$, provided that $0 < \hat{\theta} < \frac{1}{2}$. The lod score is then quadratic in θ,

$$Z(\theta) \approx c - \frac{m(\theta - \hat{\theta})^2}{2\sigma^2}, \qquad (8.8)$$

where c is a constant additive term and $m = 1/\ln(10) = 0.4343$. On the θ axis, any three points θ_i with their corresponding lod scores Z_i determine (8.8), as shown below. The first and second derivatives of (8.8) with respect to θ are given by

$$Z' \approx \frac{-m(\theta - \hat{\theta})}{\sigma^2} \qquad \text{and} \qquad (8.9)$$

$$Z'' \approx \frac{-m}{\sigma^2}. \tag{8.10}$$

Now, pick $\theta_1 < \theta_2 < \theta_3$ with respective lod scores, Z_1, Z_2, and Z_3, such that Z_2 is the largest of the three (this is to ensure numerical stability). From the three pairs of (Z_i, θ_i), derivatives may be numerically approximated as

$$Z' \approx \frac{Z_3 - Z_1}{\theta_3 - \theta_1} \quad \text{and} \tag{8.11}$$

$$Z'' \approx 2 \frac{\dfrac{Z_3 - Z_2}{\theta_3 - \theta_2} - \dfrac{Z_2 - Z_1}{\theta_2 - \theta_1}}{\theta_3 - \theta_1}. \tag{8.12}$$

The standard error may now be approximated by rearranging (8.10),

$$\sigma^2 \approx \sqrt{-m/Z''}, \tag{8.13}$$

and inserting (8.12) for Z'' in (8.13). Furthermore, it can be shown that, by virtue of (8.11), Z' is the exact first derivative of the quadratic (8.8) at the point $\frac{1}{2}(\theta_1 + \theta_3)$. Inserting this for θ in (8.9) and equating (8.9) with (8.11) leads to

$$\hat{\theta} \approx \frac{1}{2}(\theta_1 + \theta_3) - Z'/Z''. \tag{8.14}$$

At small θ values, the lod score curve is often not well approximated by a quadratic, particularly when the points of θ_i are not closely spaced. Then, it is advisable to transform the θ values such that the lod score curve on the transformed scale, x, is quadratic. Consider the power transformation, $x = \theta^\lambda$ (Box and Cox 1964), for example, $x = \sqrt{\theta}$ for $\lambda = \frac{1}{2}$, where λ is a real-valued exponent of θ. For the binomial case of scoring k recombinants and $n - k$ nonrecombinants, the appropriate value of λ can be determined as shown below. One requires that, on the transformed scale, $Z(x) = n \log 2 + k \log \theta + (n - k)\log(1 - \theta)$, with $\theta = x^{1/\lambda}$, is quadratic at $\theta = \hat{\theta}$, which is equivalent to postulating that the third and higher derivatives be equal to zero. Lengthy algebraic manipulations lead to the simple result,

$$\lambda = \frac{1}{3} \frac{1 + \hat{\theta}}{1 - \hat{\theta}}, \tag{8.15}$$

where $\hat{\theta} = k/n$. Thus, the appropriate transformation is given by the observed recombination fraction estimate. For example, $\lambda = \frac{1}{3}$ for $\hat{\theta} = 0$, and $\lambda = \frac{1}{2}$ for $\hat{\theta} = 0.20$. Equations (8.11) through (8.14) are then used with $x_i = \theta_i^\lambda$ instead of θ_i, and the resulting value, $\hat{x}$, is transformed back into $\hat{\theta} = \hat{x}^{1/\lambda}$. All of these manipulations have been incorporated into the VARCO programs.

Applying analogous considerations to the bivariate case, the likelihood $L(s, t)$ is taken to represent a bivariate normal density, where, for example, s and t stand for the male and female recombination fractions. The log likelihood is then quadratic in s and t,

$$\ln L(s, t) = c - 1/2 \frac{S^2 - 2\rho ST + T^2}{(1 - \rho^2)}, \qquad (8.16)$$

where $S = (s - \hat{s})/\sigma_s$, $T = (t - \hat{t})/\sigma_t$, and c is a constant additive term. The six parameters c, $\hat{s}$, $\hat{t}$, σ_s, σ_t, and ρ in (8.16) can be determined by six suitably chosen points (L_i, s_i, t_i). A particular layout of six such points in the (s, t) plane has been incorporated in the VARCO6 program.

Only one additional utility program shall be mentioned here: the VaryPhen program (Xie and Ott 1990) varies the disease phenotype of each individual in a family, for example, by temporarily setting it to unknown. For each such change, a linkage analysis is run and the resulting change in lod score and $\hat{\theta}$ (due to making the ith individual unknown) is recorded. The resulting list provides an investigator with an overview of which of the family members' diagnostic accuracy is most crucial for the analysis.

8.6. Paternity Calculations

In cases of disputed paternity, when an alleged father of a child claims not to be the father, the traditional approach has been to compare blood groups and other genetic markers among mother, alleged father, and child. When this comparison does not clearly exclude the man as the child's father, statistical methods are used to assess the probability with which the man might be the father. Several types of statistical analyses have been used for paternity calculations (Weir 1990). Here, only the so-called paternity index will be considered (Baur et al. 1986; Rao 1989). Also, discussion of genetic systems will be restricted to those with a clearly mendelian mode of inheritance. The statistical treatment of DNA fingerprinting data (Jeffreys, Wilson, and Thein 1985) is beyond the scope of this book (see Brookfield 1989).

Consider the two rival hypotheses, that the man is the father and that he is not the father, and assume that marker typing has been carried out on the man, the mother, the child, and perhaps other relatives of the child and/or the man. Under each of the two hypotheses, a pedigree likelihood can be computed. If the markers are unlinked, the likelihood for all markers is just the product of the likelihoods for the individual markers; when they are linked, the likelihood must be calculated in a multipoint fashion, for example, with the aid of a linkage program. When the man is not the father, he still has to appear (as an individual unrelated to the child) in the calculations. Denote the likelihoods under the two hypotheses by $P(F|\text{father})$ and $P(F|\text{not father})$, where F stands for the observed phenotypes. The likelihood ratio, $R = P(F|\text{father})/P(F|\text{not father})$, is called the *paternity index*.

When it is known or can be assumed with what probability an alleged father is the biologic father, then the posterior probability of his being the father can be expressed as

$$P(\text{father}|F) = \frac{R \times P(\text{father})}{1 - P(\text{father}) + [R \times P(\text{father})]},$$

where $P(\text{father})$ is the prior probability (frequency) that an alleged father is the biologic father. In practice, prior probabilities are not usually specified. Instead, the value $\frac{1}{2}$ is chosen, which leads to the posterior "probability," $P(\text{father}|F) = R/(1 + R)$.

8.7. Computer Simulation Methods

Computer simulation is a numerical technique that is often used as a substitute for analytical calculations that are too complex to be carried out. Computer simulation then yields approximate solutions. For example, to model traffic flow in cities, computer simulation is the method of choice to predict the effect of a temporary street closure. This section provides examples of computer simulation methods applied in human linkage analysis. Its technical aspects will be discussed first, followed by a review of the rationale and purposes of computer simulation.

Monte Carlo or computer simulation methods are based on pseudo-random numbers, which are uniformly distributed in the interval $(0, 1)$. With these methods, real-life events are simulated on the computer so that the simulated and real events share their most important properties. In human pedigree analysis, the process most often simulated is the flow of alleles and gametes from founding members of the pedigree to children and grandchildren, etc. Such a simulation usually starts with a founder, that is, an individual assumed to be randomly drawn from the population. Assume that, at a single locus, the three genotypes a/a, a/b, and b/b occur with the respective frequencies 0.04, 0.32, and 0.64. These numbers are also the probabilities with which an individual randomly drawn from the population will show any of the three respective genotypes. To simulate picking a random individual, one draws a pseudo-random number on the computer and assigns to the "individual" the genotype a/a when the number is less than 0.04, assigns a/b when the number is between 0.04 and 0.36, and assigns the genotype b/b when the number exceeds 0.36. Analogously, one can simulate passing a single-locus or multilocus gamete from parents to offspring. Computer simulation methods were proposed for certain problems in pedigree analysis many years ago (Ott 1974b, 1979a), but only recently were practical applications developed.

In chapter 5, expected lod scores $E[Z(\theta)]$ (5.11) were calculated for some family types. These calculations could be carried out analytically, since the phenotypes in those families occur in a limited number of classes with known probability of occurrence. For general pedigrees, analogous calculations could be approximated by Monte Carlo methods, as shown below. One starts by randomly assigning genotypes at, say, two loci to the founders in the pedigree, as described above. With given genotypes of two founders and an assumed ("true") recombination fraction r between the two loci, a haplotype (gamete) is randomly produced for each founder. The two haplotypes then represent the genotype of a child. This process is repeated for each child and each parental mating.

Given the genotype of each individual, a phenotype is assigned which may be the same as the genotype in the case of codominant loci, or it may have to be produced randomly in the case of incomplete penetrance. Knowing everybody's phenotypes (including the "unknown" phenotype), one computes lod scores $Z(\theta)$ at various values of θ as if these phenotypes had been observed in reality. This completes one *replicate* of the simulation. To obtain a representative random sample of phenotype arrays in the family members, a reasonably large number of replicates is required, for example, $n = 500$. Being randomly sampled, each such generated array has probability of occurrence $P_i = 1/n$ in the sample. In analogy to equation (5.11), at each θ, an expected lod score can now be calculated as the average of the lod scores generated. Once this is done at each θ value, one obtains the expected lod score curve. It should have its maximum at the true recombination fraction $\theta = r$ under which the replicates were generated. In many applications, not the whole curve but only the ELOD (chapter 5) is of interest, that is, the expected lod score at $\theta = r$. As its approximation by computer simulation is subject to random error, one should also compute its sampling variance and standard error, or bootstrap (Weir 1990) lod scores in sets of n to approximate the sampling distribution of $E[Z(r)]$. The ELOD obtained in this manner is representative of the informativeness for linkage of the given family structure.

While randomly generating genotypes for family members is relatively straightforward, it is more difficult to generate genotypes at one locus given observed phenotypes at another locus, when the two loci are genetically linked. In that case, as pointed out by Boehnke (1986), sampling must be carried out from the conditional distribution of the genotypes given phenotypes, $P(g|x)$, which replaces $P(g)$ in equation (5.11). Conditional sampling is relevant, for example, if one requires an answer to the question, given a set of families with known disease phenotypes already collected, what maximum lod score can one expect from these families if marker typing is to be carried out on family members? Answers to such questions are obviously of importance in the planning of a linkage study. A computer program, SIMLINK, has been developed to carry out the required simulations. Its original version (Boehnke 1986) required knowing the disease genotypes for each individual, but an extension of it is applicable to more general situations (Ploughman and Boehnke 1989). Another program, SLINK, is discussed below.

Instead of predicting lod scores, one may also be interested in knowing, before marker typing is carried out, what genetic risks one can expect for a particular proband in an observed family. This question was addressed by Sandkuyl and Ott (1989), who developed a corresponding computer program applicable to families with dominant diseases.

A very general method of generating conditional genotypes was described by me (Ott 1989b). It is based on iteratively calculating the "risk" of having a particular marker genotype at one locus given phenotypes at the same and other loci. This method lends itself to implementation in linkage programs as it exploits the capability of calculating risks built into most of these programs. Based on the LINKAGE programs, the SLINK program (Weeks, Ott, and Lathrop 1990) implements a particular form of these principles. It is applicable to a wide range of situations, for example, that, at the locus for which genotypes are to be generated, marker types of some individuals are already known. Given that some but not all individuals in a particular family are typed and only a portion of the remaining untyped individuals can still be investigated, one may ask who should be typed next. One way of answering this question would be to determine the increase in expected lod score due to typing each one of the remaining untyped individuals, which can be evaluated with SLINK. One would then choose that individual leading to the highest increase in ELOD. Owing to its generality, this method of generating marker genotypes is relatively slow compared with the more specialized genotype simulation procedures discussed above.

In addition to the methods discussed thus far, other approaches to computer simulation in linkage analysis have been developed. For example, Lange and Matthysse (1989) described a method based on random walks. Practice will show which of the various approaches is most suitable for particular tasks.

Two important applications of Monte Carlo methods will now be discussed: (1) power analysis, that is, an investigation of the capabilities of a given family material to detect linkage given linkage exists, and (2) determination of the p-value associated with an apparent finding of linkage (given absence of linkage).

The first of these applications was already alluded to above, that is, the prediction of lod scores in a set of families before marker typing is carried out, when phenotypes at some disease or other locus are known. To use one of the available programs such as SIMLINK or SLINK, one will have to specify an assumed true recombination fraction r between disease and a linked marker locus, which one hopes to find. With the present distribution of markers on the human gene map, one may safely assume a small value such as $r = 0.02$. Also, characteristics of the marker must be specified, for example, that it has four alleles of equal frequency (corresponding to a heterozygosity of 0.75). A simulation then usually yields various quantities that can be interpreted as follows: The ELOD, that is, the expected lod score at the recombination fraction r (section 5.2), is the statistic most often used for comparisons of linkage information content of different bodies of data. Notice, however, that it is an average; the actual lod score at $\theta = r$ found in the families investigated may be higher or lower, with about equal chances for these two possibilities. Another quantity usually furnished by the simulations is the distribution of the maximum lod score, Z_{max}. It is obtained by recording in each replicate the maximum lod score over the θ values (instead of $Z(\theta)$ at $\theta = r$ for the ELOD). Two statistics are often calculated from the Z_{max} values, their mean and the proportion of them exceeding a certain threshold such as $Z_0 = 2$ or 3. The former statistic will generally be somewhat higher than the ELOD (but its use is discouraged, see end of section 5.2), whereas the latter approximates the probability, p_0, that the maximum lod score will be as high or higher than Z_0. To generate means (also the ELOD), a few hundred replicates is usually sufficient; to approximate p_0 reliably, however, larger numbers are generally required (at least 1,000 if possible).

The two most important statistics obtained from these simulations are the ELOD and the probability p_0 that the maximum lod score exceeds a certain threshold Z_0 (see section 5.2). The ELOD is additive over families (which is not true for the mean of the Z_{max} values). For example, if the given families yield an ELOD of 0.75, one will need four times as many families of the same kind for an ELOD of 3. On the other hand, p_0 has a direct probabilistic interpretation, but it lacks the property of additivity over families. Sometimes, the largest of all the Z_{max} values generated is also reported. When the number of replicates is large enough, this overall maximum represents the highest lod score one is able to obtain from the given data. It may, however, be very unlikely to ever find this high a lod score, so that reporting that overall maximum lod score might be misleading. In these calculations, the mode of inheritance is assumed to be known, which may not be realistic for complex diseases.

The second important application of Monte Carlo methods concerns the empirical significance level p associated with an observed maximum lod score, which in this section shall be denoted by Z_{obs} while Z_{max} refers to the maximum lod score obtained in a randomly generated replicate. It is customary to declare a linkage significant when $Z_{obs} \geq 3$ (≥ 2 in the sex-linked case). As pointed out in section 4.4, the corresponding significance level is at most equal to 0.001 (0.01 in the X-linked case). However, particularly in linkage analyses of complex traits (chapter 11), researchers often make several equally plausible assumptions on the mode of inheritance of the trait and carry out a linkage analysis under each of these assumptions. For example, in a linkage analysis between schizophrenia and chromosome 5 markers (Sherrington et al. 1988), three diagnostic schemes and a range of different penetrance values under each diagnostic scheme were tried. The crucial question is then how the results of the different analyses are reported. A cautious investigator may report the lowest maximum lod score found under any of the different model assumptions, or one might think of averaging the maximum lod score over models. In practice, one usually reports and quotes the overall maximum lod score. This practice amounts to maximizing the lod score over model parameters. The resulting distribution of Z_{max} must be inflated as compared to the distribution of Z_{max} values evaluated under fixed parameter values (maximized only over θ values), which was indeed shown by Weeks et al. (1990) and by Clerget-Darpoux, Babron, and Bonaïti-Pellié (1990).

Computer simulation methods allow approximating the empirical significance level p associated with an observed Z_{obs}, even when the maximum lod score is probably inflated and hence cannot be interpreted in the usual manner (an example is shown below). Assume that a linkage study has been carried out resulting in a maximum lod score Z_{obs}. The corresponding p-value is defined as the probability, under absence of linkage, that the maximum lod score reaches or exceeds Z_{obs}, $p = P(Z_{max} \geq Z_{obs}; r = \frac{1}{2})$. To approximate this probability, one randomly generates marker data of the same kind as those used in the real analysis (Weeks et al.

1990). Notice that under $r = \frac{1}{2}$, the marker data are independent of the disease phenotypes so that the generating of marker genotypes can be carried out without conditioning on disease phenotypes (much simpler programs than SIMLINK or SLINK are sufficient for this purpose; see below for an example). When genotypes of family members have been randomly assigned, one carries out an analysis of the simulated data, applying the exact same steps as was done in the real analysis. This completes one replicate of the simulation, resulting in one value of Z_{max}. After a sufficient number n of replicates, one determines the proportion of Z_{max} values equal to or larger than Z_{obs}, which approximates p. If $p \le 0.001$ (0.01 in the X-linked case), the observed Z_{obs} can be considered significant. However, the argument is not complete without the additional step given in the subsequent paragraph.

What number of replicates shall one choose? Since high lod scores are rare, particularly under absence of linkage, a rather large number of replicates will be required for an accurate estimation of p. If n is too small, either because simulating and analyzing a replicate is time consuming or because the investigator has no interest in finding Z_{max} values exceeding his or her Z_{obs}, p will often be estimated to be zero (no Z_{max} exceeds Z_{obs}). It is therefore important to determine the sample-based confidence interval for p (section 3.6). A linkage should then be declared significant when not only p but also the upper bound of its confidence interval is smaller than 0.001. Confidence intervals are conveniently determined using the BINOM program. For example, let k denote the number of maximum lod scores generated which exceed Z_{obs}, and assume that $n = 500$ replicates have been carried out. With $k = 0$, the estimated p-value is equal to zero and its 95 percent confidence interval extends from zero through 0.006, which is larger than 0.001. Hence, one will even in the best situation ($k = 0$) never be able to declare a linkage significant when only 500 replicates are used. As outlined in section 3.6, with $k = 0$ out of n replicates, the upper endpoint of the $100(1 - \alpha)$ percent confidence interval is equal to $p_U = 1 - a^{1/n}$. Solving this for n yields $n = \log(\alpha)/\log(1 - p_U)$, which is the number of replicates required such that, with $k = 0$, the confidence interval for the p-value extends from 0 through p_U. For example, with $\alpha = 0.05$ (95 percent confidence interval), at least $n \approx 3,000$ (300 in the X-linked case) replicates are required for the upper confidence limit of p to be smaller than 0.001 (0.01 in the X-linked case).

If a real linkage has been found, simulations carried out under absence of linkage ($r = \frac{1}{2}$) will generally result in a small p-value, that is, the high lod score Z_{obs} is a rare event under free recombination. One may now also carry out a simulation under the assumption of linkage, generating the marker genotypes under a true recombination rate equal to that estimated in the real data. One would then expect that finding as high a lod score as that observed in reality (Z_{obs}) is no longer a rare event. In other words, if linkage is what causes the high value of Z_{obs}, the p-value resulting from this simulation should be much larger than 0.001. Otherwise, one has to suspect that there are reasons other than linkage which have led to the high value of Z_{obs} in the data. Such a reason could be that the model for the disease is incorrect (although that would not generally be expected to lead to false evidence for linkage); that the observations were subject to some sort of bias, for example, preferential scrutiny of recombinants (but not nonrecombinants), which tends to eliminate true recombinants; that the disease model was chosen to fit the data; or that the lod score in reality was maximized over model parameters and this was partially (or not at all) taken into account in the simulation. A simulation under $r < \frac{1}{2}$ can thus serve as a check for the plausibility of the observations but, to my knowledge, no such analysis has yet been carried out.

As an example of a simulation under absence of linkage, consider the report (Vilkki et al. 1991) of an X-linked gene linked to DXS7, which is hypothesized to be required for the expression of optic atrophy in individuals susceptible to Leber's disease (i.e., in individuals [women] carrying the appropriate mitochondrial DNA mutation). The X-linked susceptibility gene was assumed to be recessive, but its gene frequency was completely unknown. Linkage analyses in the six families (Vilkki et al. 1991) were thus carried out with gene frequencies ranging from $q = 0.05$ through 0.95 and, for each gene frequency, two penetrance values (1 and 0.9) were tried. A total of $2 \times 19 = 38$ different models were tried. The overall maximum lod score obtained was $Z_{obs} = 2.32$ at $\theta = 0$, $q = 0.35$, and a penetrance of 1. To verify that Z_{obs} was this high not only because of maximizing the lod score over the thirty-eight model parameters, computer simulation was carried out under absence of linkage using a modification of the GENRISK program (Sandkuyl and Ott 1989). In $n = 2000$ replicates, Z_{max} exceeded Z_{obs} three times. The corresponding empirical significance level is $p = 3/2000 = 0.0015$ with an upper 95 percent confidence limit of 0.0038, which is lower than 0.01. The observed Z_{obs} of 2.32 is thus significant. The effect of maximizing the lod score over model parameters can be seen in figure 8.3, which shows the graph of the distribution of the 2,000 maximum lod scores generated, where $Z1_{max}$ refers to maximization over θ only, at fixed $q = 0.5$ and penetrance 1, and $Z2_{max}$ refers to maximization over all parameters considered. In many cases, $Z2_{max} = Z1_{max}$ (points on the diagonal), that is, maximization over

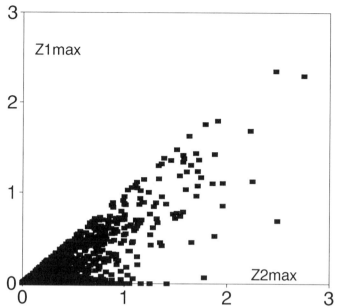

Figure 8.3. Distribution of 2,000 randomly generated lod scores, $Z1_{max}$ maximized over θ and $Z2_{max}$ maximized over θ and model parameters (based on Vilkki et al. 1991).

model parameters did not lead to an increase in Z_{max}. On the other hand, there were several instances (points along the abscissa, at $Z1_{max} = 0$) in which Z_{max} is zero when maximized only over θ but is positive when q and/or the penetrance are varied; the highest such maximum lod score was close to $Z2_{max} = 1.5$.

The Monte Carlo methods presented here are all based on so-called simple random sampling. When the calculation of a replicate is time consuming, one may want to generate only a small number of replicates and apply to them one of the numerical resampling techniques such as the jackknife or the bootstrap (Efron 1982; Weir 1990; Terwilliger and Ott 1991).

Problems

Problem 8.1. Write down the lod score corresponding to the likelihood given in equation (8.1).

Problem 8.2. For family B5 covered in section 8.1, write down the lod scores for the two limiting cases, $p = 0$ and $p = 1$.

9.

The Variability of the Recombination Fraction

Thus far, variation in the estimates, $\hat{\theta}$, of the recombination fraction have been attributed to random fluctuation about the true unknown recombination rate, r. In this section, situations will be discussed in which r is not constant but depends on other variables. Two principally different situations will be distinguished: (1) r varies between recognizable classes of families and is constant within each class and (2) families with different values of r form a mixture and cannot be differentiated as to which ones share the same r value. In statistics, the two cases are referred to as fixed effects and random effects, respectively. Sections 9.1 through 9.3 address case 1, section 9.4 covers the mixture case, and section 9.5 discusses the mixed situation, in which random effects occur within fixed categories of families. Section 9.6 addresses the effect on efficiency of analyses due to incorporation of biologic variables.

9.1. Male and Female Recombination Fractions

According to a rule by Haldane (1922), crossing over is more frequent in the homogametic sex (e.g., XX) than in the heterogametic sex (e.g., XY). This rule applies in many animal species. An extreme case is that of the fruit fly *Drosophila*, where the male does not show any recombination at all. In humans, a clear sex difference in the recombination fraction was first shown for the linkage between *ABO* and the locus for the nail-patella syndrome (NPS1), with a lower estimate of the recombination rate in males, $\hat{\theta}_m = 0.084$, than in females, $\hat{\theta}_f = 0.146$ (Renwick and Schulze 1965). Since then, the ratio θ_f/θ_m of female to male recombination rate has been found to vary in the human genome from region to region (Donis-Keller et al. 1987). On some chromosomes, there is a male excess at one or both telomeres and a female excess elsewhere, for example, on chromosome 12 (O'Connell et al. 1987) and on chromosome 16 (Keith et al. 1990); on other chromosomes, recombination in females is uniformly more frequent, on chromosome 21 for example (Warren et al. 1989). Differences in recombination rate between the two sexes are a form of *heterogeneity*, which should be taken into account in the analysis. It is thus important to estimate θ_m and θ_f separately. The two-point case will be considered first.

It is easiest to obtain separate two-point estimates of θ_m and θ_f from a set of families when one can separate the families in which only fathers are informative for linkage (doubly heterozygous) from those with only mothers as the informative parents. The former families will yield lod scores $Z_m(\theta_m)$ for the recombination fraction in males, and the latter will result in "female" lod scores, $Z_f(\theta_f)$. Bivariate lod scores with respect to male and female recombination rates are then simply the sum,

$$Z(\theta_m, \theta_f) = Z_m(\theta_m) + Z_f(\theta_f). \tag{9.1}$$

The graph of the joint lod score (9.1) can be pictured as a mountainous surface above a plane with coordinates, θ_m and θ_f, with $Z(\theta_m, \theta_f)$ being the height above the plane at the point (θ_m, θ_f). An example of a graph of bivariate lods can be found as figure 8 in Conneally and Rivas (1980).

Generally, matings cannot be separated by the sex of the informative parent, so instead one must estimate sex-specific recombination rates by calculating joint lod scores, $Z(\theta_m, \theta_f)$, for example, by using the LIPED program. Consider the results shown in table 9.1, which were obtained in a linkage analysis of a large multigenerational family (Vogel and Motulsky 1986). The values along the diagonal (italicized) are lod scores calculated under the assumption of equal male and female recombination fractions, $Z(\theta, \theta)$, $\theta = \theta_m = \theta_f$, with a maximum lod of $Z(\theta, \theta) = 6.48$ at $\theta = 0.10$. The overall maximum lod score is 7.88, the sex-specific recombination fraction estimates being $\hat{\theta}_m = 0.05$ and $\hat{\theta}_f = 0.20$.

Table 9.1. Sex-specific Lod Scores in a Pedigree with Dentinogenesis Imperfecta and GC Blood Types

θ_m	Female Recombination Fraction, θ_f				
	0.05	0.10	0.20	0.30	0.50
0.50	0.28	0.70	1.19	1.01	*0*
0.30	2.74	3.98	4.73	*4.68*	3.42
0.20	4.30	5.62	*6.42*	6.37	5.08
0.10	5.50	*6.84*	7.64	7.59	6.26
0.05	*5.74*	7.08	**7.88**	7.83	6.48

Source: Table A9.3 in Vogel and Motulsky 1986.

The significance of the observed heterogeneity in recombination fraction estimates is determined by the difference between the maximum lod scores achieved under the two hypotheses, H_0: homogeneity ($\theta_m = \theta_f$), and H_1: heterogeneity ($\theta_m \neq \theta_f$). Asymptotically,

$$X^2 = 2 \times \ln(10) [Z(\hat{\theta}_m, \hat{\theta}_f) - Z(\hat{\theta}, \hat{\theta})] \qquad (9.2)$$

follows a chi-square distribution on 1 df. For the example in table 9.1, one finds $X^2 = 4.6 \times (7.88 - 6.84) = 4.784$, with an associated empirical significance level of $p = 0.029$ (obtained from the CHIPROB program). The difference between male and female recombination fraction estimates is thus significant at the 5 percent level but not at the 1 percent level.

Table 9.1 demonstrates that it is generally easier to find a high lod score when θ_m and θ_f are distinguished then when they are kept equal. Hence one should in such cases set a higher critical lod score. This situation is analogous to multiple comparisons (two comparisons in this case) discussed in section 4.7. The appropriate critical lod score should thus be raised from $Z_0 = 3$ to $Z_0 + \log(2) = 3.3$. In practice, this is not often done. When in fact a strong difference between male and female recombination rates exists, the lod scores at $\theta = \theta_m = \theta_f$ may all be much lower than the overall maximum. One may thus miss detecting a linkage by not allowing for a difference between θ_m and θ_f.

Male and female recombination fraction estimates are independent when the bivariate lods can be represented as the sum of two terms,

$$Z(\theta_m, \theta_f) = Z(\theta_m, \tfrac{1}{2}) + Z(\tfrac{1}{2}, \theta_f) \qquad (9.3)$$

which is analogous to equation (9.1). The first term on the right side of (9.3) corresponds to the lod scores in the rightmost column (at $\theta_f = \tfrac{1}{2}$) of table 9.1, and the second term corresponds to the top row (at $\theta_m = \tfrac{1}{2}$). If θ_m and θ_f are independent, the two terms on the right side of (9.3) represent male and female lod scores, respectively, and lod scores at any point in the plane should be the sum of the corresponding two marginal lods. This condition can serve as a useful verification for the independence of male and female recombination rates. For example, one would expect that $Z(0.05, 0.20)$ should be equal to $Z(0.05, \tfrac{1}{2}) + Z(\tfrac{1}{2}, 0.20) = 6.48 + 1.19 = 7.67$. In fact, it is equal to 7.88, so that the estimates are not independent but nearly so. Nonindependence of the estimates may occur, for example, when an offspring demonstrates a recombination, but it is unknown in which parent it occurred. In such cases, one cannot estimate θ_m without specifying θ_f, and vice versa.

In practice, tables of bivariate lods such as table 9.1 are not usually published. Instead, one records the univariate lods, $Z(\theta, \theta)$, at the usual θ values. In addition, one indicates the overall maximum lod score and the values of θ_m and θ_f at which it occurred. Sometimes, male and female lods are read off a table such as table 9.1 along the margins, that is, as $Z(\theta_m, \frac{1}{2})$ and $Z(\frac{1}{2}, \theta_f)$. As pointed out by Morton (1978), when the estimates are in any way correlated, this manner of defining sex-specific lods is inappropriate. He proposed reading off male and female lod scores at axes running through the overall maximum and adjusting the resulting values so that they are again equal to zero at $\theta = \frac{1}{2}$: $Z_m(\theta_m) = Z(\theta_m, \hat{\theta}_f) - Z(\frac{1}{2}, \hat{\theta}_f)$ and $Z_f(\theta_f) = Z(\hat{\theta}_m, \theta_f) - Z(\hat{\theta}_m, \frac{1}{2})$. However, at the estimates of θ_m and θ_f, the sum of the adjusted male and female lods is not necessarily equal to the overall maximum lod score. To ensure that this is the case, a correction factor, d, is required so that corrected male and female lod scores may be given by

$$\left. \begin{aligned} Z_m(\theta_m) &= d[Z(\theta_m, \hat{\theta}_f) - Z(\frac{1}{2}, \hat{\theta}_f)] \\ Z_f(\theta_f) &= d[Z(\hat{\theta}_m, \theta_f) - Z(\hat{\theta}_m, \frac{1}{2})], \end{aligned} \right\} \tag{9.4}$$

where $d = Z(\hat{\theta}_m, \hat{\theta}_f)/[2Z(\hat{\theta}_m, \hat{\theta}_f) - Z(\frac{1}{2}, \hat{\theta}_f) - Z(\hat{\theta}_m, \frac{1}{2})]$. For the values in table 9.1, the correction factor is calculated as $d = 7.88/(2 \times 7.88 - 1.19 - 6.48) = 0.974$. With this, at $\theta = 0.05, 0.1, 0.2,$ and 0.3, one finds male lods of $Z_m = 6.52, 6.28, 5.09,$ and 3.45 and female lods of $Z_f = -0.72, 0.58, 1.36,$ and 1.31. The latter are quite different from the $Z(\frac{1}{2}, \theta_f)$ in the top row of table 9.1. As a verification of the correctness of your calculations, apart from rounding errors, the sum $Z_m(\hat{\theta}_m) + Z_f(\hat{\theta}_f)$ should be equal to the overall lod score, $Z(\hat{\theta}_m, \hat{\theta}_f)$: $6.52 + 1.36 = 7.88$.

As pointed out in section 8.3, the LINKAGE programs use a different parametrization from that described above; they work with the two parameters θ_m and R, where $R = x_f/x_m$ is the ratio of female to male map distance. Equations (8.6) and (8.7) provide conversion formulas between θ_f and R. In multipoint linkage analysis, one must be prepared to allow for a different ratio R in each interval between loci.

9.2. Recombination Fraction and Age

Several methods have been used to investigate whether the recombination fraction changes with age. These have been reviewed by Elston, Lange, and Namboodiri (1976) and by Conneally and Rivas (1980), but the question of age dependency of the recombination fraction has not received much attention since then.

A thorough analysis for the ABO-NPS1 linkage was carried out by Elston, Lange, and Namboodiri (1976), who estimated by maximum likelihood the parameters of regression lines, regressing the recombination fraction on age a, $\theta = \alpha + \beta a$, separately for males and females. In fifteen large families comprising a total of 289 individuals, achieving a maximum lod score of 15.5, they found that age was more significant than sex in its effect on the recombination fraction, but neither factor was formally significant; the empirical significance level was much larger than 0.05. The age effect observed by Elston, Lange, and Namboodiri seemed to be limited to males. Under the restriction $0 \le \theta \le \frac{1}{2}$, they estimated a decrease in θ_m of $\beta = 0.003$ per year. This means that, for example, in twenty years, θ_m for ABO versus NPS1 is expected to drop by 6 cM.

9.3. Heterogeneity between Classes of Families

A phenotype, in particular a disease, is genetically heterogeneous when it has a genetically different etiology in different individuals, for example, when in some individuals or families a disease is due to a single gene, while in other individuals the same disease phenotype is caused by an environmental agent. In the context of linkage analysis, two types of heterogeneities are distinguished, allelic and nonallelic heterogeneity; the latter is also referred to as locus heterogeneity. With allelic heterogeneity, individuals differ from each other by having different alleles at the same locus responsible for the disease; in nonallelic heterogeneity, however, the disease is caused by different loci. The two types of heterogeneity may be characterized as outlined below. Assume that some pathway of biochemical steps leads to the production of an enzyme which, when missing, results in disease. If several of the steps in the pathway are susceptible to being interrupted, the disease may show locus heterogeneity. On the other hand, if all but one of the steps are stable, but the single step accumulates different mutations, each leading to an interruption of the pathway, the disease may exhibit allelic heterogeneity. An example of the latter is cystic fibrosis: a fairly large number of different mutant alleles have been found in affected individuals, all at the same locus on chromosome 7 (Davies 1990). An example of a disease with locus heterogeneity is Charcot-Marie-Tooth disease, which can be caused by at least a locus on chromosome 1 or a locus on chromosome 17 (Vance et al. 1989) and is discussed further in section 9.4. Also, retinitis pigmentosa may be caused by various loci; even on the X chromosome there are at least two different loci for this eye disease (Ott et al. 1990a). Another well-known case of locus heterogeneity is that between elliptocytosis and the Rh blood group (Morton 1956).

A striking example for locus heterogeneity was reported by Trevor-Roper (1952) (quoted by McKusick 1990, MIM no. 203200, autosomal recessive albinism). Two albino parents had four normally pigmented children, which suggests the presence of two different genes for albinism in the parents.

When a disease is relatively rare and mutation rates are low, individuals within a family are generally homogeneous. Locus heterogeneity then leads to the situation that the recombination fraction between disease phenotype and marker will be different in different families, whereas allelic heterogeneity does not lead to such differences. Hence, only locus heterogeneity, not allelic heterogeneity, can be detected through linkage analysis. In the absence of any biochemical clues for heterogeneity, linkage analysis has more than once proved to be a powerful tool for unraveling such situations.

In this section, the rather simple case of heterogeneity between recognizable classes of families is discussed. The next section covers the more complex situation in which heterogeneity in θ is the only means of differentiating between families. The principles will be outlined below for two-point linkage analysis.

By various criteria, families may be grouped into a number c of classes, among which the recombination fraction may vary. For example, families may have been contributed to an analysis by different investigators or they may come from different countries; one may distinguish simplex from multiplex families (families with one or several affecteds); or $c = 2$ classes may be formed based on whether a disease is associated with HLA haplotypes or not (as in Hodge et al. 1983). Analogously, recombination events can be distinguished as to whether they occurred in males or females (section 9.1). Of course, each family may be considered to form its own class so that c is equal to the number of families, which is the situation originally considered by Morton (1956). To test whether the recombination fraction varies between classes, one compares the likelihood under homogeneity with that under heterogeneity. The hypothesis H_1 of linkage and homogeneity specifies $r_1 = r_2 = \ldots = r_c < \frac{1}{2}$, where r_i denotes the true value of the recombination fraction in the ith class. Under heterogeneity, H_2: $r_1 \neq r_2 \neq \ldots$, the recombination fraction is potentially different in each class. Notice that H_1 is obtained from H_2 by imposing $c - 1$ linear restrictions, for example: $r_2 = r_1, r_3 = r_1, \ldots$, $r_c = r_1$. To test H_1 against H_2, Morton (1956) introduced the likelihood ratio test (described below) into linkage analysis. To distinguish it from other homogeneity tests discussed later, Morton's test is in this book called the *M-test*.

Let $Z_i(\theta)$ denote the total lod score of the families in the ith class, and let $\hat{\theta}_i$ be the MLE of the recombination fraction in the ith class, that is, that value of θ at which $Z_i(\theta)$ is largest. Adding up the lod scores at given θ values over classes leads to the grand total $Z(\theta) = \sum_{i=1}^{c} Z_i(\theta)$, with an associated maximum at the estimate $\hat{\theta}$ of the overall recombination fraction. With this, one computes

$$X^2 = 2 \times \ln(10) \left[\sum Z_i(\hat{\theta}_i) - Z(\hat{\theta}) \right]. \tag{9.5}$$

Asymptotically, under the assumption of homogeneity (H_1), X^2 follows a chi-square distribution with $(c - 1)$ df, that is, the test is considered significant, and homogeneity is rejected, when X^2 is larger than the appropriate critical chi-square value. The test is easy to carry out by hand, or one may make use of the MTEST computer program.

As has been previously pointed out (Ott 1983) and extensively documented (Risch 1988), although under most conditions the M-test is conservative (actual significance level smaller than or equal to the one predicted on the basis of the chi-square distribution), it tends to be nonconservative for medium values of the true recombination fraction ($r \approx 0.20$) and large family sizes. For example, with $c = 10$ families of eight recombination events each, the formal critical value of χ^2_{c-1} is 16.9 for a significance level of 5 percent. However, when the true recombination fraction is equal to 0.20 in each family, the test will be significant with a probability of roughly 10 percent. Similarly, at the 5 percent significance level, with 40 families of eight members each and a true recombination fraction of 0.20 in each family, the test is significant in over 10 percent of all cases.

As an example, consider the lod scores in 29 families between polycystic kidney disease and the 3'HVR locus on chromosome 16, which are displayed in table 9.2. Inspection of the table shows that the θ estimates in each family range from 0–0.20, with one family having all negative lod scores ($\hat{\theta} = 0.50$). Application of the M-test yields a sum of the twenty-nine maximum lod scores of 64.28, and the maximum of the sum of lod scores at the same θ values over families is equal to 56.96. With this, application of equation (9.5) results in $X^2 = 33.71$ with 28 df, which approximately corresponds to a p-value of 0.21. This result suggests that no difference in the true recombination fractions in the twenty-nine fami-

Table 9.2. Two-Point Lod Scores of Polycystic Kidney Disease (PKD1) versus the Marker 3'HVR and Conditional Probability w of Being of the Linked Type

Family	0	0.001	0.05	0.10	0.20	0.30	0.40	w_i
				Recombination Fraction				
1	−2.15	−1.46	0.04	0.23	*0.28*	0.19	0.07	0.963
2	*5.19*	5.19	4.76	4.30	3.31	2.19	0.93	1.000
3	−∞	0.25	1.69	*1.71*	1.41	0.90	0.30	0.999
4	*2.92*	2.91	2.66	2.39	1.81	1.18	0.49	0.999
5	*1.09*	1.09	0.99	0.88	0.64	0.38	0.12	0.995
6	*2.24*	2.24	2.03	1.81	1.32	0.78	0.24	0.999
7	−∞	−1.13	0.37	*0.46*	0.37	0.20	0.05	0.982
8	*0.90*	0.90	0.81	0.72	0.52	0.30	0.09	0.993
9	*0.26*	0.26	0.24	0.22	0.15	0.08	0.02	0.976
10	*1.28*	1.28	1.17	1.04	0.73	0.40	0.10	0.997
11	*2.61*	2.61	2.33	2.06	1.50	0.90	0.30	0.999
12	−∞	0.02	2.51	*2.78*	2.27	1.54	0.72	0.999
13	*0.60*	0.60	0.53	0.46	0.32	0.17	0.05	0.987
14	*1.77*	1.77	1.59	1.41	1.01	0.59	0.21	0.998
15	−∞	7.26	*8.04*	7.37	5.62	3.63	1.51	1.000
16	−∞	0.53	2.04	*2.11*	1.84	1.31	0.62	0.999
17	*2.93*	2.92	2.66	2.38	1.77	1.09	0.38	0.999
18	−∞	0.50	1.94	*1.97*	1.67	1.17	0.53	0.999
19	*0.60*	0.60	0.53	0.46	0.32	0.17	0.05	0.987
20	*2.71*	2.70	2.44	2.17	1.61	1.02	0.42	0.999
21	−∞	−0.71	0.82	*0.95*	0.88	0.66	0.36	0.993
22	−∞	0.06	2.99	*3.08*	2.60	1.76	0.76	1.000
23	−∞	−0.41	1.10	*1.20*	1.05	0.74	0.45[a]	0.996
24	*3.50*	3.49	3.21	2.92	2.27	1.55	0.77	1.000
25	−∞	1.76	4.59	*4.59*	3.87	2.72	1.25	1.000
26	−∞	−2.14	1.09	1.47	*1.52*	1.38	0.56	0.996
27	−∞	0.23	3.23	*3.38*	2.96	2.11	0.99	1.000
28	*3.61*	3.16	3.32	3.02	2.38	1.67	0.89	1.000
29	−∞	−9.29	−2.76	−1.68	−0.72	−0.28	−0.06	0.040
Sum	−∞	27.19	*56.96*	55.86	45.28	30.50	13.17	

Sources: Families 1–28 from Reeders et al. 1987; family 29 from Romeo et al. 1988.
[a] Value interpolated.

lies exists. Further analysis of these families is presented in the next section.

In practice, one often investigates several linked marker loci simultaneously and calculates multipoint lod scores or location scores (section 6.1) for various positions of a disease locus along a map of marker loci. The M-test may then be carried out as before, using equation (9.5), where the constant, ln(10), must be dropped if natural logarithms instead of logarithms to the base 10 are used. Notice, however, that multipoint lod scores are generally multimodal, and it is unclear whether the same asymptotic approximations hold as in the two-point case. With multipoint lod scores, therefore, asymptotic empirical p-values have to be taken to be very approximate, or they should not be used at all. Instead one may simply report the observed likelihood ratio R between the two hypotheses H_1 and H_2, which may be obtained from equation (9.5) as

$$R = \exp(\tfrac{1}{2}X^2). \tag{9.6}$$

Of course, R may have to be interpreted differently depending on the number of classes (degrees of freedom) investigated, for it is easier to obtain a large likelihood ratio with an increased number c of classes. For example, $X^2 = 33.71$ obtained from the twenty-nine families in table 9.2 translates into a likelihood ratio of approximately $R = 2.09 \times 10^7$, which appears impressive. Per degree of freedom, however, one obtains $X^2/\text{df} = 33.71/28 = 1.204$, corresponding to a likelihood ratio of only $\exp(1.204/2) = 1.8$. This result can also be obtained as the geometric mean per degree of freedom of $R = 2.09 \times 10^7$: $(2.09 \times 10^7)^{1/28} = 1.8$.

With a single degree of freedom, various critical levels R_0 have been used as thresholds for determining "significance" or "meaningful difference." Table 9.3 lists the R_0 values commonly used along with the corresponding differences $\Delta\ln(L)$ and $\Delta\log_{10}(L)$, where L stands for likelihood. Parameter values with an associated $\ln(L)$ larger than $\ln(L_{\text{max}}) - \Delta\ln(L)$ then belong to the "$\Delta\ln(L)$"-unit support interval. Edwards (1984) recommended constructing two-unit support intervals ($\Delta\ln(L) = 2$, see section 3.6). In human genetics, the narrowest support interval generally used is that corresponding to a critical level of $R_0 = 10$, but often more stringent criteria may have to be applied.

Tests for heterogeneity are usually carried out at the 5 percent or 1 percent level of significance. In tests for linkage, however, one requires more stringent criteria, that is, a maximum lod score of at least 3, corresponding to a p-value of 0.001 or less (equation [4.10]). Assume now that, for a particular set of families, the maximum of the total lod score

Table 9.3. Likelihood Ratios R_0 and Corresponding Differences $\Delta\ln$(likelihood) and $\Delta\log_{10}$(likelihood)

R_0	$\Delta\ln L$	$\Delta\log L$
10	2.3	1.0
20	3.0	1.3
50	3.9	1.7
100	4.6	2.0
1000	6.9	3.0

(under homogeneity) stays below 3 yet a test of homogeneity results in a p-value of 0.02. Declaring the heterogeneity significant would amount to saying that in some of the families the recombination fraction is significantly smaller than 0.5. This is the same as accepting a significant linkage for some families, which contradicts the conclusion of no significant linkage based on a maximum lod score of less than 3. The solution to this dilemma is that, in the absence of a proven linkage, the test for heterogeneity should only be declared significant when the empirical p-value is no larger than 0.001 or when the likelihood ratio (perhaps on a per df basis) is at least 1000:1.

The M-test requires the estimation of a separate parameter, θ_i, in each of the c families (or classes). A more powerful (bayesian) approach was proposed by Risch (1988) in the form of the so-called *B-test*. For this test, the θ values in the different families are assumed to follow a beta distribution with two parameters. These two parameters are then estimated from the posterior distribution of θ. The test statistic is constructed on the basis of the difference of the maximum log likelihoods under H_1 and H_2 and is associated with 1 df (a computer program to carry out the B-test is available from Dr. Risch). The B-test is generally conservative and often more powerful than the M-test (Risch 1988).

An example of two distinct disease forms are Usher's syndrome types I and II, where type I is characterized by a profound hearing loss and absence of vestibular functions, and type II has a milder hearing loss and normal vestibular function. The two forms are genetically heterogeneous, since Usher's syndrome type II is linked with markers on chromosome 1 but type I is not (Kimberling et al. 1990). In this case, clinical heterogeneity runs parallel to genetic heterogeneity. As will be seen below, however, in other diseases this is not necessarily the case.

9.4. Heterogeneity due to a Mixture of Families

In the homogeneity tests considered thus far, the alternative to the hypothesis of homogeneity is that the recombination fraction is potentially different in each family (or family class). In many situations, however, a more plausible alternative is the presence of two types of families, those with linkage ($\theta_1 < \frac{1}{2}$) and those without ($\theta_2 = \frac{1}{2}$) (Smith 1961), where the two family types are mixed such that an unequivocal assignment of a given family to one or the other type is impossible. A common situation leading to this kind of heterogeneity is that in some families a disease is caused by a gene located in the vicinity of a marker locus, while in other families the same disease phenotype is due to a disease gene located elsewhere, or the disease is not due to a single gene. In this situation, linkage will exist only in the first type of family and not in the others.

Smith (1963) considered still other cases, for example, three family types, one with recombination fraction $\theta_1 < \frac{1}{2}$, another with θ_2 ($\theta_1 < \theta_2 < \frac{1}{2}$), and a third with $\theta_3 = \frac{1}{2}$, and treated the hypotheses of homogeneity and heterogeneity in a bayesian framework. In this book, the various hypotheses are evaluated by maximum likelihood rather than by bayesian methods (Ott 1983). A simple introduction to the test procedures will be given first, followed by some theoretical explanations towards the end of this section.

In the presence of a mixture of two types of families, it may be tempting to separate the families into two groups, corresponding to the two family types, and to analyze the two groups under a known classification scheme as in section 9.3. This would be fallacious, however, since an investigator uses his judgment to form the groups from the mixture of families, thereby adding extra information not contained in the data. This additional information may well inflate the evidence for the presence of two family types. Instead of separating families, it is better to analyze the families as a whole under a model allowing for a mixture. In the simplest such model, two family types exist, with α denoting the proportion of type 1 families and $1 - \alpha$ the proportion of type 2 families. The recombination fraction in the type 1 families is equal to θ_1 and that in the type 2 families is $\theta_2 = \frac{1}{2}$. The bivariate likelihood of the ith family is then given by (Smith 1961)

$$L_i(\alpha, \theta_1) = \alpha L_i(\theta_1) + (1 - \alpha)L_i(\frac{1}{2}), \tag{9.7}$$

where $L_i(\theta_1)$ is the likelihood, evaluated at $\theta = \theta_1$. Without loss of generality, one may divide (9.7) by $L_i(\frac{1}{2})$ and thereby adjust the bivariate likelihood to be equal to 1 at $\theta = \frac{1}{2}$. Thus, one obtains

$$L_i^*(\alpha, \theta_1) = \alpha L_i^*(\theta_1) + (1 - \alpha), \tag{9.8}$$

where $L_i^*(\theta_1)$ is the antilog of the usual lod score in the ith family. The overall adjusted log likelihood is then given by

$$\log L(\alpha, \theta_1) = \sum_i \log [L_i^*(\alpha, \theta_1)], \tag{9.9}$$

which is a function of the two parameters, α and θ_1. Graphically, the log likelihood (9.9) may be represented as the height above a plane with co-ordinates α and θ_1. The hypothesis of heterogeneity is then formulated as H_2: $\alpha < 1$, $\theta_1 < \frac{1}{2}$, and homogeneity is obtained from H_2 by a single

Table 9.4. Log$_e$ Likelihoods for the Twenty-nine Families in Table 9.2

				Recombination Fraction, θ				
α	0	0.001	0.05	0.10	0.20	0.30	0.40	0.50
1.00	$-\infty$	62.61	*131.16*	128.62	104.26	70.23	30.33	0
0.99	10.09	80.49	132.82	128.76	104.06	70.02	30.17	0
0.98	19.42	81.82	133.18	128.78	103.86	69.81	30.02	0
0.97	24.86	82.66	133.30	128.74	103.65	69.60	29.87	0
0.96	28.70	83.28	*133.32*	128.66	103.44	69.38	29.71	0
0.95	31.65	83.76	133.28	128.55	103.22	69.17	29.56	0
0.94	34.04	84.15	133.19	128.42	103.00	68.95	29.40	0
0.92	37.75	84.72	132.95	128.10	102.55	68.51	29.08	0
0.90	40.56	85.13	132.62	127.73	102.09	68.05	28.76	0
0.80	48.64	85.77	130.42	125.42	99.56	65.65	27.06	0
0.70	52.51	85.21	127.59	122.53	96.64	62.96	25.21	0
0.50	55.24	81.91	120.08	114.94	89.29	56.39	20.92	0
0.30	53.48	75.39	108.71	103.50	78.47	47.12	15.38	0
0.10	44.25	60.93	85.89	80.66	57.53	30.41	7.18	0
0.01	24.20	35.84	48.15	43.48	26.47	9.96	0.99	0

restriction, H_1: $\alpha = 1$, that is, the families share a common recombination fraction.

The evaluation of (9.9) for given lod scores is straightforward but somewhat time consuming. The HOMOG computer program may conveniently be used to evaluate (9.9) for various values of α and θ_1. Under H_2, estimates of α and θ_1 are obtained as that pair of points for which (9.9) is a maximum. Under H_1, the restricted estimate, $\hat{\theta}_r$, is obtained assuming homogeneity. For example, for the twenty-nine families in table 9.2 with polycystic kidney disease (PKD1) versus the 3'HVR locus on chromosome 16 (Reeders et al. 1987; Romeo et al. 1988), the HOMOG program evaluates the ln likelihoods (9.9) as given in table 9.4. The unrestricted estimates are $\hat{\alpha} = 0.96$ and $\hat{\theta}_1 = 0.05$. Under homogeneity ($\alpha = 1$), one obtains $\hat{\theta}_r = 0.05$, which happens to be equal to $\hat{\theta}_1$; generally, $\hat{\alpha}$ and $\hat{\theta}_1$ are positively correlated so that $\hat{\theta}_r > \hat{\theta}_1$. For more accurate estimates, one may apply quadratic interpolation using the VARCO3 and VARCO6 programs. The test of the hypothesis of homogeneity is carried out by calculating

$$X^2 = 2[\log_e L(\hat{\alpha}, \hat{\theta}_1) - \log_e L(1, \hat{\theta}_r)], \qquad (9.10)$$

which asymptotically has a chi-square distribution with 1 df with probability ½ and is equal to 0 with probability ½ (one-sided test). From table 9.4, one evaluates $X^2 = 2 \times (133.32 - 131.16) = 4.32$. The corresponding p-value is approximately equal to $p = 0.019$ (half of the 2p

value obtained from the CHIPROB program). Heterogeneity of θ among the PKD1 families is thus significant at the 5 percent level but not at the 1 percent level. Declaring the test result significant on the basis of the usual significance levels is warranted because the test for linkage is highly significant (lod score exceeds 3, see section 9.3). Heterogeneity of PKD1 has been confirmed by other investigators (e.g., Kimberling et al. 1988). Notice that the M-test carried out in the previous section was not significant.

The homogeneity test based on (9.10) has been termed the A-test (Hodge et al. 1983; Ott 1983), A standing for *Admixture*. It is conservative and, under the hypothesis of a mixture of linked and unlinked families, more powerful than the M-test (Risch 1988). For two-point data, the p-value obtained from the asymptotic chi-square distribution seems to be quite accurate (Ott 1989b). In multipoint situations, however, when in some families a disease is linked to a map of markers and in other families it is unlinked to the markers, it is unknown whether these asymptotic properties still hold (see discussion of this point in the previous section). In such multipoint cases, the parameter θ_1 is usually replaced by x_1, denoting the map position of the disease locus. Lod scores with respect to θ_1 are then replaced by multipoint lod scores relative to x_1 values.

Given good estimates of α and θ_1, one may compute the estimated conditional probability, given the observations, that the ith family belongs to the linked type,

$$w_i(\hat{\alpha},\ \hat{\theta}_1)\ =\ \frac{\hat{\alpha}L_i^*(\hat{\theta}_1)}{\hat{\alpha}L_i^*(\hat{\theta}_1)\ +\ 1\ -\ \hat{\alpha}},\tag{9.11}$$

which for $\hat{\alpha} = 0.96$ and $\hat{\theta}_1 = 0.05$ is given in the last column of table 9.2. For known parameter values, $w_i > \frac{1}{2}$ can be shown to represent an optimal classification rule to identify families of the linked type (Goldstein and Dillon 1978). However, with estimates for α and θ_1, in small samples, the classification rule

$$w_i(\hat{\alpha},\ \hat{\theta}_1)\ >\ \hat{\alpha}\tag{9.12}$$

is generally more reliable (Ott 1983). Inequality (9.12) is equivalent to $Z_i(\hat{\theta}_1) > 0$, where Z_i is the lod score of the ith family evaluated at the estimate for θ_1 obtained from all families together. Inequality (9.12) is intuitively appealing: when a family provides no information on linkage, then $w_i = \alpha$; evidence for linkage (i.e., for belonging to the linked family type) raises w_i above α. All but one family in table 9.2 exhibit very high conditional probabilities of linkage. The evidence for heterogeneity apparently stems from family 29, whose lod scores are equivalent to approximately four recombinants in eight phase-known meioses (as obtained from the EQUIV program). To be confident of heterogeneity, it is thus important to verify the recombination events in that family.

The number of families required to detect heterogeneity has been investigated for various situations (Cavalli-Sforza and King 1986; Ott 1986b). In particular, consider the problem that several families with linkage have been observed, and one is interested in knowing how many families are required to detect a small proportion of unlinked families. For the case of no recombination ($\theta = 0$) in linked families and n phase-known families with m meioses each, a simple solution is obtained, as shown below. Owing to tight linkage in linked families, any recombination is, by assumption, evidence for the presence of unlinked families. Thus, the question is reduced to asking how many families are required to find, with probability (power) P, at least one family with one or more recombinations? The probability that in a family with m offspring none of them is a recombinant is given by $\alpha + (1 - \alpha)(\frac{1}{2})^m$. Therefore, the probability that in n families at least one will have one or more recombinants is given by $P = 1 - [\alpha + (1 - \alpha)(\frac{1}{2})^m]^n$, which is the probability to detect heterogeneity and is easily solved for n (Ott 1986b). For example, with a power of 90 percent and families of size $m = 4$, forty-eight families are required to detect the presence of a proportion of 5 percent families with $\theta = \frac{1}{2}$. In the analysis of common diseases, allowing for incomplete penetrance makes the required numbers of families substantially higher (Clerget-Darpoux, Babron, and Bonaïti-Pellié 1987).

To establish linkage on the basis of a single family, the maximum lod score Z_{max} must exceed the critical limit of 3. If, in a number n of families, all have shown good evidence for linkage between a disease and a marker (no apparent heterogeneity), a smaller critical value for Z_{max} should be sufficient to decide whether a new family is also of the linked type. A heuristic argument may be given as follows (Ott 1986c): Let a new family be classified as linked when the predicted conditional probability of linkage w_i (9.11) is at least 0.95. Based on the current estimate of the proportion of linked families, $\hat{\alpha} = 1$, the predicted probability of linkage is also equal to 1. Therefore, judgment is based on the lower endpoint of the confidence interval for α, which will also represent the lower endpoint of the confidence interval for w_i. If at least $n = 7$ clearly linked families have been investigated, the 95 percent confidence interval for α extends from 1 down to $(0.05)^{1/n} = 0.65$ (section 3.6). What is the minimum lod score, at the overall $\hat{\theta}$, for a new family so that $w_i \geq 0.95$? Solving equation (9.11) yields $L_i^* = w(1 - \alpha)/[(1 - w)\alpha]$ for the likelihood ratio, which, with $w_i = 0.95$ and $\alpha = 0.65$, translates into a minimum lod score of $Z = 1$. Thus, a lod score of 1 at the θ estimate for all linked families together is sufficient for a new family to be classified as linked, provided that a sufficient number of families (at least seven) have already given unequivocal evidence for linkage homogeneity.

In some applications, the model for heterogeneity considered above is not realistic. Instead, a disease may be caused by either of two disease loci, where the two loci are within measurable distance of each other on the same chromosome. With respect to a particular marker locus, one will then have to estimate not one, but two recombination fractions, θ_1 and θ_2, where θ_1 refers to the disease locus segregating in type 1 families (occurring in the sample with proportion α), and θ_2 refers to the disease locus in type 2 families (proportion $1 - \alpha$). In analogy to equation (9.7), the likelihood for the ith family is then given by

$$L_i(\alpha, \theta_1, \theta_2) = \alpha L_i(\theta_1) + (1 - \alpha)L_i(\theta_2). \qquad (9.13)$$

Under heterogeneity, the three parameters α, θ_1, and θ_2 are estimated by maximum likelihood in a manner analogous to that described above. Under homogeneity, the restriction $\alpha = 1$ implies $\theta_1 = \theta_2$ so that the dimensionality of the parameter space drops from 3 to 1. This is a situation commonly encountered in the analysis of mixtures of distributions and is known to lead to unusual distributions of the test statistics. For the given situation of a mixture of two linked disease loci, the asymptotic null distribution of the test statistic,

$$X^2 = 2[\log_e L(\hat{\alpha}, \hat{\theta}_1, \hat{\theta}_2) - \log_e L(1, \hat{\theta}_r)], \qquad (9.14)$$

has not been investigated. It is sometimes said that a chi-square distribution with 2 df should be conservative, but investigations corroborating this speculation have not yet been done. It is thus best simply to quote the likelihood ratio R (9.6) obtained from X^2 (9.14) and declare a result significant when R exceeds a threshold R_0. Maximizing the likelihood over the different parameters is tedious but may conveniently be carried out using the HOMOG2 program. An example of an analysis along these lines was the investigation of multiple loci for retinitis pigmentosa on the X chromosome (Ott et al. 1990a).

The basic model of heterogeneity may be extended in still other ways, but only one model of particular importance in practice will be pursued here further. It refers to the situation where a disease (or any other phenotype) is caused in some families by one locus and in other families by another locus, with the two disease-causing loci being located on different chromosomes, each linked with a marker locus on the respective chromosome. An example is osteogenesis imperfecta, which may be due to a disease gene on chromosome 7 (OI4) or 17 (Sykes et al. 1990). This situation may in principle be handled by the HOMOG2 program, but the specialized approach implemented in the HOMOG3R program is preferable. As the disease gene may be linked to one of two marker loci, it may be sufficient to consider a corresponding mixture of two family types. However, it is prudent also to allow for a third family type, in which the disease is due to a hypothetical third gene unlinked to either of the two marker loci. Hence, three family types are distinguished with the respective sample proportions of α_1, α_2, and $\alpha_3 = 1 - \alpha_1 - \alpha_2$. The recombination fraction between disease locus 1 and the marker linked with it is θ_1, and that between disease locus 2 and its linked marker is θ_2.

With these assumptions, in analogy to (9.7) the likelihood for the ith family is derived as outlined below. For clarity, this derivation is given here in detail; the less mathematically inclined reader may proceed directly to equation (9.16). Let y, x_1, and x_2 denote the respective phenotypes for the disease, marker 1 and marker 2. For any family, the joint likelihood for the three phenotypes is obtained by conditioning on each of the three family types:

$$\begin{aligned}
P(y, x_1, x_2; \alpha_1, \alpha_2, \theta_1, \theta_2) &= \alpha_1 P(y, x_1; \theta_1)P(x_2)\\
&+ \alpha_2 P(y, x_2; \theta_2)P(x_1) \qquad (9.15)\\
&+ \alpha_3 P(y)P(x_1)P(x_2).
\end{aligned}$$

Now, define the likelihood with respect to θ_1, adjusted to be equal to 1 at $\theta_1 = \frac{1}{2}$, as $L(\theta_1) = P(y, x_1; \theta_1)/P(y, x_1; \frac{1}{2}) = P(y, x_1; \theta_1)/[P(y)P(x_1)]$. Hence, we can write $P(y, x_1; \theta_1) = L(\theta_1)P(y)P(x_1)$ and, analogously, $P(y, x_2; \theta_2) = L(\theta_2)P(y)P(x_2)$. With this, the right side of equation (9.15) can be rewritten as $\alpha_1 L(\theta_1)P(y)P(x_1)P(x_2) + \alpha_2 L(\theta_2)P(y)P(x_2)P(x_1) + \alpha_3 P(y)P(x_1)P(x_2)$. Dividing through by the common terms shows that the likelihood is proportional to

$$L(\alpha_1, \alpha_2, \theta_1, \theta_2) = \alpha_1 L(\theta_1) + \alpha_2 L(\theta_2) + 1 - \alpha_1 - \alpha_2. \qquad (9.16)$$

Expression (9.16) refers to a single family and is analogous to (9.7). The overall log likelihood is then proportional to the sum of the logarithm of (9.16) over all families. Maximum likelihood estimates of the four parameters may be obtained by an exhaustive search of the parameter space, by varying each parameter in a number of steps (this is how the HOMOG3R program works).

For the example of osteogenesis imperfecta referred to above, thirty-five of the thirty-eight families reported by Sykes et al. (1990) allow the calculating of lod scores with respect to θ_1 and θ_2, where θ_1 refers to

Table 9.5. Log$_e$ Likelihoods, ln$L$ − 90, for Thirty-five Families from Sykes et al. (1990) with Respect to a Mixture of Three Family Types

α_1	α_2										
	.20	.30	.35	.40	.45	.50	.55	.60	.65	.70	.80
.80	21.1										
.70	19.2	**25.0**									
.65	18.1	**23.8**	**26.0**								
.60	16.9	22.6	**24.8**	**26.6**							
.55	15.7	21.3	**23.4**	**25.3**	**26.9**						
.50	14.3	19.8	22.0	**23.8**	**25.4**	**26.9**					
.45	12.7	18.2	20.3	22.2	**23.8**	**25.2**	**26.5**				
.40	11.0	16.4	18.5	20.4	22.0	**23.4**	**24.7**	**25.8**			
.35	9.1	14.4	16.5	18.3	19.9	21.3	22.6	**23.7**	**24.8**		
.30	6.9	12.2	14.2	16.0	17.6	19.0	20.2	21.3	22.3	**23.2**	
.20	1.2	6.4	8.4	10.1	11.6	12.9	14.1	15.2	16.1	17.0	18.4

linkage between osteogenesis imperfecta and COL1A1 on chromosome 17, and θ_2 refers to OI4 versus COL1A2 on chromosome 7. With α and θ values incremented between 0 and 1 (or ½) in steps of 0.05 each, maximum likelihood estimates are obtained under various hypotheses. Under heterogeneity, parameter estimates are $\hat{\alpha}_1 = 0.55$, $\hat{\alpha}_2 = 0.45$ (hence, $\hat{\alpha}_3 = 0$), $\hat{\theta}_1 = 0$, and $\hat{\theta}_2 = 0$.

If one is interested only in the α values, for each pair (α_1, α_2), one may simply look at the likelihood maximized over θ_1 and θ_2 with α_1 and α_2 kept fixed. The resulting ln likelihoods for α_1 and α_2 are displayed in table 9.5. A 3.9-unit support interval (likelihood ratio of 50:1) includes all parameter values with ln(L) equal to or larger than 26.9 − 3.9 = 23.0; the corresponding log likelihoods in table 9.5 are boldfaced. As one can see, $\hat{\alpha}_1$ and $\hat{\alpha}_2$ are strongly negatively correlated (the support interval is deliberately chosen stringently so that it becomes rather wide and is better visible in the table). Corresponding to the support interval chosen, the support limits for α_1 as well as α_2 extend from 0.30 through 0.70 (for support intervals of α_3, see problem 9.1).

If one is convinced that the genetic markers are candidate loci, one may compute likelihoods only at $\theta_1 = \theta_2 = 0$. In this case, since the recombination fraction estimates turned out to be equal to zero, restricting the parameter space to $\theta_1 = \theta_2 = 0$ furnishes the same estimates for α_1 and α_2 as above, where estimation was carried out over the full parameter space including $0 \leq (\theta_1, \theta_2) \leq$ ½. There is, however, in this case one difference between the two approaches: if the parameter space is restricted to $\theta_1 = \theta_2 = 0$, the evidence for heterogeneity is inflated, which may be seen from table 9.6, which presents results obtained by the HOMOG3R

Table 9.6. Parameter Estimates and Evidence for Heterogeneity in Mixture of Osteogenesis Imperfecta Families

Hypothesis	Estimates for Parameters					$\ln L$	$\Delta \ln L$
	α_1	α_2	α_3	θ_1	θ_2		
Estimating θ							
Heter.	0.55	0.45	0	0	0	116.9	76.5
Homog.	1	0	0	0.15	½	27.9	
Homog.	0	1	0	½	0.15	40.4	
Homog.	0	0	1	½	½	0	
Setting $\theta = 0$							
Heter.	0.55	0.45	0	0	0	116.9	116.9
Homog.	1	0	0	0	½	$-\infty$	
Homog.	0	1	0	½	0	$-\infty$	
Homog.	0	0	1	½	½	0	

program. Allowing θ_1 and θ_2 to vary between 0 and ½, one will find at least some evidence for homogeneity, although it is comparatively small. The difference in log likelihood between heterogeneity and that hypothesis of homogeneity with the highest likelihood turns out to be equal to $\Delta \ln L = 76.5$. With θ_1 and θ_2 fixed at 0, the corresponding evidence for heterogeneity is $\Delta \ln L = 116.9$, which is much higher than 76.5. Of course, in both cases the conclusion of strong evidence for heterogeneity is the same, but table 9.6 does show that it is generally prudent to allow θ_1 and θ_2 to vary.

Before turning to some theoretical aspects of genetic heterogeneity, another well-known example is mentioned here. For Charcot-Marie-Tooth disease (CMT1), a form of hereditary motor and sensory neuropathy, linkage to the Duffy (FY) blood group locus had been found by Bird, Ott, and Giblett (1982) and confirmed by Guiloff et al. (1982) and Stebbins and Conneally (1982). Soon thereafter, however, families with clear absence of linkage were found, thus demonstrating genetic heterogeneity (Bird et al. 1983; Dyck et al. 1983). Over the years, a rather large number of families were investigated and those with linkage to FY appeared to be quite rare, so that questions were raised whether the FY linkage was real or an artifact of the statistical test for heterogeneity (Middleton-Price et al. 1989). Heterogeneity now seems clearly established after linkage to chromosome 17 markers has been detected (Vance et al. 1989), and additional families linked to chromosome 1 have turned up (Defesche et al. 1990; Chance et al. 1990). In the vast majority of CMT1 families, the disease seems to be due to a defect in the chromosome 17 locus.

Thus far, heterogeneity as a mixture of two or more disease loci was considered between families but was assumed to be excluded within families. For more common diseases, however, so-called bilineal pedigrees are observed in which a disease enters a family through more than one individual. Such cases cannot be handled by the methods outlined above. They require that the likelihood be calculated under a model of heterogeneity for individuals in the same family. Such approaches will be discussed in section 11.3.

For mathematically inclined readers, a few theoretical aspects of mixtures of families will now be discussed in the remainder of this section. As was mentioned above, in a mixture of linked and unlinked families the estimates of α and θ are often correlated. For a known distribution of the estimates, this correlation can be calculated. For example, consider n families with m phase-known meioses each. A family is of the linked type with probability α and of the unlinked type with probability $1 - \alpha$. Hence, in any family, the probability of occurrence of k recombinants is given by

$$P(k; \alpha, r) = \alpha P(k; r) + (1 - \alpha)P(k; \frac{1}{2}), \qquad (9.17)$$

where $P(k; r)$ is the binomial probability, $\binom{m}{k}r^k(1 - r)^{m-k}$, and r is the true recombination rate. As an example, $P(k = 2; \alpha, r) = 3[\alpha r^2(1 - r) + \frac{1}{8}(1 - \alpha)]$. Using the methods of section 5.3, it is then easy to compute the asymptotic variance-covariance matrix (5.8). For $n = 10$ phase-known families of size $m = 3$ each and given parameter values α and r, table 9.7 shows some resulting values of the correlation $\rho(\hat{\alpha}, \hat{\theta})$ and the standard error $\sigma(\hat{\theta})$. The correlation is small for $\alpha = 1$ and small recombination rates, but it increases rapidly with decreasing α and increasing r. With a decreasing α, the standard error of $\hat{\theta}$ increases, partly owing to the smaller number of families present with linkage.

In most applications, $\hat{\alpha}$ and $\hat{\theta}$ have to be found numerically. The sub-

Table 9.7. Asymptotic Correlation ρ between $\hat{\alpha}$ and $\hat{\theta}$ and Standard Error $\sigma(\hat{\theta})$ for $n = 10$ Families of Size $m = 3$ Each

	$r = 0.01$[a]		$r = 0.05$		$r = 0.10$		$r = 0.30$	
α	ρ	σ	ρ	σ	ρ	σ	ρ	σ
1.0	.07	.018	.03	.042	.51	.064	.91	.204
.9	.58	.037	.53	.060	.63	.087	.91	.235
.8	.65	.053	.60	.075	.66	.104	.92	.271
.5	.75	.126	.73	.151	.76	.187	.93	.449
.1	.88	.829	.88	.916	.89	1.052	.94	2.244

Note: r = true recombination rate.

lytic solution nicely shows the structure of such
usible that the test for heterogeneity should in-
hough values of $\alpha > 1$ are inadmissible. Con-
es with $m = 2$ offspring each. In each family,
ay occur with the respective trinomial proba-
$p_0 - p_1$. The maximum likelihood estimates
en by $\hat{p}_i = k_i/n$, where k_i denotes the number
nt offspring, $k_0 + k_1 + k_2 = n$. Since $p_0 +$
unknown probabilities that are specified as

$$1 - \alpha), \tag{9.18}$$

$\upsilon.\prime$ a... $= 0.1$ lead to $p_1 = 0.276$, $p_2 = 0.082$, and
0.642. Since the number of parameters to be estimated is equal to
the number of degrees of freedom (independent multinomial probabili-
ties), the MLEs of α and r can be obtained from $\hat{p}_1$ and $\hat{p}_2$ simply by
solving equations (9.18) (Weir 1990, 53). Hence, one obtains

$$\hat{\theta} = \tfrac{1}{2}(\hat{p}_1 - 2\hat{p}_2)/(\hat{p}_0 - \hat{p}_2), \tag{9.19}$$
$$\hat{\alpha} = (\hat{p}_0 - \hat{p}_2)^2/(\hat{p}_0 - \hat{p}_1 + \hat{p}_2);$$

for $\hat{\theta} = \tfrac{1}{2}$, define $\hat{\alpha} = 0$ and vice versa.

Equations (9.19) demonstrate that many estimates of p_i result in val-
ues of $\hat{\alpha}$ and $\hat{\theta}$ outside their range of definition. For example, $\hat{p}_0 = 0.55$,
$\hat{p}_1 = 0.40$, and $\hat{p}_2 = 0.05$ lead to $\hat{\alpha} = 1.25$ and $\hat{\theta} = 0.30$. Restricting $\hat{\alpha}$
to the range between 0 and 1 clearly introduces a bias, which, however,
tends to vanish with increasing numbers of observations, that is, the estimates will be asymptotically unbiased (and consistent).

9.5. Hierarchical and Mixed Models of Heterogeneity

Often, families are grouped in hierarchical classifications. For example, several investigators may each have contributed some families.
With fixed classifications, the overall X^2 (9.5) can then easily be parti-
tioned into components corresponding to the different levels of hierarchy
(see, e.g., Morton 1956). In a similar manner, Rao et al. (1978) analyzed
heterogeneity between studies within each sex and heterogeneity between
sexes.

In many cases, male and female recombination fractions are different.
Taking them to be equal when in fact they are not may introduce an apparent heterogeneity when in some families many more male than female

parents are informative for linkage. The appropriate remedy is either to work with the known female-to-male map distance ratio or to allow for heterogeneity both between families and between sexes. The latter possibility has been implemented in the HOMOG1a and HOMOG1b programs, which extend the model of a mixture of linked and unlinked families to allow for a sex difference in each of the family types.

A situation with important practical applications shall be demonstrated with an example. Childhood-onset spinal muscular atrophy (SMA) is recessively inherited and may be divided into two classes, an acute form (Werdnig-Hoffmann disease, SMA type I) with onset in infancy and death within the first years of life and chronic forms (e.g., Kugelberg-Welander disease) with onset between six months and seventeen years of age. Chronic SMA shows clear linkage to chromosome 5 markers (Brzustowicz et al. 1990; Melki et al. 1990). Acute SMA seems linked to about the same region on chromosome 5, although the latter linkage is not as well supported (Gilliam et al. 1990). Each of the two forms seems to be heterogeneous in the sense that each may contain unlinked families. For a test of homogeneity between the two forms, one would like to allow for the fact that the forms themselves may be heterogeneous; assuming homogeneity within each form and carrying out the M-test between them can lead to strongly biased results, for example, when the proportion of unlinked families in the two forms is very different. A solution to this problem is included in Gilliam et al. (1990) and proceeds as outlined below.

To evaluate the log likelihood (adjusted by a constant) under heterogeneity, one computes the log likelihood in each form of SMA independently, allowing for a mixture of linked and unlinked families in each form. This may be done by applying the HOMOG program to each form. Thus, the likelihood is maximized over the parameters x_1, x_2, α_1, and α_2, where x_i is the map position and α_i is the proportion of linked families in each form, with $i = 1$ for the chronic and $i = 2$ for the acute form. The resulting $\log_{10}$ likelihoods turn out to be 8.94 and 2.47 for chronic and acute families, respectively, leading to a total $\log_{10}$ likelihood under heterogeneity of 11.41. For homogeneity of map position (but possible heterogeneity within each form), one introduces the single constraint that the map locations of the two forms should be at the same position, $x = x_1 = x_2$. At each value of x, for each form, the likelihood is maximized over the other parameter (α_1 or α_2, depending on the family form analyzed) (the current version of the HOMOG program provides such maximized likelihoods as intermediate results). Thus, the likelihood is maximized over the parameters x, α_1, and α_2. The sum of the two log likelihoods,

maximized separately in each form, constitutes the log likelihood at the
map posit.____ T̄
resents the max..
and turns out to be equ
difference, $11.41 - 11.2$,
geneity. There is thus very little evidence for heterogeneity in map position between the two forms of SMA.

9.6. Covariates in the Test for Admixture

The mixture of linked and unlinked families represents a difficult
problem. Statistically, as was shown in the previous section, estimates of
α and θ may be strongly correlated so that good quasi-independent estimates of α and θ can be obtained only with a high proportion of linked
families and tight linkage in these families. Another problem is that germinal mosaicism or similar effects, when not recognized as such, may
mimic heterogeneity. A case in point is an apparent heterogeneity in families with agammaglobulinemia (Ott et al. 1986), which was recognized as
an instance of aberrant segregation upon examination with molecular genetics techniques (Hendriks et al. 1989). Another example was reported
by Arveiler et al. (1990). In the face of these problems, it would be beneficial to know biologic variables (covariates), which could help in assigning families to one or the other type. A particular such variable is the age
at disease onset; the discussion below is restricted to this important case.

As outlined in section 7.4, age at disease onset may be regarded as
the disease phenotype (or as part of it). If the observed age at onset is a,
the conditional likelihood given some genotype is then equal to $f(a)$, the
density of the age-of-onset curve. Consider now the investigation of familial osteoarthrosis (Palotie et al. 1989) discussed in section 7.4. In that
analysis, a mixture of two types of individuals in the same large pedigree
was assumed: (1) individuals in whom the disease was due to a single
gene (genetic or susceptible cases) and (2) individuals whose disease was
the consequence of environmental factors (nongenetic or nonsusceptible
cases, phenocopies). Genetic cases had an associated age-of-onset curve
with low mean and 100 percent lifetime penetrance, whereas the corresponding curve for nongenetic cases had an increased mean and less than
100 percent lifetime penetrance. Hence, the age at onset helps discriminate between genetic and nongenetic cases. In this example, the mixture
is between individuals in the same pedigree. The discussion below focuses
on a mixture of linked and unlinked families, with homogeneity within
families.

In conditions with onset after birth, mean onset age can be quite different for different diseases. For example, Alzheimer's and Parkinson's diseases generally are characterized by high age at onset, while Huntington's disease tends to manifest in mid-life (average age at onset at thirty-six to forty-five years of age; Folstein 1989), and still other diseases occur shortly after birth. In the presence of heterogeneity such as in familial osteoarthrosis, it appears plausible to assume that age at onset is later in life for nonmendelian conditions. In two recent linkage analyses, families with low mean age of onset exhibited linkage to a genetic marker, whereas families with high onset age did not (St George-Hyslop et al. 1990; Hall et al. 1990). If this difference is indicative of genetic heterogeneity, onset age may be used as a presumably powerful discriminator between family types. A maximum likelihood analysis would proceed by defining two age-of-onset distributions, one with a low mean μ_1 and one with a high mean μ_2, both perhaps having a common variance σ^2. Families of the linked type (proportion α) are assumed to have mean μ_1 and families of the unlinked type have mean μ_2. Under heterogeneity, the likelihood must be maximized over the five parameters α, θ, μ_1, μ_2, and σ^2; under homogeneity, however, the restriction $\alpha = 1$ is equivalent with $\mu_1 = \mu_2 = \mu$, so that only three parameters have to be estimated.

Problems

Problem 9.1. In table 9.5 (section 9.4), with the support region as indicated by the italicized log likelihood values, what is the support interval for α_3? If a less stringent support region is defined, for example, by $\Delta \ln L = 3.0$ (likelihood ratio $= 20:1$), what are then the support limits for α_1, α_2, and α_3?

Problem 9.2. With $n = 10$ phase-known families of $m = 3$ meioses each, given that $\alpha = 0.9$ and $\theta = 0.05$ (table 9.7), the estimate of θ has a certain precision. How many families does one have to investigate to obtain a θ estimate of equal precision when linked and unlinked families are mixed with a proportion $\alpha = 0.5$ of linked families?

10.

Inconsistencies

The example at the end of section 9.4 demonstrated a general property of maximum likelihood estimates (MLEs)—they are biased. However, in most cases of practical importance, both the bias and the variance of the estimate tend to disappear as sample size increases. This statistical property of an estimate is called consistency (section 3.3). As long as MLEs are consistent, the presence of a bias is not too serious a problem because it can be remedied by increasing the number of observations. In human linkage analysis, MLEs may be inconsistent because of biased sampling or assuming a wrong parameter value in the analysis. The degree of the statistical inconsistency may be measured by the *asymptotic bias*, that is, the limit of the bias when sample size tends to infinity. In this chapter, examples of inconsistent estimates are outlined. The first half of each section will introduce the particular problem covered, with the remainder of the section covering more theoretical aspects of it.

To prove consistency, one must show that the expected log likelihood attains its maximum at the true parameter value, which is simple to do for categorical data. The tilde sign will be used to indicate at what parameter value (e.g., $\theta = \tilde{\theta}$) the expected log likelihood is highest. When in a formula both true and variable parameter values of the recombination fraction occur, the true value will be denoted by r, while θ will be the symbol for the variable parameter.

10.1. Ascertainment Bias

Owing to their easily recognizable mode of inheritance, X-chromosomal loci were among the first to be analyzed for linkage. Since most X-linked diseases are rare recessives, implying that sons can be affected while daughters may or may not be carriers (Vogel and Motulsky 1986), a common way of analyzing families has been to score sons only. Also, to be able to count recombination events, sometimes only those families are used in which it is known or can be deduced that the mother is doubly heterozygous. Many of these ascertainment schemes have been shown to lead to biased estimates of the recombination fraction, and appropriate ascertainment corrections have been devised (Edwards 1971). Nowadays, since families are routinely analyzed in an unselected manner, there is less of a need (or easy applicability) for these ascertainment corrections.

Observing the following two rules ensures unbiased estimation of the recombination fraction:

1. Sequential sampling. On the basis of the data already collected, one may freely decide which individuals to ascertain next. However, once ascertained, each individual so selected must be included in the analysis, and no individual can be deleted from the analysis (Cannings and Thompson 1977).

2. Selection at a single locus. One may select and possibly remove from the analysis any individual as long as such a decision is based on the phenotype at only one of the loci between which recombination is to be estimated (Fisher 1935b). For example, with respect to a monogenic disease, one may ascertain family pedigrees containing a minimum of two or three affecteds. This will not bias the results as long as this selection is carried out irrespective of the phenotypes at the marker loci. There are some caveats, however. For analyses involving diseases, one often ascertains so-called high-density pedigrees containing as many affecteds as possible. If in such pedigrees penetrance is estimated in a direct manner, the estimates are bound to be much higher than in pedigrees ascertained from a single proband only. Using an inflated penetrance estimate may very well lead to a bias in the recombination estimate. This is not to say that rule 2 is violated; rather, rule 2 cannot be invoked in this case as it does not apply to segregation analysis (it applies only to linkage analysis).

Even when rule 2 is applied properly, one should recognize that different sampling strategies may yield different degrees of informativeness for linkage. For example, in a dominant disease with incomplete penetrance, when a sibship contains a high proportion of affecteds, one of the parents may well be homozygous for the disease allele and thus uninformative for linkage. In recessive diseases, too, when a high number of affected individuals occurs in a pedigree, some of them may be parents but will be uninformative for linkage (when only one parent is affected, the other is still informative, of course). Owing to assortative mating, situations in which one or both parents are uninformative for a recessive disease are not too infrequent; examples may be found in families with Usher's syndrome (e.g., Smith et al. 1989). The question of sampling strategies in linkage analysis was addressed in more detail by Cox et al. (1988).

In a linkage analysis between two loci, when individuals are deleted on the basis of the phenotypes at *both* loci, an ascertainment bias may well occur. Consider, for example, a family of the CEPH type (Dausset et al. 1990), in which both parents are doubly heterozygous with known phase. Assume two codominant loci with alleles *A* and *B* at locus *1* and alleles *1* and *2* at locus *2*, the mating being *A1/B2* × *A1/B2* (section 5.5). All but one offspring type can be scored unambiguously for two recombination events in each offspring. The ambiguous type is the result of either two recombinations or two nonrecombinations and occurs with probability $\frac{1}{2}[r^2 + (1 - r)^2]$ (table 5.4). Not trusting maximum likelihood estimates except when known recombinations and nonrecombinations can be counted, rather than analyze all the observations, researchers have often felt safer deleting ambiguous offspring from the analysis so that the recombination fraction can be estimated as the proportion of recombinants among all unambiguous meioses. This is not a good strategy, which is demonstrated below.

When all offspring are analyzed, no bias exists, and the expected lod scores $E_0[Z(r)]$ are as shown in table 10.1. When only unambiguous offspring are analyzed (first three classes in table 5.4), one must distinguish

Table 10.1. Asymptotic Bias b of Recombination Estimates and ELODs $E_i[Z(\hat{\theta})]$ for Some Ascertainment Schemes in Phase-known Double Intercross Families

		Ambiguous Offspring are:				
		Disregarded			Nonrecombinants	
r	E_0	b	E_1	E_2	b	E_3
0.001	0.44	0.001	0.59	0.30	≈ 0	0.60
0.010	0.41	0.010	0.52	0.26	≈ 0	0.55
0.020	0.37	0.018	0.46	0.24	≈ 0	0.52
0.050	0.30	0.039	0.34	0.19	-0.001	0.43
0.100	0.21	0.061	0.22	0.13	-0.005	0.33
0.200	0.10	0.073	0.09	0.06	-0.020	0.19
0.300	0.04	0.059	0.03	0.02	-0.045	0.11
0.500	0	0	0	0	-0.125	0.03

Note: E_0 = unbiased ascertainment; E_1 = ambiguous offspring are supplanted by unambiguous offspring; E_2 = ambiguous offspring are lost for the analysis.

two cases: (1) ambiguous offspring are supplanted by unambiguous off-spring so that, in the end, the same number of offspring are analyzed but a larger number of families has to be collected to find them; (2) ambiguous offspring are lost to the analysis so that one has fewer individuals available to study. The two cases will differ in the amount of linkage information furnished (calculated below), but the offspring types (table 5.4) will occur in the same proportions under the two ascertainment schemes. Disregarding ambiguous offspring from the analysis introduces an inconsistency in the θ estimate (the same for the two cases), which can be shown by computing the value, $\tilde{\theta}$, at which the expected lod score E is a maximum (problem 5.2). Deriving $dE/d\theta$ (note that r is a constant in the derivative with respect to θ), setting this derivative equal to zero, and solving for θ leads to the asymptotic estimate

$$\tilde{\theta} = r + b, \, b = \frac{r(1 - r)(1 - 2r)}{1 + 2r(1 - r)}. \tag{10.1}$$

The asymptotic bias, b, is equal to 0 for $r = 0$ and $r = \frac{1}{2}$ and is otherwise positive, with a maximum value of $d = 0.073$ at $r = 0.19$. The relative asymptotic bias, b/r, tends to 100 percent as $r \to 0$; that is, with a large number of observations, deleting ambiguous offspring will lead to an apparent recombination estimate, which is approximately twice the true recombination rate. For larger values of r, the apparent recombination rate is no longer twice the true value, but the bias may still be considerable. For example, a true recombination rate of 5 percent will be observed as 9 percent. It is thus invalid to delete ambiguous offspring from family data.

To compute ELODs for the two cases distinguished above, one calculates the weighted average of the lod score for the different offspring types and evaluates it at $\theta = \tilde{\theta}$. When discarded ambiguous offspring are replaced by the same number of unambiguous offspring (case 1 above), the probabilities in table 5.4 for the first three classes have to be scaled to sum to 1. The ELOD is then given by

$$E_1 = \log(4) + \frac{(1 - r^2)\log(1 - \tilde{\theta}) + r(2 - r)\log(\tilde{\theta})}{\frac{1}{2} + r(1 - r)}, \tag{10.2}$$

where all logarithms are to the base 10. When ambiguous offspring are lost to the analysis (case 2 above), the proportion of available offspring and, thus, of available linkage information is equal to the sum of the probabilities of the first three offspring classes in table 5.4. The "available" ELOD, E_2, is then calculated by multiplying E_1 by that sum. For small values of r, about half of all offspring are ambiguous, so deleting them results in a drastic loss of linkage information (table 10.1). When as many unambiguous offspring are collected as ascertained in an unbiased manner, that ascertainment scheme yields more linkage information than does unbiased ascertainment (E_1 versus E_0), but (as shown above) this gain is purchased at the expense of an asymptotic bias.

To researchers who routinely analyze all of their data in an unbiased manner, the discussion in the previous paragraphs may appear somewhat academic. Its main purpose is to outline in detail how such problems can be investigated statistically. It also shows, however, that well-intended selection may have undesirable properties. In this vein, one may consider yet another ascertainment strategy. Since, at least at small recombination rates, ambiguous offspring most likely are nonrecombinants, why not simply pretend that they are nonrecombinants? The effect of this scheme is again investigated by calculating the expected lod score,

$$E_3[Z(\theta)] = \log(4) + [1+(1 - r)^2]\log(1 - \theta) \qquad (10.3)$$
$$+ r(2 - r)\log(\theta),$$

and evaluating it at $\theta = \bar{\theta}$ (the derivation of $\bar{\theta}$ is deferred to problem 10.1). Indeed, the asymptotic bias, $b = \bar{\theta} - r$, is very small for small to moderate recombination rates and the gain in ELOD is considerable, but the asymptotic bias becomes relatively large when r approaches ½ (table 10.1). Furthermore, it is negative so that this ascertainment scheme tends to mimic linkage when none is present. At $r = $ ½, with $E_3 = 0.03$, 100 offspring will yield an expected lod score of 3, whose maximum occurs at $\bar{\theta} = 0.375$. For known small recombination rates, this ascertainment scheme may be useful, but it cannot be generally recommended. It may appear counterintuitive that, for at least some recombination rates, a deliberately biased ascertainment scheme performs much better (E_3 versus E_2 in table 10.1) than the cautious approach dictated by analyzing unambiguous offspring only.

As already pointed out by Morton (1955, 304), it is essential that data be published without regard for whether they indicate linkage. Naturally, investigators prefer reporting positive linkage findings. In principle, this might lead to a bias of the recombination fraction estimate in the direction of linkage. However, it is often only the initial report of a positive finding which is made because linkage has been observed. If the subsequent reports on the same relation are made without regard to the linkage outcome, then in the long run no harm is done.

In marker typing, an error rate of one to several percent is often quoted (see section 10.5). For tight linkage, the rate of typing error may be larger than the recombination rate, which is probably the reason why many people scrutinize apparent recombinants but not nonrecombinants.

This practice tends to lead to a downward bias in the recombination fraction. To scrutinize typing results in an unbiased manner, one must review all observations, not just the apparent recombinants. These questions will be discussed more generally in section 10.5.

10.2. Misclassification

While recombination occurs at the genotypic level, the phenotypic observations are often several steps removed from direct observation of genotypes, even for codominant loci. A discordance between a phenotype and the underlying genotype may be viewed as a misclassification, whose probability of occurrence is a general form of incomplete penetrance. In this section, a very simple model of misclassification in connecting phenotypes with genotypes will be introduced (Ott 1977a). Two consequences of misclassification will be considered: (1) loss of linkage information owing to misclassification, which in itself does not lead to a bias, and (2) the bias introduced by using a wrong value for the misclassification rate in the analysis, in particular, by disregarding misclassification although it exists. Some situations in real life which can lead to misclassifications will be discussed in section 10.5.

Consider recombinants and nonrecombinants occurring with respective probabilities r and $1 - r$. Assume that, with a small probability, s, a recombinant is misclassified as a nonrecombinant and, with the same misclassification probability, a nonrecombinant is mistakenly scored as a recombinant. Thus, an apparent recombinant is either a true recombinant, occurring with probability $r(1 - s)$, or a false recombinant, occurring with probability $(1 - r)s$. Therefore, apparent recombinants occur with probability

$$p = r(1 - s) + (1 - r)s = r + s(1 - 2r). \qquad (10.4)$$

The proportion of apparent recombinants is a consistent estimator of p rather than of r. To obtain $\hat{\theta}$ from $\hat{p}$, assuming a known value s of the misclassification probability, solving (10.4) for r yields $\hat{\theta} = (\hat{p} - s)/(1 - 2s)$. In a linkage analysis of family data, in which one cannot necessarily count (apparent) recombination events, the usual lod score analysis will automatically furnish $\hat{\theta}$, if misclassification is allowed for via incomplete penetrance. For example, consider a dominant disease locus with two alleles, a disease allele D and a normal allele d. The misclassification probability, s, may then be used as shown in table 10.2.

The presence of misclassification blurs our view of the genotypes and represents random noise, which reduces linkage information, even

Table 10.2. General Misclassification Probability s, Incomplete Disease Penetrance $1 - s$, and Probability s of Occurrence of Phenocopies as Special Cases of Penetrances

Genotype	Misclassification		Incomplete Penetrance		Phenocopies	
	A	N	A	N	A	N
D/D	$1 - s$	s	$1 - s$	s	0	1
D/d	$1 - s$	s	$1 - s$	s	0	1
d/d	s	$1 - s$	0	1	s	$1 - s$

Note: Phenotypes: A = affected, N = unaffected.

Table 10.3. Relative ELOD of the Recombination Fraction Estimate in the Presence of Misclassification, s

s	Recombination Fraction, r						
	0.001	0.01	0.05	0.10	0.20	0.30	0.50[a]
0	1	1	1	1	1	1	1
0.01	0.92	0.94	0.95	0.95	0.96	0.96	0.96
0.05	0.72	0.74	0.77	0.78	0.80	0.80	0.81
0.10	0.53	0.55	0.58	0.60	0.62	0.63	0.64
0.20	0.28	0.29	0.31	0.33	0.34	0.35	0.36

[a]Limiting values.

when misclassification is allowed for in the linkage analysis. For counts of recombinants and nonrecombinants, without the presence of misclassification, the ELOD is given by $E_0 = r \times \log(2r) + (1 - r) \times \log[2(1 - r)]$ (equation [5.3]). If misclassification occurs and is allowed for based on (10.4), the ELOD is

$$E_s = \log(2) + p \times \log[r + s(1 - 2r)] \qquad (10.5)$$
$$+ (1 - p)\log[1 - r - s(1 - 2r)].$$

For the simple model defined above, the relative informativeness of a linkage analysis in the presence of misclassification as opposed to one without misclassification is given by $R = E_s/E_0$. Table 10.3 shows the relative ELOD for selected values of s and r. For example, with a misclassification rate of $s = 0.05$, at a recombination fraction of $r = 0.01$, the relative ELOD is approximately $R = \frac{3}{4}$. Therefore, to obtain as much linkage information under this level of misclassification as one would have with fully informative meioses, one must increase sample size by a factor of $1/R = 4/3$, that is, by approximately 33 percent.

An investigator may be unaware of the presence of misclassification and may in the analysis assume $s = 0$ although in reality, $s > 0$. This misspecification introduces a statistical inconsistency, as shown below. The proportion of apparent recombinants consistently estimates $r + s(1 - 2r)$ (equation [10.4]) rather than r. Hence, the asymptotic bias is given by $b = s(1 - 2r)$. No bias exists for $r = \frac{1}{2}$, but b increases with decreasing r and is largest for $r = 0$. For example, at $r = 0$, when misclassification is not allowed for in the analysis, the recombination fraction estimated in such linkage analyses will tend to be equal to s rather than 0. For the assumed mating type, the ELOD is the same whether or not misclassification is allowed for. In other family types this is not the case (see section 10.5).

10.3. Misspecification of Penetrance

Incomplete disease penetrance (introduced in section 7.1) may be viewed as a special form of misclassification in which only the genotypes susceptible to disease are subject to misclassification. The occurrence of phenocopies (sporadic cases) is a form of misclassification of nonsusceptible genotypes (see table 10.2).

Relative efficiency in the presence of incomplete penetrance is covered in section 7.2. Here, we will investigate the effect of assuming full penetrance while in reality it is incomplete (assuming absence of phenocopies). Applying the methods used previously, one finds that, in this case, the ELOD has its maximum at

$$\tilde{\theta} = r + s(\tfrac{1}{2} - r), \tag{10.6}$$

where $s = 1 - f$ (f = disease penetrance). The asymptotic bias in (10.6) is only half as large as in the case of disregarding misclassification under the model discussed in the previous section. This is plausible because, under the misclassification model of section 10.2, no known recombination events can be recognized; with incomplete penetrance, however, some genotypes can be identified unambiguously from the phenotypes.

When full penetrance is assumed while in fact it is incomplete, the ELOD is somewhat smaller than when incomplete penetrance is properly built into the analysis. The corresponding calculations are easy to carry out but are not shown here. The more general case of a true penetrance, $f < 1$, with a possibly different penetrance assumed in the analysis, requires somewhat more elaborate calculations but shows similar results (Clerget-Darpoux, Bonaïti-Pellié, and Hochez 1986).

10.4. Misspecification of Heterogeneity

In a mixture of linked and unlinked families (section 9.4) with proportions α and $1 - \alpha$, respectively, joint maximum likelihood estimation of α and r (the recombination fraction in linked families) ensures consistent estimates, that is, the expected log likelihood is highest at the true parameter values (assuming the absence of any biases). However, owing to the correlation between $\hat{\alpha}$ and $\hat{\theta}$, a misspecification of α will lead to an asymptotic bias in the estimate of r. Assume the particular case that an investigator is unaware of the presence of families of the unlinked type, that is, he or she assumes $\alpha = 1$ in the analysis while in reality, $\alpha < 1$. The resulting bias can be obtained by evaluating the point $\bar{\theta}$ at which the expected lod score attains its maximum. For the example of families with $m = 3$ meioses used in section 9.4, the expected lod score is given by

$$E[Z(\theta)] = \sum_{k=0}^{3} P(k; \alpha, r) Z_k(\theta), \tag{10.7}$$

where $P(k; \alpha, r)$ is the probability of observing k recombinants in a mixture of families as given by equation (9.17) and $Z_k(\theta)$ is the corresponding lod score when homogeneity is assumed in the analysis. For example, $Z_2(\theta) = \log[8\theta^2(1 - \theta)]$. To find that value of θ at which $E[Z(\theta)]$ (equation [10.7]) is maximized, one computes the first derivative, $dE/d\theta$ (note that r is a constant in this context), sets it equal to zero, and solves this equation for θ. The result turns out to be equal to

$$\bar{\theta} = r\alpha + \tfrac{1}{2}(1 - \alpha) = r + (1 - \alpha)(\tfrac{1}{2} - r). \tag{10.8}$$

In other words, $\bar{\theta}$ is the θ estimate one tends to obtain when α is falsely assumed to be equal to 1 (i.e., when heterogeneity is disregarded in the analysis, although it exists). For example, with $\alpha = 0.80$ and $r = 0.05$, assuming homogeneity in the analysis will, in large samples, lead to an estimate of $\bar{\theta} = 0.14$. Equation (10.8) also says that the asymptotic bias is largest for $r = 0$, in which case the apparent recombination rate tends to be equal to one half the proportion of unlinked families, assuming families of equal size $m = 3$. Of course, no inconsistency occurs for $r = \tfrac{1}{2}$, since then the value of α is clearly 0.

If calculations analogous to the ones above are carried out with phase-unknown (rather than phase-known) double backcross families of size $m = 3$ each, a result analogous to (10.8) is found as

$$\bar{\theta} = r\sqrt{\alpha} + \tfrac{1}{2}(1 - \sqrt{\alpha}). \tag{10.9}$$

For example, with $\alpha = 0.80$ and $r = 0.05$, one tends to find $\bar{\theta} = 0.10$.

In the previous paragraphs, a particular case of misspecification of α was considered, namely, that α is taken to be equal to 1 in the analysis while in reality it is less than 1. One may be interested in the more general question: if α is the true value of the proportion of linked families and one assumes in the analysis a value α', what is then the asymptotic estimate $\tilde{\theta}$ of the recombination fraction? Calculations analogous to the ones above are no longer straightforward but, for given true parameter values, α and r, one can compute the expected lod score for α' and θ and numerically maximize it over θ. For $m = 3$ offspring of a phase-known double back-cross mating, table 10.4 shows the probability of occurrence of a family with k recombinants (equation [9.17]) and the corresponding lod score. Using a spreadsheet program, it is then easy to calculate the weighted average of the lod score and find its maximum over θ.

For a true value of $\alpha = 0.5$ and several true recombination rates r, table 10.5 shows asymptotic estimates $\tilde{\theta}$ and the maximum of the expected lod score at $\tilde{\theta}$, when the analysis is carried out assuming a proportion α' of linked families. Owing to the positive correlation between the estimates for α and r, too high a value of α leads to an overestimate of r, and vice versa. As table 10.5 demonstrates, the bias in $\tilde{\theta}$ is quite strong. Normally, one estimates α along with r, but in small samples the α estimates may be

Table 10.4. Probability $P(k; \alpha, r)$ of Occurrence of k Recombinants and Associated Lod Score $Z(\theta; \alpha')$ in a Family with m Meioses

k	$P(k; \alpha, r)$	$Z(\theta; \alpha')$
0	$\alpha(1 - r)^3 + \frac{1}{8}(1 - \alpha)$	$\log[8\alpha'(1 - \theta)^3 + 1 - \alpha']$
1	$3[\alpha r(1 - r)^2 + \frac{1}{8}(1 - \alpha)]$	$\log[8\alpha'\theta(1 - \theta)^2 + 1 - \alpha']$
2	$3[\alpha r^2(1 - r) + \frac{1}{8}(1 - \alpha)]$	$\log[8\alpha'\theta^2(1 - \theta) + 1 - \alpha']$
3	$\alpha r^3 + \frac{1}{8}(1 - \alpha)$	$\log[8\alpha'\theta^3 + 1 - \alpha']$

Note: α = true proportion, α' = proportion assumed in the analysis.

Table 10.5. Maximum Z of the Expected Lod Score and Value $\tilde{\theta}$ at Which That Maximum Occurs When a Proportion α' of Linked Families Is Assumed in the Analysis While True Parameter Values Are $\alpha = 0.5$ and r

α'	$r = 0.01$		$r = 0.05$		$r = 0.10$	
	$\tilde{\theta}$	Z	$\tilde{\theta}$	Z	$\tilde{\theta}$	Z
0.7	0.08	0.210	0.13	0.166	0.18	0.123
0.6	0.04	0.219	0.09	0.172	0.14	0.127
0.5	*0.01*	*0.222*	*0.05*	*0.174*	*0.10*	*0.129*
0.4	0	0.217	0.01	0.172	0.06	0.127
0.3	0	0.164	0	0.162	0.01	0.121

quite different from the true values, which in turn leads to biased estimates of r. The table also shows that the maximum lod scores obtained under wrong values α' are somewhat smaller than those obtained under the true value of α. This result is analogous to results found for misspecifying penetrance or gene frequencies (Clerget-Darpoux, Bonaïti-Pellié, and Hochez 1986) and will be discussed further in section 11.3.

10.5. Pedigree Errors

Thus far, the effect of specific analysis errors has been investigated. In section 10.2, the effects of misclassification and misspecification of misclassification errors were treated in a theoretical manner. This section, however, covers sources of errors in the gathering of family data.

On the basis of typing results for seven polymorphic enzyme markers in close to 2,000 individuals, Lathrop et al. (1983) set up a mathematical model for two classes of errors: (1) pedigree error (nonpaternity and other misidentification of individuals and relationships) and (2) typing errors of marker systems. From the observed distribution of genetic marker inconsistencies in data from a South Pacific island population, they estimated the error of nonpaternity at 4 percent and the overall system typing error at 1 percent. A third error category, "field error," might be distinguished (e.g., mislabeling of blood samples) but was not separately taken into account in that study. Below, attention is focused on errors in marker typing.

In simulation studies, misreading an allele as the next largest or next smallest on a Southern blot results in overestimation of the recombination fraction and a loss in expected lod score (Terwilliger, Weeks, and Ott 1990). For detecting linkage with a locus with unknown map position, loss of linkage information is a much larger problem than a bias in $\hat{\theta}$, while the latter is serious for fine mapping of linked markers. Such simulation studies also show that, of all typing errors generated in family data, a sizeable portion may be undetectable because they will not lead to genetic inconsistencies (but they still result in the negative consequences mentioned above). This conclusion was also reached by Lathrop et al. (1983).

In multipoint analysis, typing errors tend to simulate double recombinants (Keats et al. 1991), which at short distances are expected to be very rare. Scrutinizing apparent double recombinants indeed tends to identify a large proportion of them as errors (Kouri and Fain 1990). Some of their effects are that the estimated map lengths will be inflated (Morton and Collins 1990) and that the ability to identify correct marker order is hampered (Jiang and Buetow 1990). In two-point analysis, a bias in $\hat{\theta}$

is not serious for detecting linkage, but this is not true in multipoint analysis (Risch and Giuffra 1990).

Assuming that precautions have been taken to reduce the occurrence of laboratory error to a minimum, recommendations for handling typing errors in the analysis are given below. The main point to be made is that errors should not simply be ignored. Rather, prior to the actual linkage analysis, it is beneficial to estimate the magnitude of the various errors, but this should be done on raw data, which have not been "cleaned up" before reaching the statistical geneticist (Lathrop et al. 1983). Based on observed error rates and simulation analyses showing the relation between observed and unobserved error rates, error rates may be incorporated in the analysis as a form of misclassification, for example, by allowing for a parameter such as s in the penetrances in table 10.2 (a simple example is also given in Keats, Sherman, and Ott 1990). Notice that marker systems are no longer codominant when misclassification is allowed for. Rather than making ad hoc error corrections, it may even be preferable to leave in errors the way they come from the laboratory and allow for them via misclassification probabilities. If the correction of an error is unique, the linkage program will know that, too, so there is no penalty for having the program make the correction. If the correction is not unique, however, an ad hoc correction may be wrong. A computer program will consider various correction possibilities with the appropriate weight if the model of typing errors is correct.

10.6. Other Model Misspecifications

Disregarding misclassifications amounts to a misspecification of the analysis model. Other model misspecifications are expected to lead to inconsistencies of various degrees (see below for an exception). For example, disregarding linkage disequilibrium (allelic association) in the analysis may result in an asymptotic bias (Clerget-Darpoux 1982).

In linkage analyses, diseases are usually assumed to result from the action of a single gene, possibly modified by random environmental effects. Other models such as oligogenic or multifactorial models may be more realistic (see section 11.3), but two-point analysis under a simple mode of inheritance seems to be quite robust for detecting linkage, although not for estimating recombination fractions (Risch, Claus, and Giuffra 1989; Risch and Giuffra 1990).

In multipoint analysis, effects of parameter misspecifications have not been much studied. One problem is that, in estimating the location of a new locus on a map of markers, that map is often assumed to be known without error, which usually is far from true. The limited work done on this subject suggests that it is better to have overestimates rather than underestimates of the interval lengths in maps on which a new locus should be placed (Ott and Lathrop 1987b). Also, possible biases as a result of unequal marker polymorphism of the markers in such maps are only now beginning to be studied (Mérette and Ott 1991).

An example of a misspecification not leading to an inconsistency is the following: In phase-unknown double backcross matings with m offspring each (section 5.9), the phase probabilities are usually taken to be equal to ½ each, as one assumes independence of the phenotypes at the two loci under study (allelic association would lead to unequal phase probabilities). Consider now a true phase probability, $c \neq ½$, while in the analysis the two phases are assumed to be equally frequent. Among the $m + 1$ possible phenotypes of the offspring, the kth phenotype occurs with a probability of $p_k = \binom{m}{k}[cr^k(1 - r)^{m-k} + (1 - c)(1 - r)^k r^{m-k}]$, where r is the true recombination fraction. Also, the $(m - k)$th phenotype occurs with probability $p_{m-k} = \binom{m}{k}[cr^{m-k}(1 - r)^k + (1 - c)(1 - r)^{m-k} r^k]$. Now, assuming equal phase probabilities in the analysis, the lod scores for the kth and $(m - k)$th phenotypes are the same. Hence, in the computation of the expected lod score, p_k and p_{m-k} appear as their sum only, $p_k + p_{m-k}$. In this sum, however, c and $1 - c$ cancel so that the expected lod score does not contain c. Consequently, with assumed phase probabilities of ½ each in the analysis, the recombination fraction estimate is consistent, irrespective of the true value c of the phase probability.

Problems

Problem 10.1. Using the expected lod score function $E_3[Z(\theta)]$ given in equation (10.3), derive the asymptotic recombination estimate $\hat{\theta}$, that is, the value of θ at which E_3 attains its maximum. The relevant offspring class probabilities are given in table 5.4.

Problem 10.2. Assume a phase-known double backcross mating and a misclassification scheme at one locus as shown on the left side of table 10.2. With $s = 1$ percent misclassification, at $r = 0.001$, by what factor does the number of offspring have to be increased for the ELOD under misclassification to be the same as without misclassification?

11.

Linkage Analysis with Disease Loci

An important aspect of the effort to obtain a dense map of markers spanning the human genome is the mapping of disease genes. The rationale in this "reverse genetics" approach is to find map locations for diseases with unknown biochemical defects and elucidate the mechanism leading to disease via identification of the gene and its molecular sequence, thereby paving the way for finding a cure. Spectacular results have already been obtained, particularly in the first step of this approach, that is, the localization and, in some cases, cloning of disease genes. Among the prime examples are Duchenne muscular dystrophy (Monaco and Kunkel 1988), cystic fibrosis (Kerem et al. 1989; Davies 1990; Kerem et al. 1990), and choroideremia (Cremers et al. 1990). For other disease genes, their genetic location has been found through linkage to genetic markers, but molecular genetic identification of the gene has not yet been possible. Among the many examples are Huntington's disease (Gusella et al. 1983), multiple endocrine neoplasia type 2A (Simpson et al. 1987), an autosomal form of retinitis pigmentosa (McWilliam et al. 1989), Usher's syndrome (Kimberling et al. 1990), and Marfan's syndrome (Kainulainen et al. 1990). This chapter covers particular aspects of linkage analysis involving disease loci. One such aspect, incomplete penetrance, was discussed in chapter 7.

11.1. Genetic Involvement

One of the first questions to be asked regarding the transmission of a disease is: Is it genetic? The main clue for an etiologic involvement of genes stems from the observation that the disease "runs in families." However, one must be aware that a concentration of disease cases among family members is not specific for genetic factors—infection is another possible cause for familiality of disease (for an overview, see Ott 1990a).

230

A case in point is *kuru*, the first human degenerative neurologic disease shown to be caused by a virus, which was pointed out to me by Dr. Mary-Claire King. The account given here is based on the booklet by Lindenbaum (1979).

Kuru occurs only among some native tribes in Papua New Guinea. It is characterized by loss of balance, incoordination of movements, and tremor and usually progresses to complete motor incapacity and death in about a year. Because it seemed to run in families, it was thought to be determined by a single autosomal gene that was dominant in females but recessive in males (Bennett, Rhodes, and Robson 1959). The estimated risk of kuru in female relatives of kuru victims was 51 percent, compared with a population prevalence of close to 1 percent. Hadlow (1959) pointed out the similarities between kuru and scrapie, a degenerative disease of the central nervous system in sheep, which was transmissible by inoculation. Gajdusek, Gibbs, and Alpers (1966) then injected the brains of chimpanzees with brain material from individuals who had died of kuru. They reported that, after incubation periods of up to four years, the chimpanzees developed a clinical syndrome very similar to human kuru (Carleton Gajdusek received the Nobel prize in medicine in 1976 for his pioneering work on kuru). Hence, kuru appeared to be a disease like scrapie, caused by a slow-acting infectious agent. The disease evidently had reached epidemic proportions as a result of cannibalism; particularly women and children used to eat the corpses of relatives. Indeed, after government and missionary intervention led to the abandonment of cannibalism, the incidence of kuru dramatically declined. It is interesting to note an analogy to Gerstmann-Sträussler syndrome and Creutzfeld-Jacob syndrome in humans and scrapie in animals, all of which belong to a class of slow, transmissible, lethal brain diseases caused by an unusual pathogen called a prion, whose composition and action are not well understood (Weissmann 1989).

It is often difficult to distinguish between genetic and cultural inheritance. For example, it is hard to determine whether food preferences are transmitted genetically or culturally (Cavalli-Sforza 1990). For other cases such as myopia, causation by a single autosomal dominant gene (MIM no. 16070) is generally accepted, but the visual image formed by the eye plays an important part in regulating the eye's growth—if the retina does not receive a visual image, the eye overgrows and becomes myopic (Judge 1990).

The relative influences of inheritance and environment are often not easy to tease apart. Transmission of an infectious disease is usually thought of as being due to environmental factors, but different individuals may react to infection differently depending on their genotypes. An interesting finding in this regard is the existence of a dominant gene for polio-virus sensitivity on chromosome 19 (Miller et al. 1974; Siddique et al. 1988). Another example is schizophrenia, for which penetrance seems to depend on recently experienced stressful life events (Snell Dohrenwend and Dohrenwend 1981). The causal relationships are unclear, however.

A well-known method for establishing genetic involvement in disease etiology is to compare the phenotypic concordance rate for a disease among monozygotic twins with that among dizygotic twins (Vogel and Motulsky 1986). Whereas monozygotic twins are genetically identical, dizygotic (fraternal) twins on average share only 50 percent of their genes. Hence, a disease that is at least partially determined genetically is ex-pected to show a higher frequency (recurrence rate) in a monozygotic cotwin than in a dizygotic cotwin of an affected person. Furthermore, the degree of reduction from 100 percent in the concordance rate among monozygotic twins is an indication of the degree to which environmental factors contribute to the disease. For behavioral and psychiatric traits, comparisons of concordance rates between monozygotic and dizygotic twins must be interpreted with caution (Kendler 1983).

As long as twins share the same family environment, effects of this environment contribute to the similarity of both monozygotic and di-zygotic twins. Investigating twins reared apart is thus important for sepa-rating genetic effects from those due to common family environment.

Genetic involvement in disease causation does not mean that a single gene is present which predisposes individuals to become affected. Various other genetic mechanisms could be acting, which will be discussed in section 11.3.

11.2. Disease Phenotype

Thus far, diseases have been assumed to be dichotomous traits. In many cases, however, such a dichotomy is arrived at after observing sev-eral variables on an individual, on the basis of which a rule is applied as to who is affected and who is unaffected. Ideally, one would use all vari-ables jointly in a linkage analysis of a multivariate phenotype, in which the observations form a mixture of two (presumably overlapping) multi-variate distributions whose two mean vectors correspond to genetically susceptible and nonsusceptible individuals. One may also try to reduce the dimensionality of the phenotypes (given by the number of variables) to a one-dimensional quantity, for example, using discriminant analysis. Multivariate analyses have indeed been carried out on patterns of psychi-atric symptoms (Kendler et al. 1987; Stassen et al. 1988).

On the other hand, forming two classes (affected/unaffected) obviates the need for parameter estimation, although dichotomization generally entails a great loss of information (Cohen 1990). As it is often unclear how to define the genetically most relevant class boundaries, investigators tend to try several alternative classification schemes, for example, by applying various degrees of stringency in their criteria for affectedness. If each such scheme is used to carry out a linkage analysis and if the overall maximum lod score under any classification scheme is reported, computer simulation may have to be used to assess the empirical significance level associated with such a maximum lod score (see section 8.7).

The choice of a threshold for affection status greatly influences linkage analyses (Kendler 1988). In psychiatric traits, the classical criterion for the definition of the "affected" category has been the extent to which potentially related clinical states show familial aggregation (Baron 1986; Kendler 1986). Using more than one threshold (Reich et al. 1979) and thus more than two classes is expected to reduce misclassification. For example, on the basis of several severity grades for osteoarthrosis, Palotie et al. (1989) formed three classes: unaffected, unknown, and affected.

A particular scheme for forming graded phenotype classes rests on a measure c of certainty that an individual is truly affected (Ott 1991). That measure may be Rice et al.'s (1987) estimated probability that an observed case is a true case, or it may simply be a clinician's opinion, expressed as a fraction between zero and one indicating his or her belief that an individual is affected. One may then form classes for the c values, for example, class 1 with $c = 1$ (clearly affected), class 2 with $1 > c \geq 0.90$ (most likely affected), etc. Now, assume a monogenic mode of inheritance with the respective penetrances f and $1 - f$ for the phenotypes "clearly affected" and "clearly unaffected." An individual with, for example, 60 percent certainty of being affected will then have penetrance $0.6 \times f + 0.4 \times (1 - f)$, that is, the penetrance is a weighted average of the penetrances of the extreme classes. Individuals midway between the extremes ($c = \frac{1}{2}$) will obtain a penetrance of $\frac{1}{2}$ irrespective of their genotype so that they are effectively coded as having phenotype "unknown." Although this scheme may appear arbitrary and subjective, it combines different diagnostic schemes into one analysis and thus does not suffer from the shortcomings of multiple analyses carried out with multiple diagnostic schemes.

A theoretical justification for the above procedure of assigning penetrances to classes of certainty of affectedness is obtained by distinguishing two levels of phenotypes, true phenotypes A (affected) and U (unaffected) and corresponding apparent phenotypes A^* and U^* (a similar approach was taken by Lathrop et al. [1983] in their investigation of pedigree errors). Given a genotype g conferring disease susceptibility, the penetrance for true affecteds is $f = P(A|g)$. Through misclassification, the phenotype A is recognized only with probability $c = P(A^*|A)$ and mistaken as phenotype U with probability $1 - c = P(U^*|A)$. Analogously, $c = P(U^*|U)$ and $1 - c = P(A^*|U)$. Consequently, the penetrances for apparent phenotypes become $P(A^*|g) = cf + (1 - c)(1 - f)$ and $P(U^*|g) = (1 - c)f + c(1 - f) = 1 - P(A^*|g)$ (cf. section 10.2 on misclassification).

The above scheme for forming disease phenotype classes is targeted towards diseases in which diagnosis is ambiguous, for example, in many psychiatric traits. In other diseases, affection status is clear-cut, but underlying genotypes may be ambiguous, either because the disease is inherited in a recessive fashion or because penetrance is incomplete. Often, concomitant variables (also called biologic markers or endophenotypes) are available, which partially reveal underlying genotypes. In Duchenne's muscular dystrophy (X-linked), for example, female carriers of the disease gene are unaffected, but their serum level of the enzyme creatine kinase (CK) is increased—about 70 percent of obligate carriers have CK values above the 95th percentile of the normal range (Vogel and Motulsky 1986). This difference in percentile can be exploited in linkage analyses. Another example, aspartyl glucosaminuria (AGU, MIM number 20840), is one of the Finnish diseases (Vogel and Motulsky 1986). While heterozygous carriers of the AGU gene do not express the disease, they can be identified through low activity of the enzyme aspartyl glucosaminidase (Grön, Aula, and Peltonen 1990); thus, AGU effectively becomes a codominant trait.

The appropriate phenotype definition may depend on the purpose of a linkage analysis. For example, the gene underlying the fragile X syndrome (Martin-Bell syndrome; Vogel and Motulsky 1986) potentially causes two distinct phenotypes: (1) mental retardation and other clinical features and (2) cytologic abnormalities (secondary restrictions in X chromosome, fragile X phenotype) (Sherman et al. 1985). For gene mapping and carrier detection, one would like to make as much use as possible of the phenotype for recognizing the underlying genotype. For that reason, one would call someone affected when that person is either is mentally retarded *or* shows cytologic abnormalities. In genetic counseling, on the other hand, one may only be interested to know whether the proband is mentally retarded or not. The cytologic status is then a covariate that should not be part of the phenotype. In that case, "affected" is taken to mean only "mentally retarded," with two penetrance classes defined by the presence or absence of cytologic abnormalities.

11.3. Mode of Inheritance

In many hereditary diseases, a simple mode of inheritance can be recognized. For example, Huntington's disease can be clearly seen to follow an autosomal dominant mode of transmission even though penetrance is age dependent. In other conditions, a mutant gene manifests itself only in special situations (strong environmental influence as in genetically determined drug reactions or alcoholism). Most traits, however, are so *complex* that direct analysis of all contributing factors becomes impossible and genetic analysis is more readily carried out by statistical rather than biologic methods (Vogel and Motulsky 1986).

Various genetic models can be proposed for the familial aggregation of diseases (Ott 1990a). Techniques to delineate the mode of inheritance of a trait fall under the heading of segregation analysis, specifically complex segregation analysis. Since families are not collected at random, proper ascertainment correction is essential for results of segregation analysis to be valid and meaningful. Unfortunately, these results tend to depend crucially on the ascertainment scheme applied, which is rarely known with certainty (Greenberg 1986). Nonsensical "evidence" for major genes in familial traits seems to be easy to obtain (McGuffin and Huckle 1990). On the other hand, somatic mutational models for the occurrence of some cancers seem to be quite realistic (Knudson 1971, 1985; see also Sager 1989 and chapter 10 on cancer genetics in Gelehrter and Collins 1990). In animal models some forms of complex inheritance have been at least partially unraveled. For example, in nonobese diabetic (NOD) mice, insulin-dependent diabetes is caused by polygenic interactions of at least three recessive loci (Prochazka et al. 1987).

Statistical investigations of mode of inheritance most often rest on comparisons of disease recurrence in different categories of relatives (see also section 4.9). The above-mentioned ratio of concordance rates in monozygotic and dizygotic twins is a statistic often used to infer genetic involvement, but it does not address the nature of the inheritance, for example, whether a single gene or polygenes are causing higher concordance rates in monozygotic twins. Comparing population incidence of a disorder with the incidence in relatives of probands, Edwards (1960) provided approximate simple statistics to discriminate among dominant, recessive, and multifactorial (polygenic threshold) inheritance. The SEDA (structured exploratory data analysis) statistics (Karlin et al. 1981) have also been used to distinguish among different modes of inheritance, particularly to detect effects of single major genes. Further, a major gene statistic has been proposed for quantitative characters such as obesity, for which weak evidence for the involvement of single genes was found (Zonta et al. 1987). Recently, Risch (1990) investigated the drop-off with degree of relationship of a particular risk ratio (the ratio of the risk to relatives of a proband versus the population prevalence of a quantitative trait; see also Ott 1990b). He found, for example, that epistatic interaction of approximately three major loci accounts best for observed prevalence rates of schizophrenia.

The current computer programs for linkage analysis basically all assume a monogenic inheritance of the trait to be mapped. Fortunately, computer simulation analyses show that analyzing oligogenic traits (small number of loci jointly responsible for disease occurrence) under an assumed monogenic mode of inheritance retains much of the information on linkage between one of the trait loci and the marker linked to it (Risch, Claus, and Giuffra 1989; Vieland et al. 1991). Also, ignoring polygenic correlation among relatives in linkage analyses does not seem to have too serious an effect (Konigsberg et al. 1990).

Oligogenic models for disease inheritance have only recently been considered. An early approach to simulate the effects of multiple genes as a second locus in a two-locus disease model were not further pursued (Mittmann 1938). A particular type of oligogenic model assumes that an individual is affected only when homozygous for a disease allele at each of a number of two-allele loci (Li 1987; Majumder 1989). Recently, two-locus disease models were implemented in the LINKAGE programs (Lathrop and Ott 1990). For many proteins and enzymes, of course, interaction of two or more genes for a final functioning product is well known, a newly detected example being that of glucose 6-phosphate dehydrogenase (G6PD) (Kanno et al. 1989). Two-locus or multilocus models for diseases are thus reasonable, but information for linkage appears to be limited when more than one of the loci has a major effect on disease inheritance (Vieland et al. 1991).

In the absence of a known mode of inheritance, in addition to trying different diagnostic schemes as pointed out above, researchers often try different plausible modes of inheritance or different parameter values in the genetic model. For example, Sherrington et al. (1988) carried out a linkage analysis of schizophrenia versus chromosome 5 markers for three different classification schemes and a variety of penetrance values and calculated the maximum lod score in each analysis. Effectively, they maximized the lod score over diagnostic schemes and penetrance values. For simple family types, analyzing the data under a false penetrance value will not inflate the lod score (Clerget-Darpoux, Bonaïti-Pellié, and Hochez 1986; Greenberg 1989; see also section 8.7). This result has sometimes falsely been interpreted to mean that maximizing the lod score over model parameters will not inflate the lod score either, but such a conclusion is fallacious. In fact, maximizing lods over diagnostic schemes *or* over penetrance values will tend to inflate the lod score, but the effect is much stronger when diagnostic classes are varied than when penetrance values are varied (Weeks et al. 1990).

The conclusions from the above theoretical investigations are that one may analyze a trait for linkage under a rather simple model and still find evidence for linkage when it is present and that one should limit analyses to a small number of models. One must be aware that estimates of the recombination fraction obtained under a wrong model tend to be much too high (Clerget-Darpoux, Bonaïti-Pellié, and Hochez 1986). This does not present a major problem in the search for linkage by two-point analysis. However, in multipoint analyses of an oligogenic trait versus a dense map of markers, when the location of a disease is constrained to be close to neighboring markers, the disease may be excluded from the true location of one of its genes (Risch and Giuffra 1990).

It was outlined in section 4.7 that a critical lod score of 3 is applicable even when a trait locus is tested for linkage versus several marker loci, the reason being that an increased prior probability of linkage counteracts the potential for an increase in the type I error. Of course, these conclusions are based on the assumption that the trait to be mapped is due to a single gene. For complex traits, this assumption is not necessarily warranted—a trait may predominantly be caused by environmental agents. Hence, it is important in such situations that the critical lod score be adjusted upward using equation (4.15) to reflect the number of marker loci tested.

Rather than working under simple and presumably wrong genetic models, one may resort to nonparametric approaches, which were briefly discussed in section 4.9. An interesting combination of parametric and nonparametric analyses was applied by Hyer et al. (1991) in an exclusion of diabetes susceptibility genes from a candidate region of chromosome 11. These authors carried out a primary analysis in a nonparametric manner by estimating two identity-by-descent probabilities, p_1 and p_2, that is, the respective probabilities that two siblings share one or two alleles identical by descent. The likelihood $L(p_1, p_2)$ can then be pictured as the height above the point (p_1, p_2) in a plane with coordinates p_1 and p_2, and a support region for the true IBD probabilities is easily constructed. Next, they considered a large number of parametric models and for each model derived its prediction of the two IBD probabilities. Depending on whether or not the predicted pair of values (p_1, p_2) was inside the support region, the parametric models could be divided into those that were compatible with the observations and those that could be rejected.

Another model-free method, also based on sib pairs, incorporates multiple measurements on each individual and estimates the linear function that results in the strongest correlation between the squared pair differences in these measurements and identity by descent at a marker locus (Amos et al. 1990).

To conclude this section, I will outline a few basic properties of simple mendelian modes of inheritance for rare diseases. *Dominant traits* such as Huntington's disease typically occur clustered in large pedigrees, with affected individuals being found in many generations. Affected individuals probably carry only one disease gene and, assuming full penetrance, unaffecteds carry none. Thus, the trait genotype is known for each individual. Usually, only one of two parents is heterozygous for the disease allele and thus potentially informative for linkage. Owing to the small gene frequencies of most dominant traits, homozygotes for the disease allele are extremely rare. Some of the few observed cases exhibit the same phenotype as heterozygotes (Nordström and Thorburn 1980; Holmgren et al. 1988).

In contrast, rare autosomal *recessive traits* are usually manifest only in a single sibship and are therefore much harder to study. Both parents of affected individuals are heterozygous (unaffected) carriers of the disease gene and thus potentially informative for linkage. On the other hand, although affected offspring are homozygous for the disease, unaffected offspring may or may not carry a disease gene. This uncertainty about their trait genotype has the effect that they provide much less information for linkage than do affected offspring (see discussion of table 11.1). Consequently, when affected children die at a young age, it becomes very hard to carry out linkage analyses for such traits. Examples of autosomal recessive conditions are phenylketonuria and cystic fibrosis. Notice that autosomal recessive inheritance may be difficult to distinguish from germline mosaicism (see section 11.8), since the occurrence of both is restricted to sibs (J. H. Edwards 1989b).

X-linked traits are most often recessive with full penetrance in (hemizygous) males. An exception is the fragile X syndrome, which is inherited as an X-linked recessive trait with incomplete penetrance in males (Sherman et al. 1985).

In linkage analyses of autosomal recessive traits, an important practical question is, how much linkage information do unaffected offspring provide? Is it useful at all to carry out marker typing for unaffected offspring? This question may be answered by calculating the ELOD for given numbers of affected and unaffected offspring. Assume that the disease is rare and that the marker locus is highly polymorphic so that the parents have four different marker alleles. At the disease locus, each parent is heterozygous, d/D, where d is the disease allele and D is the normal allele. The joint genotype of parent 1 is $d1/D2$ or $d2/D1$ and that of parent 2 is $d3/D4$ or $d4/D3$. Four different phase combinations can be distinguished among the parents, each occurring with prior probability ¼. It is then straightforward although somewhat tedious to calculate the expected lod score, $E[Z(r)]$, where r is the true recombination fraction between disease and marker genes (Leal and Ott 1990). The results shown in table 11.1 suggest that an affected offspring provides approximately five times as much linkage information as an unaffected offspring. With tight linkage, each affected offspring independently contributes 0.602 and each unaffected contributes 0.125 towards the ELOD. For an ELOD of 3, for example, one needs five affected offspring or twenty-four unaffected offspring or a total of three affected and ten unaffected offspring.

For rare recessive traits, the parents of an affected individual tend to be related more often than in the general population because they have an increased probability of sharing two copies of the same ancestral disease allele (the two copies are said to be identical by descent, IBD). The two disease alleles in an affected child are then also IBD, and the two alleles of a marker locus tightly linked with the disease gene tend to be IBD as well. This situation was discussed by Smith (1953) and shown to depend critically on close linkage and a high degree of polymorphism of the marker. As pointed out by Lander and Botstein (1986b), a dense map

Table 11.1. Increase δ in Expected Lod Score at Given True Value r of the Recombination Fraction due to Adding One Affected (δ_a) or One Unaffected (δ_u) Offspring, Given a Sibship of n Affected and No Unaffected Offspring, for Autosomal Recessive Disease and Highly Polymorphic Marker

	$r = 0$			$r = 0.05$		
n	δ_a	δ_u	R^a	δ_a	δ_u	R
1	0.602	0.125	4.8	0.329	0.055	6.0
2	0.602	0.125	4.8	0.383	0.066	5.8
3	0.602	0.125	4.8	0.415	0.075	5.5

Source: Leal and Ott (1990).
[a]R = ratio of ELOD for an affected over that for an unaffected offspring.

of genetic markers will satisfy these conditions. These authors further showed that, under ideal conditions, a single affected child born of first cousins is roughly as informative as a nuclear family with three affected children. The term *homozygosity mapping* was introduced by Lander and Botstein (1986b) to denote the fact that an increased degree of homozygosity for marker alleles in affected children of related parents is indicative of linkage between the marker and the disease. To apply homozygosity mapping in practice, a regular linkage analysis may be carried out with one of the available computer programs. If the program is informed of the relationship between the parents (and perhaps other pedigree members), it will automatically make use of the increased informativeness inherent in the family.

11.4. Associations between Phenotypes and Alleles

An association is said to exist between two phenotypes when they occur together in the same individual more often than expected by chance. For example, assume that in the population p_1 is the proportion of individuals with stomach ulcer and p_2 is the proportion of individuals with the A blood type. If these two characteristics occur independently of each other one expects a proportion $p_1 \times p_2$ of individuals to have both stomach ulcer and the A blood type. One finds, however, that the A blood type is clearly associated with cancer of the stomach (Vogel and Motulsky 1986), but the nature of the association is still unclear (Beckman and Ängqvist 1987).

To investigate whether phenotypes are associated, one usually collects two groups of individuals, for example, patients (in this case with stomach ulcers) and a control sample. In each group the proportion of interest is then determined. The usual chi-square test for 2×2 tables is then applied to determine significance. The strength of an association is often measured by the relative incidence or relative risk,

$$R = \frac{n_1(n_2 + n_4)}{n_2(n_1 + n_3)},$$

where n_1 is the number of patients with the characteristic, n_2 is the number of control individuals with the characteristic, and n_3 and n_4 are the corresponding numbers without the characteristic. Often, the odds ratio,

$$R_1 = \frac{n_1 n_4}{n_2 n_3},$$

is used as an approximation to the relative risk and is referred to as approximate relative risk or simply as relative risk (Armitage and Berry 1987). For example, the odds ratio for the association between blood type A and stomach ulcer is $R_1 = 1.2$ and is highly significant (Vogel and Motulsky 1986). Another measure for the strength of an association is the correlation coefficient,

$$\rho = \frac{n \times n_1 - (n_1 + n_2)(n_1 + n_3)}{\sqrt{(n_1 + n_2)(n_3 + n_4)(n_1 + n_3)(n_2 + n_4)}},$$

where $n = n_1 + n_2 + n_3 + n_4$, and $n\rho^2$ is identical with the usual formula for the chi-square statistic in a 2×2 table whose cells contain n_1, n_2, n_3, and n_4 observations.

Various mechanisms can cause phenotypic associations, of which four are discussed here.

1. *Clustered sampling* can lead to association. For investigations of an association, one must collect unrelated individuals for the chi-square test to be valid. Assume now that in the population no association between two phenotypes exists (null hypothesis in the significance test). In the absence of a sufficient number of unrelated individuals affected with a rare trait, investigators sometimes collect related individuals for the patient group. However, the presence of relatives amounts to a deviation from the null hypothesis of independence of the observations, which the chi-square test may detect. In other words, the lack of independence among individuals tends to inflate chi-square, but the effect is entirely due to clustered sampling. For tests of Hardy-Weinberg equilibrium, Sing and Rothman (1975) showed that the average value of chi-square is inflated by a factor of $1 + \rho(n - 1)$, where ρ is the average correlation between any two of the n individuals sampled. Cohen (1976) obtained a similar result for chi-square tests in contingency tables.

2. *Interaction* between the two loci, either on the phenotypic level or on the allelic level (epistasis), will lead to an association of phenotypes. The association between ABO blood types and stomach ulcer mentioned above is thought to be due to some form of interaction, for example, to a protective effect of the O blood type. In linkage analysis, phenotypic interactions are assumed absent. One way of allowing for phenotypic interactions in linkage analysis is to make the penetrances at one locus depend on the phenotypes at the other locus (Ott and Falk 1982).

3. *Admixture* is another statistical artifact that can cause phenotypes to appear associated. Consider admixture between two populations (or a mixture of two samples from different populations), where a disease and a particular characteristic both occur in higher frequency in one population than in the other but in both populations disease and characteristic occur

independently of each other. It is then easy to show that in the mixed population the disease and the characteristic appear correlated. The correlation is positive when in one population the frequencies of disease and characteristic are both increased or both decreased; it is negative when one of the two frequencies is increased and the other is decreased; and it is zero otherwise. Specifically, let p and q be the proportions of individuals in the total (mixed) population carrying the disease and the characteristic, respectively. Further, p_1 and q_1 denote the analogous proportions in population 1 before the mixture took place, whereas c stands for the proportion of individuals in population 1, that is, the proportion of individuals in the mixed population originating from population 1. Then, in the population as a whole, the disease and the characteristic of interest are correlated with

$$\rho = [c/(1 - c)] \frac{(p_1 - p)(q_1 - q)}{\sqrt{p(1 - p)q(1 - q)}}.$$

Analyzing stratified data in an unstratified manner is well known possibly to lead to paradoxical results. It can be shown, for example, that the relative risk in each of two portions of a population can be larger than 1 while for the total population it is smaller than 1 (see example 12.5 in Armitage and Berry 1987). This phenomenon is known as Simpson's paradox (Louis 1982).

Now, consider the effects of population admixture at the genotypic level. Assume two loci that are in Hardy-Weinberg equilibrium (HWE) in each population before admixture. Clearly, after one generation of random mating in the mixed population, each locus will again be in HWE. Let p_i and q_i denote the gene frequencies at loci 1 and 2, respectively, in the mixed population. For simplicity, assume two alleles only at each locus. If the alleles from the two loci occur independently in haplotypes, the haplotype carrying allele 1 at locus 1 and allele 1 at locus 2 occurs in the population with frequency

$$P_{11} = p_1 q_1, \tag{11.1}$$

where P_{ij} is the population frequency of the haplotype with allele i at locus 1 and allele j at locus 2. However, this equilibrium frequency is not reached after one generation of random mating but only gradually in successive generations (see below). The deviation from equilibrium is measured by the linkage disequilibrium parameter (Hartl 1988),

$$D = P_{11} - p_1 q_1. \tag{11.2}$$

The equilibrium state (11.1) is characterized by $D = 0$ and is called gametic phase equilibrium or linkage equilibrium, and a deviation from it is termed *linkage disequilibrium*. Note that this term does not necessarily imply linkage between the two loci considered. Linkage disequilibrium is derived here as a consequence of population admixture, but it may be due to other factors as well. As will be seen below, tight linkage can also lead to linkage disequilibrium. As a matter of fact, it has become common among human geneticists to take linkage disequilibrium to mean association among alleles due to close linkage. Therefore, Edwards (1980) proposed the neutral term *allelic association* for a deviation from gametic phase equilibrium, without any implication as to the nature of the deviation.

The linkage disequilibrium parameter (often simply called linkage disequilibrium) D can take only a limited range of values (Hartl 1988):

$$D_{min} = \max(-p_1 q_1, -p_2 q_2), D_{max} = \min(p_1 q_2, p_2 q_1). \qquad (11.3)$$

Because of these bounds, the strength of an allelic association is often indicated as the proportion, D/D_{max} or D/D_{min}. Here, only one disequilibrium parameter (equation [11.1]) is considered. In general, several disequilibrium parameters must be distinguished (Elandt-Johnson 1971), and gametic disequilibria at multiple loci require consideration of higher-order disequilibrium parameters (Weir 1990).

4. *Tight linkage* between two loci may be the explanation of why their alleles (and thus their phenotypes) are associated. Imagine a piece of DNA at which a disease-causing mutation occurs, and consider a genetic marker 5 cM away. Initially, the mutant allele is in coupling with the marker allele on the same chromosome. As time goes by, the disease allele may increase in frequency, and occasionally recombination occurs between disease and marker so that in some individuals the disease gene will be in coupling with a marker allele other than the one on the chromosome where the disease-causing mutation originally occurred. Initially, there is complete linkage disequilibrium between disease and marker but, as outlined below, it tends to disappear due to recombination. With tight linkage (little recombination), the linkage disequilibrium can persist for many generations. Hence, tight linkage is not really the cause of the disequilibrium (the original mutation is), but it maintains it at a high level.

With recombination between two loci, an existing disequilibrium D is reduced by a factor of $1 - r$ in each generation, where r is the recombination fraction between the two loci (Hartl 1988; Elandt-Johnson 1971). Hence, after t generations, the disequilibrium D is changed to a value

$$D_t = (1 - r)^t D. \qquad (11.4)$$

The half-life of a disequilibrium value, that is, the number of generations it takes for D to fall to one half of its value, is obtained by setting $D_t/D = \frac{1}{2}$ and solving (11.4) for t, which yields

$$t = \frac{\log(\frac{1}{2})}{\log(1 - r)}. \tag{11.5}$$

Decay of D is most rapid when two loci are unlinked ($r = \frac{1}{2}$). For tightly linked loci, allelic association may exist for a long time in a population, which is the basis for "disequilibrium mapping," discussed below.

The presence of allelic association is often interpreted as evidence for linkage between two loci, but as one can see from the above discussion, several factors other than tight linkage can be responsible for allelic association. For verification of linkage between loci showing allelic association, the most direct procedure would be to carry out a linkage analysis in which haplotype frequencies instead of gene frequencies are specified (most computer programs can accommodate allelic association). Allelic association, as long as it is not due to an interaction among loci, is relevant only for individuals marrying into a pedigree but not for other family members, whose genotypes are determined by the genotypes of their parents and not by population haplotype frequencies. Experience shows that linked loci tend to show allelic association when the recombination fraction between them is smaller than 2 percent. A well-known example of allelic association due to tight linkage is that at the MN and Ss blood groups. Each of the two loci is in HWE, but linkage disequilibrium is present and equal to $D = 0.07$, which is one half of its maximum value (Hartl 1988).

For genetic marker loci, haplotype frequencies may be estimated on the basis of a random sample of individuals. Consider alleles A and a at locus *1* and alleles B and b at locus *2*. Many individuals (2-locus genotypes) will allow direct observation of their haplotypes. For example, the genotype AB/aB necessarily contains the haplotypes AB and aB. Which haplotypes are contained in a double heterozygote, however, depends on the gametic phase. Since that is generally unknown, phase has to be estimated. An elegant iterative estimation procedure (a form of the EM algorithm; Dempster, Laird, and Rubin 1977) is based on the gene counting technique (Ceppellini, Siniscalco, and Smith 1955; Smith 1957; Ott 1977b) and works as follows: assuming preliminary values for the haplotype frequencies, one determines the probabilities of the two phases and uses these as weights in counting haplotypes from each assumed phase. This count yields improved estimates for the haplotype frequencies, with which the phase probabilities are again determined, etc. This procedure has been implemented in various computer programs, for example, in the ASSOCIATE program, one of the linkage utility programs (section 8.5).

Based on a random sample of individuals, for two codominant autosomal loci the ASSOCIATE program partitions the chi-square for genotype associations into two portions, one due to allelic associations and the other due to all other associations, for example, deviations from HWE at locus *1* depending on the genotypes at locus *2*. The program cannot indicate the causes leading to either of these two categories of associations. Also, the reader should be aware that allelic association in unrelated individuals cannot be assessed for VNTR markers with more than approximately five alleles if these cannot uniquely be identified across families.

Estimates of haplotype frequencies involving disease genes are usually based on a sample of families segregating the disease. Care must be taken to adjust estimated frequencies for ascertainment biases (Chakravarti, Li, and Buetow 1984). Provisional haplotype frequencies may be obtained from pedigree data by use of the ILINK program. The estimated frequencies then refer to the haplotypes in the individuals marrying into the pedigrees analyzed and must be normalized by the population gene frequencies as shown below. In many cases, it is possible to obtain preliminary direct counts of haplotypes. As an example, consider the data for cystic fibrosis (CF) reported by Beaudet et al. (1989), which are based on close linkage to two DNA probes XV-2c and KM-19 (not on direct recognition of the mutant gene). Each marker has two alleles, which are jointly coded as four haplotypes *A* through *D*. Because of tight linkage among these two and other markers analyzed, it was possible in most cases to recognize the most likely phase in the doubly heterozygous parents of affected offspring, which allowed a count of marker haplotypes in coupling with either a disease allele or a normal allele at the CF locus.

Table 11.2. Counts of Marker Haplotypes *A* through *D* on CF and Normal (NL) Chromosomes

Marker Haplotype	Chromosome Count		Estimated Haplo-Type Frequency			Expected under Equilibrium	
	CF	NL	CF	NL	Sum	CF	NL
A	17	74	0.00135	0.290	0.29135	0.0058	0.2855
B	218	35	0.01730	0.137	0.15430	0.0031	0.1512
C	7	110	0.00056	0.431	0.43156	0.0086	0.4230
D	10	31	0.00079	0.122	0.12279	0.0025	0.1203
Sum	252	250	0.02	0.98	1	0.02	0.98

Source: Beaudet et al. (1989).

The result of known counts of CF haplotypes is shown in table 11.2. The preliminary counts are adjusted to proportions reflecting the population frequencies of the CF and NL (normal) alleles. For example, the population frequency of the *A-CF* haplotype is estimated as $0.02 \times 17/252 = 0.0013$. Also shown in table 11.2 are the corresponding frequencies expected under the assumption of linkage equilibrium. For example, the haplotype *B-CF* is observed with population frequency of 0.0173 but would be expected with a frequency of only $0.1543 \times 0.02 = 0.0031$.

With tight linkage between a disease and marker loci, one rarely finds recombinants, which would allow assigning the disease locus to one of the intervals between markers. In this situation, the presence of allelic association is sometimes used to localize a disease gene more accurately, the idea being that the disease gene is closest to that marker showing the highest degree of allelic association with it (Edwards 1980). This approach has been applied to homogeneous diseases such as cystic fibrosis and Huntington's disease (Sneel et al. 1989), but estimates of map location based on allelic association are generally imprecise and may not really represent an improvement over linkage analysis (Weir 1989). Furthermore, this method must be unreliable when several disease-causing mutations occurred at different times because the disequilibrium depends on the recombination fraction and on the number of generations passed since a single mutation occurred. Also, selection at the disease locus may influence gene frequencies at nearby markers (Weir 1989).

Several multifactorial diseases such as insulin-dependent diabetes and multiple sclerosis are associated with specific HLA alleles or haplotypes. These associations are usually measured as a relative risk on the basis of two samples, a disease and a control sample, where determination of an appropriate control sample may be a difficult task. In contrast to this classical approach, the so-called haplotype relative risk (HRR) statistic does not require a control sample but uses an "internal" control (Rubinstein et al. 1981; Falk and Rubinstein 1987). In this method, the parental alleles transmitted to an affected offspring are compared with those not transmitted. The unit of observation is then a single affected offspring. The HRR statistic has different statistical properties than the usual relative risk based on two independent samples (Ott 1989a). In practice, one may often have more than a single affected offspring, but the statistical properties of the HRR statistic have not been worked out for these cases and the method may be difficult to extend to more than one affected offspring.

11.5. Candidate Loci

Candidate loci are genes that, for some a priori reason, have been implicated as possible causes of a disease; for example, their function may be suggestive of their being involved in the disease etiology. Usually, candidate loci are the first loci with which linkage analysis is carried out in the attempt to map a given diease. Only rarely, however, has this approach uncovered a disease linkage. Examples of successfully applied candidate loci are the nerve growth factor receptor and neurofibromatosis (Seizinger et al. 1987); a collagen gene, *COL2A1* on chromosome 12, which was implicated as a candidate gene for familial osteoarthrosis (Palotie et al. 1989); and the prion protein *PRIP* on the tip of the short arm of chromosome 20, which was suspected to be the cause of Gerstmann-Sträussler syndrome (Hsiao et al. 1989). Sometimes, investigators feel that the prior probability of linkage is larger for candidate genes than just for any marker gene so that a lower critical lod score than 3 should be allowed as proof for linkage. Although this reasoning appears sound, the relatively poor record of the candidate gene approach suggests that the increase in prior probability of linkage is rather modest and does not warrant a strong deviation from the classical critical lod score level of 3.

In linkage analyses with candidate genes, one is often interested in knowing how many meioses one must investigate to *dis*prove that a particular candidate gene is the real disease-causing gene? Throughout this section, assume that you have phase-known matings such that recombinations and nonrecombinations can be scored in the offspring. Disproving a candidate gene then amounts to finding an obligate recombinant. Further assume that the true recombination fraction is equal to $r = \frac{1}{2}$. What number n_1 of recombination events does one have to inspect such that, with probability P, that number will contain at least one recombination? By the binomial formula, one has $P = 1 - (\frac{1}{2})^{n_1}$, or

$$n_1 = \frac{\log(1 - P)}{\log(\frac{1}{2})}.$$

For probabilities $P = 0.95$ and 0.99, one has $n_1 = 4$ and 7, respectively. Furthermore, as given by the mean of the geometric waiting time distribution (Elandt-Johnson 1971), one will on average have to inspect two nonrecombinants before the first recombinant is found.

One may not want to reject a candidate gene based on only a single recombination but may want to see at least two recombinations before excluding a candidate gene. Under absence of linkage, the probability of finding two or more recombinations is given by $P = 1 - (\frac{1}{2})^{n_2}(1 + n_2)$. This equation cannot be solved directly for n_2, but the following equation provides an iterative solution:

$$n_2 = \frac{\log(1 - P) - \log(1 + n_2)}{\log(\frac{1}{2})}.$$

For $P = 0.95$ and 0.99, $n_2 = 8$ and 10, respectively. On average, under absence of linkage, four recombination events must be investigated before the second recombination is found (mean of negative binomial distribution; Elandt-Johnson 1971).

As another criterion for excluding a candidate gene, one may want to require the observation of as many recombination events as necessary so the expected lod score at a given value of θ falls below the classical boundary of -2. As long as only nonrecombinants are seen, the lod scores will be positive. So, this criterion can be applied only when at least one recombination has already been observed. The expected lod score is then equal to $-\infty$ at $\theta = 0$ and rises to perhaps positive values for larger θ values. At a given value of θ, assuming absence of linkage, the expected lod score for a single opportunity for recombination is equal to $\frac{1}{2}[\log(2 - 2\theta) + \log(2\theta)]$. The condition that the expected lod score should be equal to or less than -2 is thus given by the inequality $(n/2)\log[4\theta(1 - \theta)] \leq -2$ or

$$n \geq -4/\log[4\theta(1 - \theta)].$$

For $\theta = 0.01, 0.05$, and 0.10, the corresponding values of n are $3, 6$, and 9, respectively. The preceding results suggest that fewer than ten meioses have to be looked at to be able to reject a candidate gene in the absence of linkage.

When nothing but nonrecombinants are being observed, one may wonder how many offspring must be investigated to be able to *prove* linkage to a candidate gene. In table 5.8, it was shown that, under a true recombination fraction of $r = 0.01$, $n = 16$ recombination events are required to obtain a maximum lod score of 3 with power of 90 percent. In other words, if one has a candidate gene, $n = 16$ recombination events provide good power to prove linkage ($r \ll \frac{1}{2}$). However, to show that one has a candidate gene requires more than that—one must show that the confidence interval for r is restricted to small values. Assume that one observes only nonrecombinants. The estimate of the recombination fraction is then zero and the $100(1 - \alpha)$ percent confidence interval ranges from 0 through $\theta = 1 - \alpha^{1/n}$ (section 3.6). Solving its upper bound for n leads to

$$n = \frac{\log(\alpha)}{\log(1 - \theta)},$$

which is the number of nonrecombinants required so that the $100(1 - \alpha)$ percent confidence interval for r extends from 0 through θ. For a small confidence interval (low value of θ), a large number of observations are required. Specifically, for $\theta = 0.01, 0.05$, and 0.10, the respective numbers $n = 298, 59$, and 29 are required.

11.6. Exclusion Mapping

In the search for a disease gene on the human genome, "negative" information is useful because it narrows the region of the genome possibly containing the gene. (Criteria for excluding candidate loci were discussed in the previous section.) Classically, for two loci, those values of θ, at which the lod score is less than or equal to -2, are considered excluded. (A lod score of -2 corresponds to a likelihood ratio of $1:100$.) The same criterion is also applied to the multipoint lod score in linkage analysis of a disease versus a map of markers. After negative linkage analyses of a disease with a set of markers, there are thus regions of exclusion around the markers; if markers on a chromosome are rather closely spaced, the region of exclusion may eventually be continuous along the whole chromosome if the disease locus is not on that chromosome. The exclusion criterion of $Z \leq -2$ is quite stringent, so linkage analyses tend to furnish small regions of exclusion, which are unlikely to contain the disease locus (a small probability for the disease to be in the excluded region remains).

In this classical approach, the exclusion criterion is always the same no matter how many markers have been investigated. A different approach makes use of the fact that a gene excluded from one region must have a higher probability of being in another region of the genome (Edwards 1987), provided that the phenotype used for mapping is indeed due to a single gene (or perhaps a small number of genes). Initially, one may assume that the disease has an equal prior probability of being in any interval of a given size. Each linkage analysis then modifies this prior density of disease location, resulting in a posterior density. The EXCLUDE program (available from Dr. J. H. Edwards) implements this approach for two-point analyses and graphically presents the likely disease locations. Researchers may then work with markers located in areas most likely to contain the disease gene.

Several examples of successful applications of exclusion mapping exist, the most recent one being that of Marfan's syndrome (Kainulainen et al. 1990). For *heterogeneous traits*, exclusion mapping is somewhat problematic. Assume that a small proportion of the families investigated segregate a gene located on the map of markers under study but the overall lod score (summed over families assuming homogeneity) is smaller than -2 at each point on the map. If exclusion is based on the total lod score, a true disease location will be excluded. A possible solution is to estimate the proportion α of families in which the disease gene is linked to a given region of the genome (estimates will often be $\hat{\alpha} = 0$), jointly with the map position x of that gene. A disease gene should then be excluded from a map only when the families appear to be homogeneous. Good evidence for heterogeneity, however, indicates that in some of the families there is a gene located on the map under study. For detecting linkage under heterogeneity, the requirements for significance were discussed in the third to last paragraph of section 9.3. Applying the same stringent criteria for significance when excluding linkage tends to exclude true locations of disease genes. Hence, for exclusion mapping under heterogeneity, a better approach is to apply less stringent criteria, for example, to declare heterogeneity significant (thus allowing for the presence of a disease gene) with a p-value of 0.01 or a likelihood ratio of 100:1. In practice, this means that one evaluates $Z(\hat{\alpha}, x)$ at each map position, x, where $\hat{\alpha}$ is determined by the maximum of $Z(\alpha, x)$ at the given x value. Only those points x are then excluded for which $Z(\hat{\alpha}, x) < 2$ and $Z(x) < -2$.

A partly nonparametric approach to exclusion mapping under possible heterogeneity via the exclusion of certain IBD probabilities was referred to above (Hyer et al. 1991; see section 11.3).

11.7. Genetic Risks

A genetic risk may be defined as the probability (usually conditional on observations on relatives) that an individual will develop a genetically inherited trait. For mendelian traits, the genetic risk is the conditional probability that an individual has the disease-predisposing genotype, given his or her phenotype and other family information, notably phenotypes at marker loci. The *proband* or counselee is the individual for whom risk is calculated.

For complex traits (exact mode of inheritance unknown), risks have to be based largely on empirically obtained estimates of recurrence risks (Murphy and Chase 1975; Vogel and Motulsky 1986), but various statistical problems make empirical risk estimation difficult (Chakraborty 1987). In this section, genetic risks are restricted to mendelian traits and risks will be calculated parametrically on the basis of a known model of disease inheritance.

As an introduction to the concept of genetic risk, consider the CK values mentioned in section 11.2 and denote a carrier by C and a noncarrier by N. If one distinguishes only between low (L) and high (H) values and the 95th percentile of the normal range is taken as a cutoff point, with probability $P(H|N) = 0.05$ a noncarrier woman has a high CK value. On the other hand, women carrying a DMD allele have elevated CK levels with probability $P(H|C) \approx 2/3$ (Vogel and Motulsky 1986). If a woman randomly drawn from the population shows an elevated CK value, what is her probability of being a carrier? By Bayes theorem, as introduced in section 3.7,

$$P(C|H) = \frac{P(H|C) \cdot P(C)}{P(H|C)P(C) + P(H|N)P(N)}, \tag{11.6}$$

where $p = P(C) = 1 - P(N)$ is the proportion of carriers in the population and $P(C|H)$ is the woman's risk of being a carrier given her CK status. With the values for $P(H|C)$ and $P(H|N)$ given above, the risk (11.6) becomes $2/3p/[2/3p + 0.05(1 - p)] = p/(0.075 + 0.925p)$. Since $p \ll 0.075$ (see below), $0.925p$ is negligibly small and the woman's risk is approximately $13p$, that is, thirteen times the population prevalence.

For mendelian traits, in which no direct molecular or cytogenetic test for the disease gene is available, risks are usually determined via a closely linked marker. For single individuals, allowing for allelic association may improve the accuracy of genotype predictions. For example, an unaffected individual has a probability of 0.0392 of being a carrier of the CF allele, but the analogous probability for an individual with the BB marker genotype is 0.199, approximately five times the population risk (Beaudet et al. 1989; see also table 11.2).

In family data, the risk to a proband may sometimes be calculated analytically. For example, consider the family shown in figure 4.1, in which the linkage relationship between Charcot-Marie-Tooth disease (CMT1) and ABO blood type is investigated. The same family was also analyzed for CMT1 versus the Duffy blood group (FY) (Dyck et al. 1983). The father (individual 3.1) was doubly heterozygous with known phase, Db/da, where D is the disease allele and a and b are the relevant two Duffy alleles. He had passed the disease allele and the Duffy b allele to each of his four offspring, so these were all nonrecombinants. Assume now that a newly born child (not shown in figure 4.1) has received the Duffy allele a from his father. What is this proband's risk of having inherited the disease allele D from his father? Given that the father passes an a allele to the proband, he transmits a D allele with probability θ and a d allele with probability $1 - \theta$. Hence, the risk to the proband is equal to the recombination fraction, $R = \theta$. Usually, the recombination fraction is not known with certainty but is known only as a more or less precise estimate around which one constructs a confidence or support interval for the true recombination fraction (section 4.4). In this case, obviously, the risk estimate is as precise as $\hat{\theta}$ is, so the support interval for θ also applies to the risk R.

There has been some debate as to whether it is meaningful to compute support intervals for genetic risks R (A. W. F. Edwards 1989). R is a probability just as is, for example, the proportion α of the linked family type in a mixture of linked and unlinked families (section 9.4), and for this and other proportions it is customary to compute support or confidence intervals. There is thus no reason why support intervals should not also be constructed for genetic risks. Knowing the support interval for a genetic risk will enable a genetic counselor to see how much faith he or she should have in the point estimate R. Of course, since it is often difficult to convey even the notion of a risk to a counselee, the concept of a support interval for the true risk is more difficult to grasp still and may best be avoided in genetic counseling sessions.

Consider again the pedigree of figure 4.1 with FY genotypes as discussed above. Assume that the grandparents are unavailable so that the phase in the father is unknown. What, then, is the risk to the proband, who received the Duffy a allele from the father? This problem is more difficult to solve by hand than the previous one. Its solution is demonstrated below as an example of how some computer programs calculate risks. In practice, a problem of this difficulty would not be solved by hand but with a computer program such as MLINK. The reader who is not interested in the mathematical derivation of a complicated risk may simply skip the next paragraph.

A general expression for genetic risks in pedigree data is

$$R = P(g|F) = P(F, g)/ \sum_h P(F, h) \qquad (11.7)$$

(Elston and Stewart 1971), where F stands for the pedigree data and g is the proband's genotype whose conditional probability is to be determined. $P(F, g)$ is the probability (likelihood) of the individuals' phenotypes and that the proband has genotype g. In the present case, let $g = D$ denote the situation that the proband receives the disease allele from the father and $g = d$ that he receives the normal allele, these two cases being the only possible ones. Considering the two phases in the father, the pedigree likelihood is obtained as $P(F, g = D) = (1 - \theta)^4\theta + (1 - \theta)\theta^4$, since under the first phase four offspring are nonrecombinants and the proband is a recombinant, and the situation is reversed for the second phase. Each phase has probability of occurrence of ½, but this term is left off as it will cancel in numerator and denominator. Similarly, $P(F, g = d) = (1 - \theta)^5 + \theta^5$. The risk of having received the D allele is then obtained from (11.7) as $R = P(F, g = D)/[P(F, g = D) + P(F, g = d)]$, which is a complicated expression in θ. Numerical evaluation shows that R is close to θ, for example, $R = 0.202$ for $\theta = 0.20$.

Kinship L, shown in figure 4.1, is one of a number of pedigrees forming a mixture of linked and unlinked families with respect to CMT1 and the Duffy locus (section 9.4). In such a situation, one may calculate a risk R_L assuming a proband's family is of the linked type and a risk R_U given that the family is of the unlinked type (generally one may have more than two types). When $R_L \approx R_U$ one does not need to go any further. If the two risks are quite different, one will in many cases recognize from the linkage analysis which of the risks is the more plausible figure. A possible rigorous statistical solution consists of calculating the overall risk as a weighted average of R_L and R_U (Weeks and Ott 1989). As an example, if the mixture analysis (e.g., furnished by the HOMOG program) yields an estimate $\hat{\theta} = 0.05$ for the recombination fraction in the linked families, the risk for the hypothetical new offspring in family L discussed above is $R_L = 0.05$ when the family is of the linked type and $R_U = 0.50$ when it is of the unlinked type. The overall risk estimate is

$$R_w = wR_L + (1 - w)R_U, \tag{11.8}$$

where w is the conditional probability that the proband's family is of the linked type. The estimated value of w may be calculated using equation (9.11); it is also furnished by the HOMOG program. For the given family, for example, at $\theta = 0.05$ and $\alpha = 0.65$, one finds $w = 0.92$ so that $R_w = 0.92 \times 0.05 + 0.08 \times 0.50 = 0.086$. A support interval for R_w would be based on the support interval of the estimated parameters, α and θ. Each pair (α, θ) inside the support region is associated with a value of R_w. Scanning a large number of pairs (α, θ) will yield a range of R_w values whose endpoints define the desired support interval.

For X-linked lethal recessive traits, the prior probability that a woman with no information about her male relatives is carrying a disease allele is equal to $q = 4\mu$ (Murphy and Chase 1975), where μ is the mutation rate.

This implies that a woman with one affected son has posterior probability $\frac{2}{3}$ of being a carrier and $\frac{1}{3}$ of not carrying the disease allele (Murphy and Chase 1975). This result is sometimes phrased as "one third of all cases are new mutations" while, of course, $\frac{1}{3}$ of the isolated cases only are new mutations. Also, under equilibrium, the gene frequency is equal to 3μ (Haldane 1935). In most computer programs, q depends on the population frequency p of the disease allele, $q = 2p(1 - p)$. Therefore, in these programs, one should not use p as the gene frequency but rather use p to set the appropriate prior carrier probability. In other words, one should choose p such that $2p(1 - p) = q$ or $p \approx \frac{1}{2}q = 2\mu$ with the mutation rate generally being in the order of $\mu = 10^{-5} = 0.00001$ (e.g., for Duchenne's muscular dystrophy (Cavalli-Sforza and Bodmer 1971).

It was mentioned in section 11.2 that the CK value of a woman can discriminate between carriers and noncarriers of the DMD gene. For this reason, CK values are used in genetic counseling. The most reliable procedure is to use the actually measured CK levels in the linkage analysis and to have good estimates for means and variances for obligate carriers and noncarriers. As a shortcut, researchers sometimes use a cutoff value, which distinguishes only normal and abnormal levels (see section 11.2). This obviates the need for specifying means and variances but is less precise than using actual CK levels.

Often, one is interested in knowing what risks might be expected before marker typing is carried out. In simple situations, hand calculations can provide the answer (Ott et al. 1990b). A more complicated example in which all possible risks can be enumerated and evaluated by computer was demonstrated in section 8.4. In most applications, however, risk distributions before marker typing must be approximated by computer simulation (Sandkuyl and Ott 1989). Briefly, given the disease status for family members at some mendelian disease locus and parameter values such as recombination fraction and gene frequencies, marker genotypes are randomly generated, which is repeated for many replicates. For each replicate, the risk to the proband is computed as if the marker genotypes had actually been observed. The resulting distribution of risks can then be represented as a histogram and risks R may be classified into informative and uninformative, where, for example, risks $R > 0.90$ and $R < 0.10$ may be called informative. The proportion of informative risks may be taken as a measure for the probability of successful counseling of the family at hand.

One might expect that theoretical risk distributions obtained before marker typing should be symmetric about 50 percent. Experience with testing for Huntington's disease (autosomal dominant) shows, however, that in many cases the risk distribution is strongly skewed towards low risk figures. Three major reasons account for this skewness: (1) Probands are often already far past the age of onset, yet are still unaffected. Hence, their risk of carrying the disease allele is less than 50 percent. (2) Genetic testing is carried out as so-called nondisclosure or nondisclosing testing (Folstein 1989), in which the proband has a risk of 50 percent or ≈ 0 percent, depending on whether the relevant gene marker was obtained from the affected or unaffected grandparent. Nondisclosure testing of a proband child is either voluntary (the unaffected parent at risk, who is potentially a carrier of the disease gene, does not want to be tested) or the consequence of insufficient information (parent at risk is uninformative for linkage). (3) Consider a mother at risk and two offspring. Of these, one is affected and the other (the proband) is unaffected. The mother is not tested and is thus not known a priori to be heterozygous. To recognize unequivocally that she is heterozygous for the marker and thus informative for linkage, one must know that the two children have received two different marker alleles from the mother. With close linkage, this situation leads either to a low risk to the proband (when the mother is heterozygous) or to a risk in the neighborhood of 50 percent (when the mother is not known to be heterozygous). An example may be found in Ott et al. (1990b).

The population-genetic consequences of genetic testing and selective abortion were long ago well investigated (Crow 1966; Motulsky, Fraser, and Felsenstein 1971). Prospects for extensive screening of all newborns for many disease genes were discussed by Vogel and Motulsky (1986, 628–29) and in chapter 4 of *Mapping Our Genes* (U.S. Congress OTA 1988). The possibility of predicting one's genetic fate at birth, envisioned more than sixty years ago by Haldane (reprinted 1985), may well have a strong influence on society, which I briefly discussed elsewhere (Ott 1990a).

11.8. Irregular Segregation

In most linkage analyses, regular mendelian inheritance is taken for granted. Sometimes, however, unusual inheritance patterns cast doubt on the mode of inheritance assumed. This section briefly points out some of these irregular segregation patterns and discusses their effect on linkage analysis. Recognition of many cases of special segregation has become possible only with the advent of molecular genetic techniques and has had a lasting effect on linkage analysis.

For a parent with marker genotype *1/2*, one expects half of the children to receive the *1* allele and half to receive the *2* allele. Segregation of the alleles deviating markedly from the 1:1 ratio has no effect on the estimate of the recombination fraction but should make investigators alert to possible errors in the data, such as sample mix-ups.

As mentioned in section 1.3, disease alleles are, for some conditions, preferentially received from the father or from the mother, which represents a form of genomic imprinting (Hall 1990). As long as one recognizes unequivocally which parent passed the disease allele(s) to the·children, this is analogous to skewed segregation (discussed in the previous paragraph) and has no negative effect on linkage analysis. Similarly, for some disorders, new mutations tend to originate preferentially in a male or a female. A recent investigation of fourteen families with a new mutation of neurofibromatosis (Jadayel et al. 1990) showed that the mutation originated in a male in twelve families and in a female in only two families.

While skewed segregation may be unlikely, it belongs to the realm of mendelian inheritance. Other segregation patterns, however, do not. For example, cases of uniparental disomy have been reported—both chromosomes of a pair were received from the same parent (Engel 1980). A recent example of such a case is a boy with cystic fibrosis, who evidently had received both his entire chromosomes no. 7 from his mother (Voss et al. 1989). Obviously, such phenomena can lead linkage analysis astray.

Another serious problem in linkage analysis is mosaicism. Consider a mother with a large number of offspring, two of whom are affected with a dominant disease. Explaining the two affecteds as two independent mutations is unsatisfactory as it has very low probability. A more plausible interpretation is germline mosaicism, also called gonadal or germinal mosaicism (Murphy and Chase 1975; J. H. Edwards 1989b), which postulates that one mutation has occurred during the formation of the germ cells so that a germline mosaic produces mutant and nonmutant gametes. Mosaicism has long been considered as a potential factor in linkage analysis (Bell and Haldane 1937), but only recently has it become possible to document clearly the rather widespread occurrence of germline mosaicism and similar phenomena. An interesting case was reported by Hendriks et al. (1989). They identified a healthy male as the source of three gametes with an agammaglobulinemia disease allele, although men with this gene are generally severely affected. Unrecognized mosaicism may be confused with genetic heterogeneity, and this can have a devastating effect on linkage analysis. Also, it may lead to wrong estimates of genetic risks. Linkage programs currently do not routinely allow for germline mosaicism. Its effect may be reduced by allowing for a rather high mutation rate, but the safest solution is to trace the origin of each chromosome as best as one can.

11.9. Planning a Linkage Analysis

Assume that you set out to find the gene locus of a particular disease. Here is a brief list of the steps you will have to take. One of the first tasks is to get a good picture of the properties of the disease—its phenotype, mode of inheritance, population frequency, etc. Also, find out what has already been published regarding linkage analysis with the disease.

If the phenotype is quantitative (e.g., if it consists of enzyme activity levels), their distributions will presumably differ in their means (and perhaps variances) depending on the genotypes of individuals. As an example, arylsulfatase A activity strongly depends on the genotype (Hohenschutz et al. 1989). At this locus, genotypes can be recognized directly so that there is no need to work with activity levels for linkage analysis. In many cases, however, gene carriers and noncarriers cannot be told apart unequivocally. Then, an analysis of a mixture of distributions is required and may be carried out with the NOCOM program (section 8.5).

You may want to estimate the number of families required to find linkage to a hypothetical marker. In terms of phase-known meioses (opportunities for recombination, offspring scorable for recombinations), $n = 20$ meioses is a reasonable number (section 5.10, table 5.8). Various complicating factors may now translate this figure into a higher number of family members. Unknown phase adds one offspring (more for loose linkage) to each sibship (section 5.8). Marker heterozygosity determines the frequency with which a parent is potentially informative for linkage. As a rough adjustment for less than 100 percent marker informativeness, the number of families required is multiplied by the inverse of the marker's heterozygosity.

Other factors reducing informativeness may be taken into account using the various tables in which ELODs or variances have been calculated. Note, however, that the adjustments to the numbers of observations based on these tables are very approximate, since the tables were calculated for a specific mating type and would presumably be somewhat different for other mating types. With incomplete penetrance, n must be multiplied by the inverse of the relative ELOD (section 7.2); with an average penetrance of 50 percent, a threefold number of offspring is required (table 7.2). Heterogeneity also reduces informativeness and may be allowed for by further multiplying the number of offspring by the inverse of the relative efficiency (ratio of variances). As a rough guideline, table 9.7 provides standard errors for θ estimates in a specific family type. As an example, when 20 percent of families are of the unlinked type ($\alpha = 0.80$), with $\theta = 0.05$, the number of offspring must be multiplied by the inverse of the ratio of the variances, that is, by $(0.075/0.042)^2 = 3.2$. Errors in marker typing may be allowed for under a simple misclassification model (section 10.2). Table 10.3 lists the corresponding relative ELODs. For example, with $\theta = 0.05$ and a misclassification rate of $s = 0.05$, the number of offspring has to be increased by a factor of $1/0.77 = 1.3$. In summary, for example, the original number of twenty meioses is increased to $20 \times 3 \times 3.2 \times 1.3 \approx 250$ meioses by a penetrance of 50 percent, a proportion of linked families of 80 percent, and a misclassification rate of 5 percent.

The complicating factors mentioned above have been assumed to be known. In reality, they have to be estimated, which further requires some increase in the number of observations. Other factors will also play a role. For example, family members may be unwilling to cooperate or some cell lines may not grow.

A more specific determination of the number of families required is possible on the basis of a sample of families already collected. Assume that a preliminary assessment of affection status has been made on the family members and that you would like to know the expected lod score for the family data at hand. Computer simulation methods are now the standard technique to approximate the ELOD before marker typing (see section 8.7). With the use of computer programs, genotypes for a hypothetical marker linked with the disease gene are randomly generated into your family members and analyzed as if they had been observed. If your families furnish an ELOD of 0.75, you will need approximately four times as many families of the same structure to obtain an ELOD of 3.

Genetic marker data for your family members may be obtained through collaboration with a molecular geneticist. One of the first steps in the analysis will be to scrutinize the data for genetic consistency. The best method to verify paternity and other relationships is to use one of the highly polymorphic probes ("molecular fingerprinting," see section 2.5). Carrying out two-point analyses between the disease and each of the markers may also point out genetic inconsistencies, which are often caused by laboratory errors.

Some marker systems such as HLA are so polymorphic that, in the linkage program, specifying a large number of alleles creates problems. A first step towards ameliorating the situation is to allow for only as many alleles as one encounters in the families analyzed plus one allele, which collectively stands for all the unobserved alleles. An additional reduction in the number of alleles may be achieved by using the same allele number for different alleles in different portions of a family while retaining knowledge of the path of alleles from parents to offspring (Ott 1978). For example, when two parents and a child have the respective genotypes *1/2*, *3/4*, and *1/3* and the child is married to an individual with genotype *5/6*, allele number *5* may be replaced by *2* and *6* by *4* in that spouse's genotype and in his or her offspring's genotypes. Additional recoding schemes were described by Lange and Weeks (1989). All of these techniques are designed to reduce computing time while leading to the same results as obtained with the unmodified data. Simply lumping several alleles into one will also reduce the number of alleles but tends to reduce heterozygosity and thus informativeness as well.

It will often be important to know the phase of a doubly heterozygous individual. Marker and disease phenotypes may be able to identify phase unequivocally. If not, nonstatistical methods have occasionally been used to determine phase. One may be able to separate the two chromosomes by somatic cell genetic methods (Zoghbi et al. 1989) or by the PCR technique (Jeffreys, Neumann, and Wilson 1990; Ruano, Kidd, and Stephens 1990).

When "high-density" pedigrees (with a large number of affected individuals) are collected, estimating penetrances from the pedigree data is bound to furnish high values. In the absence of good estimates, one possibility is to try a limited number of reasonable-appearing values or simply to work with a penetrance of, say, 0.5 for susceptible genotypes.

In the analysis, it will be important to allow for errors that are known from experience to occur. Such errors might be misreading of alleles in marker typing or changes of disease diagnostic state over time. They may be taken into account via incomplete penetrance models.

Problems

Problem 11.1. In section 11.2, 70 percent of obligate carriers of the X-linked recessive Duchenne's muscular dystrophy (DMD) gene are said to have CK values above the 95th percentile of the normal range. Taking that 95th percentile as a cutoff point to distinguish between low and high CK values, set up the penetrance model for the various male and female DMD phenotypes, assuming that genotypes cannot be identified by DNA analysis. Note: disregard female homozygous carriers.

Problem 11.2. Consider two (unaffected) parents who had a child affected with cystic fibrosis, which has passed away. The wife is pregnant again, and marker typing with the haplotypes *A* through *D* (table 11.2) has been carried out. The father is *BC*, the mother *AB*, and the fetus is *BB*. What is the risk to the fetus of being affected with cystic fibrosis (1) without knowledge of marker types and (2) with the given marker types? For simplicity, assume zero recombination among the loci.

Problem 11.3. Consider a healthy male, who had a sister with cystic fibrosis. His sister as well as his parents are no longer alive. (1) What is his risk of being a carrier for the disease allele? (2) He was tested for the most common disease-causing mutation (ΔF_{508}) and turned out to be negative. That mutation is known to occur on 75 percent of the CF chromosomes, and 25 percent of chromosomes carrying a CF gene do not show the mutation. What is now his risk of carrying a cystic fibrosis gene?

Problem 11.4. Assume two loci with two alleles each. What is the highest possible value of the linkage disequilibrium parameter *D* for the two loci?

Problem 11.5. Assume that the two loci in problem 11.4 are unlinked but that in the current generation a disequilibrium of $D = 0.18$ exists. How many generations does it take for the disequilibrium to be smaller than 0.10? After how many generations will it be zero?

Solutions to Study Problems

Solution 1.1. One proceeds as shown in section 1.4 for the Haldane mapping function. From (1.3) one finds $x_{12} = \frac{1}{4} \ln[(1 + 2\theta_{12})/(1 - 2\theta_{12})]$ and the analogous expression for x_{23}. The sum, $x_{12} + x_{23}$, is obtained as $\frac{1}{4} \ln\{(1 + 2\theta_{12})(1 + 2\theta_{23})/[(1 - 2\theta_{12})(1 - 2\theta_{23})]\}$ and represents the map distance between loci *1* and *3*. The corresponding recombination fraction is obtained by substituting $x_{12} + x_{23}$ for x in the inverse of (1.3) so that, with $\exp[4(x_{12} + x_{23})] = (1 + 2\theta_{12})(1 + 2\theta_{23})/[(1 - 2\theta_{12})(1 - 2\theta_{23})]$, one obtains $\theta_{13} = (\theta_{12} + \theta_{23})/(1 + 4\theta_{12}\theta_{23})$.

Solution 1.2. In analogy to the previous problem, one finds $x_{12} + x_{23} = [\frac{1}{2}/(2 - k)] \ln\{[1 + 2\theta_{12}(2 - k)/(1 - 2\theta_{12})][1 + 2\theta_{23}(2 - k)/(1 - 2\theta_{23})]\}$ and $\exp[2(x_{12} + x_{23})(2 - k)] = [1 + 2\theta_{12}(2 - k)/(1 - 2\theta_{12})][1 + 2\theta_{23}(2 - k)/(1 - 2\theta_{23})]$. A somewhat lengthy calculation then leads to $\theta_{13} = (\theta_{12} + \theta_{23} - 2k\theta_{12}\theta_{23})/[1 + 4(1 - k)\theta_{12}\theta_{23}]$. Solving this expression for the interference parameter yields $k = [\theta_{12} + \theta_{23} - \theta_{13}(1 + 4\theta_{12}\theta_{23})]/[2\theta_{12}\theta_{23}(1 - 2\theta_{13})]$.

Solution 1.3. The map distances in the three intervals are calculated as 0.14, 0.04, and 0.19 Morgans (Haldane), which are expressed in terms of recombination fractions 0.1221, 0.0384, and 0.1581 (perhaps obtained using the MAPFUN program). These recombination fractions are then converted to map distances in Kosambi-Morgans: 0.1246, 0.0385, and 0.1637. From these interval widths, the map positions of the four loci are obtained as 0, 0.1246, 0.1631, and 0.3268 Morgans (Kosambi) or, approximately, as 0, 12, 16, and 33 cM (Kosambi).

Solution 1.4. Under complete interference, there is at most one crossover. Assuming that there is always one crossover, half the strands (chromatids) are recombinant and half are nonrecombinant. According to the definition of map distance, therefore, the expected number of crossovers per strand is equal to $\frac{1}{2}$.

Solution 2.1. Subtracting equation (2.4) from (2.2) yields $(n - 1)/n^3$ as the difference between H and PIC. The inequality, $(n - 1)/n^3 < 0.01$ leads to a cubic equation which, after rearranging terms, may be solved iteratively as $n = [(n - 1)/0.01]^{1/3}$. The solution is 9.46, that is, with $n \geq 10$ equally frequent alleles, the difference between H and PIC is smaller than 0.01.

Solution 2.2. If markers were equally spaced, ten markers would be sufficient because the distance between adjacent markers would be 10 cM; thus, any new locus is never more than 5 cM away from the nearest marker. With random placement of markers, equation (2.5) with $L = 100$, $d = 5$, and $P = 0.95$ must be used. The result is $n \approx 29$ markers.

Solution 3.1. Based on the phenotype, the genotype must contain at least one A allele. If one of the parents has phenotype A$-$ (genotype a/a), that tells us that a child with phenotype A$+$ must have genotype A/a.

Solution 3.2. Each parent has two possible genotypes, A/A with conditional probability $p^2/[p^2 + 2p(1 - p)] = p/(2 - p)$ and A/a with conditional probability $1 - p/(2 - p) = 2(1 - p)/(2 - p)$. For each of the $2 \times 2 = 4$ possible genotypic matings of mother and father, it is easy to determine the probability of their having an A$+$ child. All matings, except $A/a \times A/a$, produce only A$+$ children. For the $A/a \times A/a$ mating, whose probability of occurrence is $[2(1 - p)/(2 - p)]^2$, the probability of an A$-$ child (a/a genotype) is equal to $\frac{1}{4}$. Hence, the parents have an A$+$ child with probability $Q = 1 - (\frac{1}{4})[2(1 - p)/(2 - p)]^2 = (3 - 2p)/(2 - p)^2$. This probability tends to 1 as $p \to 1$ (the parents are both A/A) and tends to $\frac{3}{4}$ as $p \to 0$ (the parents are both A/a).

The answer to the second question is No, Q does not necessarily stay the same but may vary with the phenotypes of the children already born. Since the parental genotypes are unknown, offspring phenotypes may give clues as to what the parents' genotypes are. For example, if the first child has phenotype A$-$, this will identify both parental genotypes as A/a; therefore, the second child (and each later child) has probability $\frac{3}{4}$ of being A$+$, which is different from Q unless $p = 0$.

Solution 3.3. Both L_1 and L_2 are correct likelihoods, but they refer to different sampling frames. L_1 is calculated for given birth order of the children, which is customary in human linkage analysis, as it is customary to calculate pedigree likelihoods for given sex of the pedigree members. L_2 refers to an event that comprises three different birth orders, each of which has likelihood L_1. In calculations of likelihoods with respect to recombination fractions, one could use either L_1 or L_2. The constant factor between L_1 and L_2 cancels in the likelihood ratio usually formed.

Solution 3.4. Following formula $1 - \alpha^{1/n}$, with $n = 10$ and $\alpha = 0.10$, one finds a confidence interval of $(0, 0.206)$.

Solution 4.1. Yes, one should. However, in this case, the grandparental mating is a phase-unknown double backcross with only one offspring. Hence, there is no information for linkage from that generation.

Solution 4.2. (1a) With $k = 1$ and $n = 5$, one has $\hat{\theta} = 1/5 = 0.20$. (1b) For unknown phase, the adjusted likelihood is $L^*(\theta) = 16[\theta(1 - \theta)^4 + \theta^4(1 - \theta)]$. Numerical evaluation of it with an accuracy of two decimal places in θ shows that its maximum, 1.3333, occurs at $\hat{\theta} = 0.21$. (2a) $\hat{\theta} = 1/4 = 0.25$. (2b) $L^*(\theta) = 8[\theta(1 - \theta)^3 + \theta^3(1 - \theta)]$ turns out to rise from 0 at $\theta = 0$ to a maximum at $\theta = \frac{1}{2}$ so that the estimate of the recombination fraction is $\hat{\theta} = \frac{1}{2}$.

Solution 4.3. The power of H_0 versus H_1 is given by $(1 - \theta)^{15}$. With $\theta = 0.01$, this yields a value of 0.86. For H_0 versus H_2, the power is given by $(1 - \theta_m)^7(1 - \theta_f)^6[1 + 7\theta_m(1 - 2\theta_f) + 6\theta_f]$. For $\theta = \theta_m = \theta_f$, this reduces to $(1 - \theta)^{14}(1 + 14\theta)$ and, with $\theta = 0.01$, results in 0.99.

Solution 4.4. For k recombinants in $n = 20$ meioses, Z_{max} is given by equation (4.11) and the upper bound to the significance level is given by $p_u = 10^{-Z_{max}}$ (4.10). The actual significance level p can be obtained using the BINOM program. One obtains the following results:

k	Z_{max}	p_u	p
1	4.30	0.00005	0.00002
2	3.20	0.0006	0.0002
3	2.35	0.0045	0.0013
4	1.67	0.0212	0.0059
5	1.14	0.0731	0.0207

Solution 4.5. Sometimes, people are impressed by the strongly negative lod score. However, since it occurs at $\theta = 0$, the unspectacular inter-

pretation of this finding goes as follows. One or more known recombinants lead to a lod score of $-\infty$ at $\theta = 0$. A strongly negative lod score at $\theta = 0$ implies that almost certainly there was at least one recombinant in the data, but one cannot tell for certain, perhaps as a consequence of incomplete penetrance.

Solution 5.1. Parent 1 can produce only two types of gametes, *A1* and *B1*, with probability ½ each, since of the four possible gametes two each are undistinguishable. Analogously, parent 2 potentially produces gametes *C1* and *C2* with probability ½ each, since the two *C* cannot be distinguished. There are then four offspring genotypes, *A1/C1*, *A1/C2*, *B1/C1*, and *B1/C2*, with probabilities of occurrence of ¼ each. These probabilities do not contain θ (or r) so that no information on the recombination fraction is available.

Solution 5.2. The crucial fact in such ascertainment problems is that the lod scores $Z(\theta)$ used after selection are the same as the ones without selection, but the class probabilities change owing to selection. When class 4 individuals are discarded, only individuals in classes 1 through 3 occur, the corresponding class probabilities being given by $f_i = p_i/(p_1 + p_2 + p_3)$, for example, $f_1 = (1 - r)^2/[1 + 2r(1 - r)]$. The expected lod score is then given by $\Sigma f_i Z_i(\theta)$. Work is simplified by omitting the "4" in each of the three lod scores—this will add a constant to the expected lod score but will not change the estimate of θ because the derivative of a constant is zero. Also, natural instead of decimal logs are preferable—this multiplies the equation by a constant factor that drops out when the derivative is set equal to zero. Once this is done, one may collect terms of θ so that the expected log likelihood is given by

$$\ln[L(\theta)] = (2f_1 + f_2)\ln(1 - \theta) + (f_2 + 2f_3)\ln(\theta).$$

The first derivative is obtained as

$$d\ln(L)/d\theta = \frac{f_2 + 2f_3}{\theta} - \frac{2f_1 + f_2}{1 - \theta}.$$

Setting this equal to zero and solving the resulting equation for θ leads to $\tilde{\theta} = \frac{1}{2}f_2 + f_3$, which is the point of θ at which the expected log likelihood, or expected lod score, has its maximum. That it is a maximum rather than a minimum may be verified by showing that the second derivative with respect to θ is negative at $\theta = \tilde{\theta}$. Substituting the f_i by the corresponding expressions in the true recombination fraction r, one finds that $\tilde{\theta} =$

$r(2 - r)/[1 + 2r(1 - r)]$, and this is larger than r except at $r = 0$ and $r = \frac{1}{2}$.

Solution 5.3. Proceeding as outlined in section 5.5, you will find that for the offspring genotypes only two distinct probabilities occur. Using the numbering scheme of table 5.3, combining phenotypes $1 + 3 + 5 + 7 + 9$ leads to a class with associated probability of $2r(1 - r)$, which is the same as the probability for one of the two classes in the phase-unknown double backcross with two offspring.

Solution 5.4. One finds the following three phenotype classes among the offspring where, for example, genotypes T/t or T/T lead to the dominant phenotype T, and q is the first derivative of p with respect to r:

Phenotype	p	q^2/p	$Z(\theta)$
T-D	$\frac{1}{4}(2 + r^2)$	$r^2/(2 + r^2)$	$\log[(4/9)(2 + \theta^2)]$
T-d, t-D	$\frac{1}{2}(1 - r^2)$	$2r^2/(1 - r^2)$	$\log[(4/3)(1 - \theta^2)]$
t-d	$\frac{1}{4}r^2$	1	$2\log(2\theta)$

	$r = 0$	0.1	0.2	0.3	0.4	0.5
$i(r)$	1	1.025	1.103	1.241	1.455	1.778
$E[Z(r)]$	0.037	0.032	0.022	0.011	0.003	0

The results presented in the preceding table show the unusual phenomenon that, for r approaching $\frac{1}{2}$, the expected lod score decreases (which is normal) while the expected information increases. Therefore, with data from this mating type, the recombination fraction estimate has smallest variance at $\theta = \frac{1}{2}$.

Solution 5.5. The second parent is $A1/A1$ or $A1/A2$ or $A2/A2$ with the respective unconditional frequencies p^2, $2p(1 - p)$, and $(1 - p)^2$. Given the first or third genotype of this parent, the ELOD is $E_1 = r\log(2r) + (1 - r)\log(2 - 2r)$. With genotype $A1/A2$, three offspring genotype classes exist, whose frequencies are $\frac{3}{4}(1 - r)$, $\frac{3}{4}r$, and $\frac{1}{4}$. The corresponding ELOD is $E_2 = \frac{3}{4}(1 - r)\log(2 - 2r) + \frac{3}{4}r\log(2r)$. The unconditional ELOD is thus obtained as $E(Z) = 2p(1 - p)E_2 + [1 - 2p(1 - p)]E_1$. This example shows a case in which gene frequencies enter the calculation of lod scores. Obviously, E_2 is smaller than E_1. The overall ELOD will be highest when the genotype $A1/A2$ of the second parent has low probability, and this is the case for small or high values of p.

Solution 5.6. Since each parent is doubly heterozygous (*1/2*, *1/2*) with unknown phase, there are four possible phase combinations, each occurring with equal probability. For each phase combination, one now has to compute the probability of the n offspring phenotypes (1/2, 1/2). For example, assuming genotypes *11/22* for both parents, one prepares a table whose marginals are given by the probabilities of the gametes (haplotypes) that each parent can produce. In the body of the table are the phenotype probabilities for one offspring.

	$P(11)$ $= \frac{1}{2}(1 - \theta)$	$P(22)$ $= \frac{1}{2}(1 - \theta)$	$P(12)$ $= \frac{1}{2}\theta$	$P(21)$ $= \frac{1}{2}\theta$
$P(11) = \frac{1}{2}(1 - \theta)$	0	$\frac{1}{2}(1 - \theta)^2$	0	0
$P(22) = \frac{1}{2}(1 - \theta)$	$\frac{1}{4}(1 - \theta)^2$	0	0	0
$P(12) = \frac{1}{2}\theta$	0	0	0	$\frac{1}{2}\theta^2$
$P(21) = \frac{1}{2}\theta$	0	0	$\frac{1}{4}\theta^2$	0

For this phase combination, the probability of a 1/2 offspring is thus $\frac{1}{2}(1 - \theta)^2 + \frac{1}{2}\theta^2$, and for n offspring it is this quantity raised to the nth power. It turns out that phase combination 12/12 × 12/12 yields the same offspring probabilities. For phase combinations 11/22 × 12/21 and 12/21 × 11/22, one finds an offspring probability of $[\theta(1 - \theta)]^n$ each. After some manipulations the likelihood ratio is then obtained as $L(\theta)/L(\frac{1}{2}) = 2^{n-1}\{[(1 - \theta)^2 + \theta^2]^n + [2\theta(1 - \theta)]^n\}$. At $\theta = 0$, this is equal to 2^{n-1}, which is equal to 1 for $n = 1$ and is larger than 1 for $n > 1$. Hence, the mating is uninformative for linkage with only one offspring but is informative for linkage with more than one offspring.

Solution 5.7. For a phase-known double backcross family of size 6, with $r = 0.10$, the calculation of $E[Z(r)] = \Sigma_k Z(k; r)P(k)$ and $E(Z_{max}) = \Sigma_k Z_{max}(k)P(k)$ proceeds as shown in the following table:

k	$Z(0.10)$	Z_{max}	$P(k)$	$Z(0.1) \times P(k)$	$Z_{max} \times P(k)$
0	1.532	1.806	0.531441	0.814	0.960
1	0.577	0.632	0.354294	0.204	0.224
2	-0.377	0.148	0.098415	-0.037	0.014
3	-1.331	0	0.014580	-0.019	0
4	-2.285	0	0.001215	-0.003	0
5	-3.240	0	0.000054	-0.000	0
6	-4.194	0	0.000001	-0.000	0
			Weighted average	0.959	1.198

For a single family of size 3 (table 5.1), one has ELOD = 0.480 and $E(Z_{max})$ = 0.676. Doubling these values for two families of size 3 each (one family of size 6) yields 2 × 0.480 = 0.960 for the ELOD, which is what the table above furnishes (the difference of 0.001 must be due to rounding errors), and 2 × 0.676 = 1.352 for $E(Z_{max})$, which is much larger than the correct value of 1.198.

Solution 6.1. Starting with $d\theta/dx = 1 - 4\theta^2$, one computes the second derivative (notice that θ is the function, not the variable with respect to which one differentiates), $d^2\theta/dx^2 = -8\theta(d\theta/dx) = -8\theta(1 - 4\theta^2) = -8\theta + 32\theta^3$. From this, the third derivative is obtained as $d^3\theta/dx^3 = -8(dr/dx) + 96\theta^2(d\theta/dx) = (96\theta^2 - 8)(1 - 4\theta^2)$, which is equal to -8 for $\theta = 0$, violating condition (6.22) for multilocus feasibility.

Solution 6.2. A set of closely linked markers is required, with a marker being located at each chromosome end. No two adjacent loci must have a recombination fraction larger than 10 percent. Then, the recombination fraction is essentially equal to the map distance, and the sum of all recombination fractions in the different intervals is equal to the total map length.

Solution 6.3. For the Haldane map function (use equation [6.13] with $c = 1$), one finds θ_{AC} = 0.122, and the Kosambi map function predicts (equation [6.18]) θ_{AC} = 0.128. The difference between the two values is 0.006, corresponding to a relative difference of approximately 5 percent.

Solution 6.4. Using equation (1.9) or the MAPFUN program, one translates θ_{AB} = 0.05 and θ_{BC} = 0.08 into map distances, x_{AB} = 0.0513 and x_{BC} = 0.0835. The map distance over the two intervals is then $x_{AC} = x_{AB} + x_{BC}$ = 0.1348, which is retransformed using equation (1.8) into θ_{AC} = 0.1257. With this, equation (6.12) furnishes c = ½(0.05 + 0.08 − 0.1257)/(0.05 × 0.08) = 0.54.

Solution 7.1. Known age at onset x is associated with penetrance $f(x)$. According to the f_{genet} curve in figure 7.3, $f(x)$ = 1/50 = 0.02. In the treatment of penetrance presented in the text, current age is irrelevant once age at onset is known. More complicated models may incorporate current age in addition to age at onset, for example, when there is a chance that affected individuals become unaffected again (as in some psychiatric traits).

Solution 7.2. One needs to find that age, x, for which $F(x) = 0.80$. Through linear interpolation between $x_1 = 5$ and $x_2 = 40$, the 80 percent value of F is found at age $x = 5 + [0.80 \times (40 - 5)] = 33$ years.

Solution 8.1. The lod score is $Z(\theta) = \log[2\theta^2 + 2(1 - \theta)^2]$.

Solution 8.2. With $p = 0$, one obtains $Z = \log[4\theta(1 - \theta)]$; with $p = 1$, the lod score is $Z = 0$. In the latter case, none of the parents is doubly heterozygous; therefore, the mating is uninformative for linkage.

Solution 9.1. When, for each of the italicized likelihood values, the value of α_3 is calculated from the values of α_1 and α_2, one finds that only the values 0, 0.05, and 0.10 occur. Hence, the 3.9-unit support interval for α_3 is equal to (0, 0.10). With a 3-unit support interval, the following support intervals are found: (0.35, 0.70) for α_1, (0.30, 0.65) for α_2, and (0, 0.05) for α_3.

Solution 9.2. The standard errors of $\hat{\theta}$ at $\alpha = 0.9$ and 0.5 are equal to 0.060 and 0.151, respectively (table 9.7). The increase in the number of observations required is given by the inverse of the ratio of the variances (section 5.10), that is, by $(0.151/0.060)^2 = 6.3$. Hence, when $\alpha = 0.5$, sixty-three families furnish a θ estimate as precise as the one obtained from ten families when $\alpha = 0.9$.

Solution 10.1. Since class 4 offspring (table 5.4) are now taken to be double nonrecombinants each, their lod score is the same as that for class 1 individuals. Hence, one has the following three classes with their probabilities p of occurrence and associated lod score Z:

Class	p	Z
1 + 4	$\frac{1}{2}r^2 + (1 - r)^2$	$\log(4) + 2 \times \log(1 - \theta)$
2	$2r(1 - r)$	$\log(4) + \log(\theta) + \log(1 - \theta)$
3	$\frac{1}{2}r^2$	$\log(4) + 2 \times \log(\theta)$

Computing the weighted average of Z over the three classes leads to $E_3 = \Sigma pZ = \log(4) + p_1\log(1 - \theta) + p_2\log(\theta)$ given in equation (10.3), where $p_1 = 1 + (1 - r)^2$ and $p_2 = r(2 - r)$. The derivative of E_3 with respect to θ is equal to $p_2/\theta - p_1/(1 - \theta)$. Setting this equal to zero and solving for θ leads to $\tilde{\theta} = r(1 - \frac{1}{2}r)$. The asymptotic bias is equal to $b = \tilde{\theta} - r = -\frac{1}{2}r^2$.

Solution 10.2. From table 10.3, a relative ELOD of 0.92 is read off. For the same ELOD, the number of offspring must be increased by a factor of $1/0.92 = 1.087$ or by close to 10 percent.

Solution 11.1. The penetrances, $P(\text{phenotype}|\text{phenotype})$, are given in the table below (d = disease allele, n = normal allele):

Genotype		Female phenotype			Male phenotype	
Female	Male	CK High	CK Low	Unaffected[a]	Affected	Unaffected
n/n	n	0.05	0.95	1	0	1
n/d	d	0.70	0.30	1	1	0

[a]CK value unknown

Solution 11.2. The sole effect of the affection status of the first (untested) child is to make the parents unequivocally known to be heterozygous carriers of the CF gene. (1) Without marker typing, the unborn child has probability ¼ of being homozygous for the CF gene. (2) With the marker types, each parent is a double heterozygote, phase unknown. The father has genotypes *CF B/+ C* or *CF C/+ B* (+ = normal allele), the mother is *CF A/+ B* or *CF B/+ A*. Based on table 11.2, the first phase in the father has probability $2 \times 0.0173 \times 0.431 = 0.014913$, and the second phase has probability $2 \times 0.00056 \times 0.137 = 0.000153$. Since these are the only two possibilities, their conditional probabilities of occurrence are obtained by scaling them so that they sum to 1, which yields 0.99 and 0.01. Analogously, the two phases of the mother have conditional probabilities of occurrence of 0.04 and 0.96. This result nicely shows how different the phase probabilities can be under allelic association (under linkage equilibrium they are ½ each). Without recombination, the parents have a child with *CF/CF* genotype only for phase I in the father and phase II in the mother. The probability that a child with marker typing *B/B* has cystic fibrosis is thus approximately obtained as $0.99 \times 0.96 = 0.95$.

Solution 11.3. (1) Each of the parents must have genotype *CF/N*, where *CF* stands for a disease allele and *N* denotes the normal allele. Their offspring is expected to have genotypes *CF/CF* (affected), *CF/N*, and *N/N* in the proportions ¼, ½, and ¼, respectively. The proband is known to be unaffected, so he can have only one of the latter genotypes. Hence, the conditional probability of being *CF/N* is obtained as

$\frac{1}{2}/(\frac{1}{2} + \frac{1}{4}) = \frac{2}{3}$. (2) This situation is easy to handle when one distinguishes two different CF alleles, $CF\Delta$ being the disease allele with the ΔF_{508} mutation and CFm being a disease allele without that mutation, where CF without an additional symbol represents any CF allele. One now writes down the possible genotypes for the proband, given that he is unaffected, as shown in the following table (above each genotype, its probability of occurrence is indicated given the genotype or phenotype further up):

	Proband		
	$\frac{2}{3}$ CF/N		$\frac{1}{3}$ N/N
$\frac{3}{4}$ $CF\Delta/N$ $\frac{1}{2}$	$\frac{1}{4}$ CFm/N 1/6		1 N/N $\frac{1}{3}$
		$\frac{1}{3}$	$\frac{2}{3}$

As calculated under (1), the proband is *CF/N* with probability $\frac{2}{3}$, and this CF allele is randomly picked from the population. Hence, with probability $\frac{1}{4}$ it does not show the ΔF_{508} mutation. The total probability of a *CFm/N* genotype is given by $\frac{2}{3} \times \frac{1}{4} = \frac{1}{6}$. Also, the *N/N* genotype has probability of occurrence $\frac{1}{3} = \frac{2}{6}$. Since these are the only two possible genotypes, normalizing their probabilities to sum to 1 yields a conditional probability of $\frac{1}{3}$ of being a CF carrier, down from $\frac{2}{3}$ without the test for the ΔF_{508} mutation.

Solution 11.4. Following equation (11.3), the highest disequilibrium $D = \frac{1}{4}$ value is obtained for gene frequencies of $\frac{1}{2}$ at each locus.

Solution 11.5. According to equation (11.5), with $\theta = \frac{1}{2}$, $D = 0.18$ is halved every generation. Hence, it only takes one generation for D to fall below 0.10. However, it theoretically takes an infinite number of generations for D to disappear completely.

References

Note: Exact references to the human gene mapping (HGM) workshops are given at the end of this reference list.

Akaike, H. 1985. Prediction and entropy. In *A celebration of statistics. The ISI centenary volume*, edited by A. C. Atkinson and S. E. Fienberg, 1–24. New York: Springer.

Ala-Kokko, L., C. T. Baldwin, R. W. Moskowitz, and D. J. Prockop. 1990. Single base mutation in the type II procollagen gene (COL2A1) as a cause of primary osteoarthritis associated with a mild chondrodysplasia. *Proc. Natl. Acad. Sci. USA* 87:6565–68.

Amos, C. I., R. C. Elston, G. E. Bonney, B. J. B. Keats, and G. S. Berenson. 1990. A multivariate method for detecting genetic linkage, with application to a pedigree with an adverse lipoprotein phenotype. *Am. J. Hum. Genet.* 47:247–54.

Anderson, S., A. T. Bankier, B. G. Barrell, M. H. L. de Bruijin, A. R. Coulson, J. Drouin, I. C. Eperon, D. P. Nierlich, B. A. Rose, F. Sanger, P. H. Schreier, A. J. H. Smith, R. Staden, and I. G. Young. 1981. Sequence and organization of the human mitochondrial genome. *Nature* 290:457–65.

Anderson, T. W., and S. L. Sclove. 1986. *The statistical analysis of data.* 2d ed. Palo Alto, Calif.: Scientific Press.

Anstee, D. J. 1990. Blood group-active surface molecules of the human red blood cells. *Vox Sang.* 58:1–20.

Armitage, P., and G. Berry. 1987. *Statistical methods in medical research.* Oxford: Blackwell.

Arnheim, N., H. Li, and X. Cui. 1990. Review: PCR analysis of DNA sequences in single cells: Single sperm gene mapping and genetic disease diagnosis. *Genomics* 8:415–19.

Arveiler, B., G. de Saint-Basile, A. Fischer, C. Griscelli, and J. L. Mandel. 1990. Germ-line mosaicism simulates genetic heterogeneity in Wiscott-Aldrich syndrome. *Genomics* 46:906–11.

Ayala, F. J., and J. A. Kiger. 1984. *Modern genetics.* Menlo Park, Calif.: Benjamin/Cummings.

Bailey, N. T. J. 1961. *Introduction to the mathematical theory of genetic linkage.* Oxford: Clarendon Press.

Barnard, G. A. 1949. Statistical inference. *J. R. Statist. Soc.* B11:115–39.

Baron, M. 1986. Genetics of schizophrenia: II. Vulnerability traits and gene markers. *Biol. Psychiatry* 21:1189–1211.

Barratt, R. W., D. Newmeyer, D. D. Perkins, and L. Garnjobst. 1954. Map construction in *Neurospora. Adv. Genet.* 6:1–93.

Bateson, W. 1913. *Mendel's principles of heredity.* Cambridge: Cambridge University Press.

Baur, M. P., R. C. Elston, H. Gurtler, K. Henningsen, K. Hummel, H. Matsumoto, W. Mayr, J. W. Morris, L. Niejenhuis, H. Polesky, D. Salmon, J. Valentin, and R. Walkers. 1986. No fallacies in the formulation of the paternity index. *Am. J. Hum. Genet.* 39:528–36.

Beaudet, A. L., G. L. Feldman, S. D. Fernbach, G. J. Buffone, and W. E. O'Brien. 1989. Linkage disequilibrium, cystic fibrosis, and genetic counseling. *Am. J. Hum. Genet.* 44:319–26.

Beckman, L., and K.-A. Ängqvist. 1987. On the mechanism behind the association between ABO blood groups and gastric carcinoma. *Hum. Hered.* 37:140–43.

Bell, J., and J. B. S. Haldane. 1937. The linkage between the genes for colour-blindness and haemophilia in man. *Proc. R. Soc. Ser. B* 123:119–50.

Bennett, J. H., F. A. Rhodes, and H. N. Robson. 1959. A possible genetic basis for kuru. *Am. J. Hum. Genet.* 11:169–87.

Berg, K., and A. Heiberg. 1976. Linkage studies on familial hyperlipoproteinemia with xanthomatosis: Normal lipoprotein markers and the C3 polymorphism. *HGM* 3:266–70.

———. 1978. Linkage between familial hypercholesterolemia with xanthomatosis and the C3 polymorphism confirmed. *HGM* 4:621–23.

Bernstein, F. 1931. Zur Grundlegung der Chromosomentheorie der Vererbung beim Menschen. *Z. Abst. Vererb.* 57:113–38.

Bird, T. D., and G. H. Kraft. 1978. Charcot-Marie-Tooth disease: Data for genetic counseling relating age to risk. *Clin. Genet.* 14:43–49.

Bird, T. D., J. Ott, and E. R. Giblett. 1982. Evidence for linkage of Charcot-Marie-Tooth neuropathy to the Duffy locus on chromosome 1. *Am. J. Hum. Genet.* 34:388–94.

Bird, T. D., J. Ott, E. R. Giblett, P. F. Chance, S. M. Sumi, and G. H. Kraft. 1983. Genetic evidence for heterogeneity in Charcot-Marie-Tooth neuropathy (HMSN-Type I). *Ann. Neurol.* 14:679–84.

Bishop, D. T. 1985. The information content of phase-known matings for ordering genetic loci. *Genet. Epidemiol.* 2:349–61.

Bishop, D. T., and E. A. Thompson. 1988. Linkage information and bias in the presence of interference. *Genet. Epidemiol.* 5:107–19.

Bishop, D. T., and J. A. Williamson. 1990. The power of identity-by-state methods for linkage analysis. *Am. J. Hum. Genet.* 46:254–65.

Blackwelder, W. C., and R. C. Elston. 1985. A comparison of sib-pair linkage tests for disease susceptibility loci. *Genet. Epidemiol.* 2:85–97.

Bodmer, W. F. 1981. HLA structure and function: A contemporary view. *Tissue Antigens* 17:9–20.

Bodmer, W. F., C. J. Bailey, J. Bodmer, H. J. R. Bussey, A. Ellis, P. Gorman, F. C. Lucibello, V. A. Murday, S. H. Rider, P. Scambler, D. Sheer, E. Solomon, and N. K. Spurr. 1987. Localization of the gene for familial adenomatous polyposis on chromosome 5. *Nature* 328:614–16.

Boehnke, M. 1986. Estimating the power of a proposed linkage study: A practical computer simulation approach. *Am. J. Hum. Genet.* 39:513–27.

Boehnke, M., N. Arnheim, H. Li, and F. S. Collins. 1989. Fine structure genetic mapping of human chromosomes using the polymerase chain reaction on single sperm: Experimental design considerations. *Am. J. Hum. Genet.* 45:21–32.

Bolling, D. R., and E. A. Murphy. 1979. Finite sample properties of maximum likelihood estimates of the recombination fraction in double backcross matings in man. *Am. J. Med. Genet.* 3:81–95.

Botstein, D., R. L. White, M. H. Skolnick, and R. W. Davies. 1980. Construction of a genetic linkage map in man using restriction fragment length polymorphisms. *Am. J. Hum. Genet.* 32:314–31.

Bowden, D. W., T. C. Gravius, P. Green, K. Falls, D. Wurster-Hill, W. Noll, H. Müller-Kahle, and H. Donis-Keller. 1989. A genetic linkage map of 32 loci on human chromosome 10. *Genomics* 5:718–26.

Bowler, P. J. 1989. *The mendelian revolution.* Baltimore: Johns Hopkins University Press.

Brookfield, J. F. Y. 1989. Analysis of DNA fingerprinting data in cases of disputed paternity. *IMA J. Math. Appl. Med. Biol.* 6:111–31.

Brzustowicz, L. M., T. Lehner, L. H. Castilla, G. K. Penchaszadeh, K. C. Wilhelmsen, R. Daniels, K. E. Davies, M. Leppert, F. Ziter, D. Wood, V. Dubowitz, K. Zerres, I. Hausmanowa-Petrusewicz, J. Ott, T. L. Munsat, and T. C. Gilliam. 1990. Genetic mapping of chronic childhood-onset spinal muscular atrophy to chromosome 5q11.2–12.3. *Nature* 344:540–41.

Buetow, K. H., D. Nishimura, P. Green, Y. Nakamura, O. Jiang, and J. C. Murray. 1990. A detailed multipoint gene map of chromosome 1q. *Genomics* 8:13–21.

Cann, R. L., M. Stoneking, and A. C. Wilson. 1987. Mitochondrial DNA and human evolution. *Nature* 325:31–36.

Cannings, C., and E. A. Thompson. 1977. Ascertainment in the sequential sampling of pedigrees. *Clin. Genet.* 12:208–12.

Cannings, C., E. A. Thompson, and M. H. Skolnick. 1978. Probability functions on complex pedigrees. *Adv. Appl. Prob.* 10:26–61.

Carter, T. C., and D. S. Falconer. 1951. Stocks for detecting linkage in the mouse and the theory of their design. *J. Genet.* 50:307–23.

Cavalli-Sforza, L. L. 1990. Cultural transmission and nutrition. In *Genetic variation and nutrition*, edited by A. P. Simopoulos and B. Childs, 35–48. Basel: Karger.

Cavalli-Sforza, L. L., and W. F. Bodmer. [1971] 1977. *The genetics of human populations.* Paperback reprint. San Francisco: Freeman.

Cavalli-Sforza, L. L., and M.-C. King. 1986. Detecting linkage for genetically heterogeneous diseases and detecting heterogeneity with linkage data. *Am. J. Hum. Genet.* 38:599–616.

Ceppellini, R., M. Siniscalco, and C. A. B. Smith. 1955. The estimation of gene frequencies in a random-mating population. *Ann. Hum. Genet.* 20:97–115.

Chakraborty, R. 1987. Further considerations of difficulties of estimating familial risks from pedigree data. *Hum. Hered.* 37:222–28.

Chakraborty, R., and E. Boerwinkle. 1990. Population genetics of VNTR polymorphisms in humans. *Am. J. Hum. Genet.* 47:A129 (abstr.).

Chakraborty, R., P. A. Fuerst, and R. E. Ferrell. 1979. Potential information in family studies of linkage. In *Genetic analysis of common disorders: Applications to predictive factors in coronary disease*, edited by C. F. Sing and M. Skolnick, 297–303. New York: Alan R. Liss.

Chakravarti, A., J. A. Badner, and C. C. Li. 1987. Tests of linkage and heterogeneity in mendelian diseases using identity by descent scores. *Genet. Epidemiol.* 4:255–66.

Chakravarti, A., C. C. Li, and K. H. Buetow. 1984. Estimation of the marker gene frequency and linkage disequilibrium from conditional marker data. *Am. J. Hum. Genet.* 36:177–86.

Chakravarti, A., and S. A. Slaugenhaupt. 1987. Methods for studying recombination on chromosomes that undergo nondisjunction. *Genomics* 1:35–42.

Chance, P. F., T. D. Bird, P. O'Connell, H. Lipe, J.-M. Lalouel, and M. Leppert. 1990. Genetic linkage and heterogeneity in type I Charcot-Marie-Tooth disease (hereditary motor and sensory neuropathy type I). *Am. J. Hum. Genet.* 47: 915–25.

Chotai, J. 1984. On the lod score method in linkage analysis. *Ann. Hum. Genet.* 48:359–78.

Clerget-Darpoux, F. M. 1982. Bias of the estimated recombination fraction and lod score due to an association between a disease gene and a marker. *Ann. Hum. Genet.* 46:363–72.

Clerget-Darpoux, F., M.-C. Babron, and C. Bonaïti-Pellié. 1987. Power and robustness of the linkage homogeneity test in genetic analysis of common disorders. *J. Psychiatr. Res.* 21:625–30.

———. 1990. Assessing the effect of multiple linkage tests in complex diseases. *Genet. Epidemiol.* 7:245–53.

Clerget-Darpoux, F., C. Bonaïti-Pellié, and J. Hochez. 1986. Effects of misspecifying genetic parameters in lod score analysis. *Biometrics* 42:393–99.

Cockerham, C. C., and B. S. Weir. 1983. Linkage between a marker locus and a quantitative trait of sibs. *Am. J. Hum. Genet.* 35:263–73.

Cohen, J. 1990. Things I have learned (so far). *Am. Psychol.* 45:1304–12.

Cohen, J. E. 1976. The distribution of the chi-squared statistic under clustered sampling from contingency tables. *J. Am. Statist. Assoc.* 71:665–70.

Conneally, P. M., J. H. Edwards, K. K. Kidd, J.-M. Lalouel, N. E. Morton, J. Ott, and R. White. 1985. Report of the committee on methods of linkage analysis and reporting. *Cytogenet. Cell Genet.* 40:356–59.

Conneally, P. M., and M. L. Rivas. 1980. Linkage analysis in man. In *Advances in human genetics*, vol. 10, edited by H. Harris and K. Hirschhorn, 209–66. New York: Plenum.

Cook, P. J. L., E. B. Robson, K. E. Buckton, P. A. Jacobs, and P. E. Polani. 1974. Segregation of genetic markers in families with chromosome polymorphisms and structural rearrangements involving chromosome 1. *Ann. Hum. Genet.* 37: 261–74.

Cooper, H. L., and R. Hernits. 1963. A familial chromosome variant in a subject with anomalous sex differentiation. *Am. J. Hum. Genet.* 15:465–75.

Cotterman, C. W. 1969. Factor-union phenotype systems. In *Computer applications in genetics*, edited by N. E. Morton, 1–19. Honolulu: University of Hawaii Press.

Cox, D. R., M. Burmeister, E. R. Price, S. Kim, and R. M. Myers. 1990. Radiation hybrid mapping: A somatic cell genetic method for constructing high-resolution maps of mammalian chromosomes. *Science* 250:245–50.

Cox, N. J., S. E. Hodge, M. L. Marazita, M. A. Spence, and K. K. Kidd. 1988. Some effects of selection strategies on linkage analysis. *Genet. Epidemiol.* 5: 289–97.

Cremers, F. P., D. J. R. van de Pol, L. P. M. van Kerkhoff, B. Wieringa, and H.-H. Ropers. 1990. Cloning of a gene that is rearranged in patients with choroideremia. *Nature* 347:674–77.

Crow, J. F. 1966. The quality of people: Human evolutionary changes. *Bioscience* 16:863–67.

Dausset, J., H. Cann, D. Cohen, M. Lathrop, J.-M. Lalouel, and R. White. 1990. Centre d'Etude du Polymorphisme Humain (CEPH): Collaborative genetic mapping of the human genome. *Genomics* 6:575–77.

Davies, K. 1990. Complimentary endeavours. *Nature* 348:110–11.

Defesche, J. C., J. E. Hoogendijk, M. de Visser, B. W. Ongerboer de Visser, and P. A. Bolhuis. 1990. Genetic linkage of hereditary motor and sensory neuropathy type I (Charcot-Marie-Tooth disease) to markers of chromosomes 1 and 17. *Neurology* 40:1450–53.

Dempster, A. P., N. M. Laird, and D. B. Rubin. 1977. Maximum likelihood from incomplete data via the EM algorithm. *J. R. Statist. Soc.* 39B:1–38.

Devlin, B., N. Risch, and K. Roeder. 1990. No excess of homozygosity at loci used for DNA fingerprinting. *Science* 249:1416–20.

Donahue, R. P., W. B. Bias, J. H. Renwick, and V. A. McKusick. 1968. Probable assignment of the Duffy blood group locus to chromosome 1 in man. *Proc. Natl. Acad. Sci. USA* 61:949–55.

Donis-Keller, H., P. Green, C. Helms, S. Cartinhour, B. Weiffenbach, K. Stephens, T. P. Keith, D. W. Bowden, D. R. Smith, E. S. Lander, D. Botstein, G. Akots, K. S. Rediker, T. Gravius, V. A. Brown, M. B. Rising, C. Parker, J. A. Powers, D. E. Watt, E. R. Kauffman, A. Bricker, P. Phipps, H. Muller-Kahle, T. R. Fulton, S. Ng, J. W. Schumm, J. C. Braman, R. G. Knowlton, D. F. Barker, S. M. Crooks, S. E. Lincoln, M. J. Daly, and J. Abrahamson. 1987. A genetic linkage map of the human genome. *Cell* 51:319–37.

Dyck, P. J., J. Ott, S. B. Moore, C. J. Swanson, and E. H. Lambert. 1983. Linkage evidence for genetic heterogeneity among kinships with hereditary motor and sensory neuropathy type I. *Mayo Clin. Proc.* 58:430–35.

Edwards, A. W. F. 1984. *Likelihood* (paperback edition). Cambridge: Cambridge University Press.

———. 1989. Probability and likelihood in genetic counselling. *Clin. Genet.* 36:209–16.

Edwards, J. H. 1960. The simulation of mendelism. *Acta Genet.* 10:63–70.

———. 1971. The analysis of X-linkage. *Ann. Hum. Genet.* 34:229–59.

———. 1972. Linkage studies. In *Perspectives in cytogenetics: The next decade*, edited by S. W. Wright, B. F. Crandall, and L. Boyer, 97–114. Springfield, Ill.: Charles C Thomas.

———. 1976. The interpretation of lod scores in linkage analysis. *HGM* 3:289–93.

———. 1980. Allelic association in man. In *Population structure and genetic disorders*, edited by A. W. Ericksson, H. R. Forsius, H. R. Nevanlinna, P. L. Workman, and R. K. Norio, 239–55. New York: Academic Press.

———. 1987. Exclusion mapping. *J. Med. Genet.* 24:539–43.

———. 1989a. The locus positioning problem. *Ann. Hum. Genet.* 53:271–75.

———. 1989b. Familiarity, recessivity and germline mosaicism. *Ann. Hum. Genet.* 53:33–47.

Efron, B. 1982. *The jacknife, the bootstrap and other resampling plans.* CBMS-NSF Regional Conference Series in Applied Mathematics, Monograph 38. Philadelphia: SIAM.

Elandt-Johnson, R. C. 1971. *Probability models and statistical methods in genetics.* New York: John Wiley.

Ellis, N., and P. N. Goodfellow. 1989. The mammalian pseudoautosomal region. *Trends Genet.* 5:406–10.

Elston, R. C. 1973. Ascertainment and age of onset in pedigree analysis. *Hum. Hered.* 23:105–12.

Elston, R. C., and K. Lange. 1975. The prior probability of autosomal linkage. *Ann. Hum. Genet.* 38:341–50.

Elston, R. C., K. Lange, and K. K. Namboodiri. 1976. Age trends in human chiasma frequencies and recombination fractions: II. Method for analyzing recombination fractions and applications to the ABO:Nail-Patella linkage. *Am. J. Hum. Genet.* 28:69–76.

Elston, R. C., K. K. Namboodiri, R. C. P. Go, R. M. Siervogel, and C. J. Glueck. 1976. Probable linkage between essential familial hypercholesterolemia and third complement (C3). *HGM* 3:294–97.

Elston, R. C., and J. Stewart. 1971. A general model for the analysis of pedigree data. *Hum. Hered.* 21:523–42.

Engel, E. 1980. A new concept: Uniparental disomy and its potential effect, isodisomy. *Am. J. Med. Genet.* 6:137–43.

Excoffier, L. 1990. Evolution of human mitochondrial DNA: Evidence for departure from a pure neutral model of populations at equilibrium. *J. Mol. Evol.* 30:125–39.

Excoffier, L., and A. Langaney. 1989. Origin and differentiation of human mitochondrial DNA. *Am. J. Hum. Genet.* 44:73–85.

Fain, P. R., E. Wright, H. F. Willard, K. Stephens, and D. F. Barker. 1989. The order of loci in the pericentric region of chromosome 17, based on evidence from physical and genetic breakpoints. *Am. J. Hum. Genet.* 44:68–72.

Falk, C. T. 1989. A simple scheme for preliminary orderings of multiple loci: Application to 45 CF families. In *Multipoint mapping and linkage based upon affected pedigree members: Genetic Analysis Workshop 6*, 17–22. New York: Alan R. Liss.

———. 1991. A simple method for ordering loci using data from radiation hybrids. *Genomics* 9:120–23.

Falk, C. T., and J. H. Edwards. 1970. A computer approach to the analysis of family genetic data for detection of linkage. *Genetics* 64:s18 (abstr.).

Falk, C. T., and P. Rubinstein. 1987. Haplotype relative risks: An easy reliable way to construct a proper control sample for risk calculations. *Ann. Hum. Genet.* 51:227–33.

Feller, W. F. 1968. *An introduction to probability theory and its applications,* vol. 1, 3d ed. New York: John Wiley.

Felsenstein, J. 1979. A mathematically tractable family of genetic mapping functions with different amounts of interference. *Genetics* 91:769–75.

Ferguson-Smith, M. A., P. M. Ellis, O. Mutchinick, K. P. Glen, G. B. Côté, and J. H. Edwards. 1975. Centromeric linkage. *HGM* 2:300–307.

Fisher, R. A. 1921. On the mathematical foundations of theoretical statistics. *Philos. Trans. R. Soc.* A202:309–68.

———. 1922. The systematic location of genes by means of crossover observations. *Am. Naturalist* 56:406–11.

———. 1925. Theory of statistical estimation. *Proc. Camb. Philos. Soc.* 22:700–725.

———. 1935a. The detection of linkage with dominant abnormalities. *Ann. Eugen.* 6:187–201.

———. 1935b. The detection of linkage with recessive abnormalities. *Ann. Eugen.* 6:339–51.

———. 1960. *The design of experiments.* Edinburgh: Oliver & Boyd.

———. 1970. *Statistical methods for research workers.* 14th ed. New York: Hafner Press.

Fishman, P. M., B. Suarez, S. E. Hodge, and T. Reich. 1978. A robust method for the detection of linkage in familial diseases. *Am. J. Hum. Genet.* 30:308–21.

Folstein, S. E. 1989. *Huntington's disease.* Baltimore: Johns Hopkins University Press.

Gajdusek, D. C., C. J. Gibbs, and M. Alpers. 1966. Experimental transmission of a kuru-like syndrome to chimpanzees. *Nature* 209:794–96.

Gedde-Dahl, T., Jr., M. K. Fagerhol, P. J. L. Cook, and J. Noades. 1972. Autosomal linkage between the Gm and Pi loci in man. *Ann. Hum. Genet.* 35:393–99.

Gelehrter, T. D., and F. S. Collins. 1990. *Principles of medical genetics*. Baltimore: Williams & Wilkins.

Gilliam, T. C., L. M. Brzustowicz, L. H. Castilla, T. Lehner, G. K. Penchaszadeh, R. J. Daniels, B. C. Byth, J. Knowles, J. E. Hislop, Y. Shapira, V. Dubowitz, T. L. Munsat, J. Ott, and K. E. Davies. 1990. Genetic homogeneity between acute and chronic forms of spinal muscular atrophy. *Nature* 345:823–25.

Goldgar, D. E., and P. R. Fain. 1988. Models of multilocus recombination: Nonrandomness in chiasma number and crossover positions. *Am. J. Hum. Genet.* 43: 38–45.

Goldgar, D. E., P. R. Fain, and W. J. Kimberling. 1989. Chiasma-based models of multilocus recombination: Increased power for exclusion mapping and gene ordering. *Genomics* 5:283–90.

Goldgar, D. E., P. Green, D. M. Parry, and J. J. Mulvihill. 1989. Multipoint linkage analysis in neurofibromatosis type I: An international collaboration. *Am. J. Hum. Genet.* 44:6–12.

Goldin, L. R., and E. S. Gershon. 1988. Power of the affected-sib-pair method for heterogeneous disorders. *Genet. Epidemiol.* 5:35–42.

Goldstein, M., and W. R. Dillon. 1978. *Discrete discriminant analysis*. New York: John Wiley.

Goss, S. J., and H. Harris. 1975. New method for mapping genes in human chromosomes. *Nature* 255:680–84.

Gough, N. M., D. P. Gearing, N. A. Nicola, E. Baker, M. Pritchard, D. F. Callen, and G. F. Sutherland. 1990. Localization of the human GM-CSF receptor gene to the X-Y pseudoautosomal region. *Nature* 345:734–36.

Green, J. R., and J. C. Woodrow. 1977. Sibling method for detecting HLA-linked genes in disease. *Tissue Antigens* 9:31–35.

Greenberg, D. A. 1986. The effect of proband designation on segregation analysis. *Am. J. Hum. Genet.* 39:329–39.

———. 1989. Inferring mode of inheritance by comparison of lod scores. *Am. J. Med. Genet.* 34:480–86.

Greenberg, D. A., and S. E. Hodge. 1989. Linkage analysis under "random" and "genetic" reduced penetrance. *Genet. Epidemiol.* 6:259–64.

Grimm, T., B. Müller, M. Dreier, E. Kind, T. Bettecken, G. Meng, and C. R. Müller. 1989. Hot spot of recombination within DXS164 in the Duchenne muscular dystrophy gene. *Am. J. Hum. Genet.* 45:368–72.

Grön, K., P. Aula, and L. Peltonen. 1990. Linkage of aspartylglucosaminuria (AGU) to marker loci on the long arm of chromosome 4. *Hum. Genet.* 85:233–36.

Guiloff, R. J., P. K. Thomas, M. Contreras, S. Armitage, G. Schwarz, and E. M. Sedgwick. 1982. Evidence for linkage of type I hereditary motor and sensory neuropathy to the Duffy locus on chromosome 1. *Ann. Hum. Genet.* 46:25–27.

Gusella, J., N. S. Wexler, P. M. Conneally, S. L. Naylor, M. A. Anderson, R. E. Tanzi, P. C. Watkins, K. Ottina, M. R. Wallace, A. Y. Sakaguchi, A. B. Young, I. Shoulson, E. Bonilla, and J. B. Martin. 1983. A polymorphic DNA marker genetically linked to Huntington's disease. *Nature* 306:234–38.

Hadlow, W. J. 1959. Scrapie and kuru. *Lancet* 2:289–90.

Haldane, J. B. S. 1919. The combination of linkage values and the calculation of distances between the loci of linked factors. *J. Genet.* 8:299–309.

———. 1922. Sex ratio and unisexual sterility in hybrid animals. *J. Genet.* 12: 101–9.

———. 1935. The rate of spontaneous mutation of a human gene. *J. Genet.* 31: 317–26.

———. 1985. The future of biology. In *On Being the Right Size and other essays—J. B. S. Haldane*, edited by John Maynard Smith. Oxford, England: Oxford University Press.

Haldane, J. B. S., and C. A. B. Smith. 1947. A new estimate of the linkage between the genes for colour-blindness and haemophilia in man. *Ann. Eugen.* 14:10–31.

Hall, J. G. 1990. Genomic imprinting: Review and relevance to human diseases. *Am. J. Hum. Genet.* 46:857–73.

Hall, J. M., M. K. Lee, B. Newman, J. E. Morrow, L. A. Anderson, B. Huey, and M.-C. King. 1990. Linkage of early-onset familial breast cancer to chromosome 17q21. *Science* 250: 1684–89.

Halloran, S. L., and A. Chakravarti. 1987. DSLINK: A computer program for gene-centromere linkage analysis in families with a trisomic offspring. *Am. J. Hum. Genet.* 41:350–55.

Harris, H., D. A. Hopkinson, and Y. H. Edwards. 1977. Polymorphism and the subunit structure of enzymes: A contribution to the neutralist-selectionist controversy. *Proc. Natl. Acad. Sci. USA* 74:698–701.

Hartl, D. L. 1988. *A primer of population genetics.* Sunderland, Mass.: Sinauer Associates.

Haseman, J. K., and R. C. Elston. 1972. The investigation of linkage between a quantitative trait and a marker locus. *Behav. Genet.* 2:3–19.

Hasstedt, S. J. 1982. Linkage analysis using the mixed, major gene with general penetrance or three-locus model. *HGM* 6:284–85.

Hasstedt, S. J., and P. E. Cartwright. 1981. PAP—pedigree analysis package, University of Utah, Department of Medical Biophysics and Computing, technical report no. 13. Salt Lake City, Utah.

Heimbuch, R. C., S. Matthysse, and K. K. Kidd. 1980. Estimating age-of-onset distributions for disorders with variable onset. *Am. J. Hum. Genet.* 32:564–74.

Hendriks, R. W., E. J. B. M. Mensink, M. E. M. Kraakman, A. Thompson, and R. K. B. Schuurman. 1989. Evidence for male X chromosomal mosaicism in X-linked agammaglobulinemia. *Hum. Genet.* 83:267–70.

Heslop-Harrison, J. S., A. R. Leitch, T. Schwarzacher, J. B. Smith, M. D. Atkinson, and M. D. Bennett. 1989. The volumes and morphology of human chromosomes in mitotic reconstructions. *Hum. Genet.* 84:27–34.

Heuch, I., and F. H. F. Li. 1972. PEDIG—a computer program for calculation of genotype probabilities using phenotype information. *Clin. Genet.* 3:501–4.

Higgins, M. J., C. Turmel, J. Noolandi, P. E. Neumann, and M. Lalande. 1990. Construction of the physical map for three loci in chromosome band 13q14: Comparison to the genetic map. *Proc. Natl. Acad. Sci. USA* 87:3415–19.

Hill, A. P. 1975. Quantitative linkage: A statistical procedure for its detection and estimation. *Ann. Hum. Genet.* 38:439–49.

Hodge, D. E. 1981. Some epistatic two-locus models of disease: I. Relative risks and identity-by-descent distributions in affected sib pairs. *Am. J. Hum. Genet.* 33: 381–95.

———. 1984. The information contained in multiple sibling pairs. *Genet. Epidemiol.* 1:109–22.

Hodge, S. E., C. E. Anderson, K. Neiswanger, R. S. Sparkes, and D. L. Rimoin. 1983. The search for heterogeneity in insulin-dependent diabetes mellitus (IDDM): Linkage studies, two-locus models, and genetic heterogeneity. *Am. J. Hum. Genet.* 35:1139–55.

Hohenschutz, C., P. Eich, W. Friedl, A. Waheed, E. Conzelmann, and P. Propping. 1989. Pseudodeficiency of arylsulfatase A: A common genetic polymorphism with possible disease implications. *Hum. Genet.* 82:45–48.

Holliday, R. 1964. A mechanism for gene conversion in fungi. *Genet. Res.* 5: 282–304.

Holmgren, G., E. Haettner, I. Nordenson, O. Sandgren, L. Steen, and E. Lundgren. 1988. Homozygosity for the transthyretin-met^{30}-gene in two Swedish sibs with familial amyloidotic polyneuropathy. *Clin. Genet.* 34:333–38.

Hsiao, K., H. F. Baker, T. J. Crow, M. Poulter, F. Owen, J. D. Terwilliger, D. Westaway, J. Ott, and S. B. Prusiner. 1989. Linkage of a prion protein missense variant to Gerstmann-Sträussler syndrome. *Nature* 338:342–45.

Huether, C. A., and E. A. Murphy. 1980. Reduction of bias in estimating the frequency of recessive genes. *Am. J. Hum. Genet.* 32:212–22.

Hultén, M., J. M. Luciani, V. Kirton, and M. Devictor-Vuillet. 1978. The use and limitations of chiasma scoring with reference to genetic mapping. *HGM* 4: 37–58.

Hyer, R. N., C. Julier, J. D. Buckley, M. Trucco, J. Rotter, R. Spielman, A. Barnett, S. Bain, C. Boitard, I. Deschamps, J. A. Todd, J. I. Bell, and G. M. Lathrop. 1991. High-resolution linkage mapping for susceptibility genes in human polygenic disease: Insulin-dependent diabetes mellitus and chromosome 11q. *Am. J. Hum. Genet.* 48:243–57.

Jadayel, D., P. Fain, M. Upadhyaya, M. A. Ponder, S. M. Huson, J. Carey, A. Fryer, C. G. P. Mathew, D. F. Barker, and B. A. J. Ponder. 1990. Paternal origin of new mutations in von Recklinghausen neurofibromatosis. *Nature* 343:558–59.

Järvelä, I., J. Schleutker, L. Haataja, P. Santavuori, L. Puhakka, T. Manninen, A. Palotie, L. A. Sandkuijl, M. Renlund, R. White, P. Aula, and L. Peltonen. 1990. Infantile form of neuronal ceroid lipofuscinoses (CLN1) maps to the short arm of chromosome 1. *Genomics* 9:170–73.

Jeffreys, A. J., R. Neumann, and V. Wilson. 1990. Repeat unit sequence variation in minisatellites: A novel source of DNA polymorphism for studying variation and mutation by single molecule analysis. *Cell* 60:473–85.

Jeffreys, A. J., V. Wilson, and S. L. Thein. 1985. Individual-specific "fingerprints" of human DNA. *Nature* 316:76–79.

Jiang, O. X., and K. H. Buetow. 1990. A simulation evaluation of high resolution meiotic gene mapping. *Am. J. Hum. Genet.* 47:A185 (abstr.).

Johnson, N. L., and S. Kotz. 1970. *Continuous univariate distributions,* vol. 2. Boston: Houghton Mifflin.

Johnson, S. M. 1963. Generation of permutations by adjacent transposition. *Math. Comp.* 17:282–85.

Judge, S. J. 1990. Does the eye grow into focus? *Nature* 345:477–78.

Julier, C., Y. Nakamura, M. Lathrop, P. O'Connell, M. Leppert, M. Litt, T. Mohandas, J.-M. Lalouel, and R. White. 1990a. A detailed genetic map of the long arm of chromosome 11. *Genomics* 7:335–45.

Julier, C., Y. Nakamura, M. Lathrop, P. O'Connell, M. Leppert, T. Mohandas, J.-M. Lalouel, and R. White. 1990b. A primary map of 24 loci on human chromosome 16. *Genomics* 6:419–27.

Juneja, R. K., L. R. Weitkamp, A. Stratil, B. Gahne, and S. A. Guttormsen. 1988. Further studies of the plasma α_1B-glycoprotein polymorphism: Two new alleles and allele frequencies in Caucasians and in American Blacks. *Hum. Hered.* 38:267–72.

Kainulainen, K., L. Pulkkinen, A. Savolainen, I. Kaitila, and L. Peltonen. 1990. Location on chromosome 15 of the gene defect causing Marfan syndrome. *N. Engl. J. Med.* 323:935–39.

Kanno, H., I. Y. Huang, Y. W. Kan, and A. Yoshida. 1989. Two structural genes on different chromosomes are required for encoding the major subunit of human red cell glucose-6-phosphate dehydrogenase. *Cell* 58:595–606.

Karlin, S. 1984. Theoretical aspects of genetic map functions in recombination processes. In *Human population genetics: The Pittsburgh symposium,* edited by A. Chakravarti, 209–28. New York: Van Nostrand Reinhold.

Karlin, S., and U. Liberman. 1978. Classifications and comparisons of multilocus recombination distributions. *Proc. Natl. Acad. Sci. USA* 75:6332–36.

Karlin, S., P. T. Williams, S. Jensen, and J. W. Farquhar. 1981. Genetic analysis of the Stanford LRC family study data: I. Structured exploratory data analysis of height and weight measurements. *Am. J. Epidemiol.* 113:307–24.

Keats, B., J. Ott, and M. Conneally. 1989. Report of the committee on linkage and gene order. *Cytogenet. Cell Genet.* 51:459–502.

Keats, B. J. B., S. L. Sherman, N. E. Morton, E. B. Robson, K. H. Buetow, H. M. Cann, P. E. Cartwright, A. Chakravarti, U. Francke, P. P. Green, and J. Ott. 1991. Guidelines for human linkage maps: An international system for human linkage maps (ISLM, 1990). *Genomics* 9:557–60.

Keats, B. J. B., S. L. Sherman, and J. Ott. 1990. Report of the committee on linkage and gene order. *Cytogenet. Cell Genet.* 55:387–94.

Keith, T. P., P. Green, S. T. Reeders, V. A. Brown, P. Phipps, A. Bricker, K. Falls, K. S. Rediker, J. A. Powers, C. Hogan, C. Nelson, R. Knowlton, and H. Donis-Keller. 1990. Genetic linkage map of 46 DNA markers on human chromosome 16. *Proc. Natl. Acad. Sci. USA* 87:5754–58.

Kendler, K. S. 1983. Overview: A current perspective on twin studies of schizophrenia. *Am. J. Psychiatry* 140:1413–25.

————. 1986. The genetics of schizophrenia: A current perspective. *Psychopharmacol. Bull.* 22:918–22.

————. 1988. The impact of varying diagnostic thresholds on affected sib pair linkage analysis. *Genet. Epidemiol.* 5:407–19.

Kendler, K. S., A. C. Heath, N. G. Martin, and L. J. Eaves. 1987. Symptoms of anxiety and symptoms of depression. *Arch. Gen. Psychiatry* 44:451–57.

Kerem, E., M. Corey, B. Kerem, J. Rommens, D. Markiewicz, H. Levison, L.-C. Tsui, and P. Durie. 1990. The relation between genotype and phenotype in cystic fibrosis—analysis of the most common mutation (ΔF_{508}). *N. Engl. J. Med.* 323:1517–22.

Kerem, B., J. M. Rommens, J. A. Buchana, D. Markiewicz, T. K. Cox, A. Chakravarti, M. Buchwald, and L.-C. Tsui. 1989. Identification of the cystic fibrosis gene: Genetic analysis. *Science* 245:1073–80.

Kidd, K. K., A. M. Bowcock, P. L. Pearson, J. Schmidtke, H. F. Willard, R. K. Track, and F. Ricciuti. 1988. Report of the committee on human gene mapping by recombinant DNA techniques. *Cytogenet. Cell Genet.* 49:132–218.

Kidd, K. K., A. M. Bowcock, J. Schmidtke, R. K. Track, F. Ricciuti, G. Hutchings, A. Bale, P. Pearson, and H. F. Willard. 1989. Report of the DNA committee and catalogs of cloned and mapped genes and DNA polymorphisms. *Cytogenet. Cell Genet.* 51:622–947.

Kidd, K. K., and J. Ott. 1984. Power and sample size in linkage studies. *HGM* 7:510–11.

Kimberling, W. J., P. R. Fain, J. B. Kenyon, D. Goldgar, E. Sujansky, and P. A. Gabow. 1988. Linkage heterogeneity of autosomal dominant polycystic kidney disease. *N. Engl. J. Med.* 319:913–18.

Kimberling, W. J., M. D. Weston, C. Möller, S. L. H. Davenport, Y. Y. Shugart, I. A. Priluck, A. Martini, M. Milani, and R. J. Smith. 1990. Localization of Usher syndrome type II to chromosome 1q. *Genomics* 7:245–49.

Kloepfer, H. W. 1946. An investigation of 171 possible linkage relationships in man. *Ann. Eugen.* 13:35–71.

Knudson, A. G. 1971. Mutation and cancer: Statistical study of retinoblastoma. *Proc. Natl. Acad. Sci. USA* 68:820–23.

————. 1985. Hereditary cancer, oncogenes, and antioncogenes. *Cancer Res.* 45: 1437–43.

Koenig, M., E. P. Hoffman, C. J. Bertelson, A. P. Monaco, C. Feener, and L. M. Kunkel. 1987. Complete cloning of the Duchenne muscular dystrophy (DMD) cDNA and preliminary genomic organization of the DMD gene in normal and affected individuals. *Cell* 50:509–17.

Konigsberg, L. W., J. Blangero, B. D. Mitchell, and C. M. Kammerer. 1990. A simulation study of quantitative trait linkage analysis under a mixed polygenic and major gene model. *Am. J. Hum. Genet.* 47:A139 (abstr.).

Kosambi, D. D. 1944. The estimation of map distances from recombination values. *Ann. Eugen.* 12:172–75.

Kouri, R. E., and P. R. Fain. 1990. Meiotic mapping panels: An efficient mapping strategy for genetic mapping. *Am. J. Hum. Genet.* 47:A186 (abstr.).

Krüger, J., and F. Vogel. 1989. The problem of our common mitochondrial mother. *Hum. Genet.* 82:308–12.

Kullback, S. 1959. *Information theory and statistics.* New York: John Wiley.

Kullback, S., and R. A. Leibler. 1951. On information and sufficiency. *Ann. Math. Statist.* 22:79–86.

Lalouel, J. M. 1977. Linkage mapping from pair-wise recombination data. *Heredity* 38:61–77.

———. 1979. GEMINI—a computer program for optimization of general nonlinear functions. University of Utah, Department of Medical Biophysics and Computing, technical report no. 14. Salt Lake City, Utah.

Lamm, L. U., and B. Olaisen. 1985. Report of the committee on the genetic constitution of chromosomes 5 and 6. *Cytogenet. Cell Genet.* 40:128–55.

Lander, E. S., and D. Botstein. 1986a. Strategies for studying heterogeneous genetic traits in humans by using a linkage map of restriction fragment length polymorphisms. *Proc. Natl. Acad. Sci. USA* 83:7353–57.

———. 1986b. Mapping complex genetic traits in humans: New methods using a complete RFLP linkage map. *Cold Spring Harbor Symp. Quant. Biol.* 51:49–62.

———. 1989. Mapping mendelian factors underlying quantitative traits using RFLP linkage maps. *Genetics* 121:185–99.

Lander, E. S., P. Green, J. Abrahamson, A. Barlow, M. J. Daly, S. E. Lincoln, and L. Newburg. 1987. MAPMAKER: An interactive computer package for constructing primary genetic linkage maps of experimental and natural populations. *Genomics* 1:174–81.

Lange, K. 1986. The affected sib-pair method using identity by state relations. *Am. J. Hum. Genet.* 39:148–50.

Lange, K., and M. Boehnke. 1982. How many polymorphic genes will it take to span the human genome? *Am. J. Hum. Genet.* 34:842–45.

———. 1983. Some combinatorial problems of DNA restriction fragment length polymorphisms. *Am. J. Hum. Genet.* 35:177–92.

Lange, K., and R. C. Elston. 1975. Extensions to pedigree analysis. I. Likelihood calculations for simple and complex pedigrees. *Hum. Hered.* 25:95–105.

Lange, K., and S. Matthysse. 1989. Simulation of pedigree genotypes by random walks. *Am. J. Hum. Genet.* 45:959–70.

Lange, K., M. A. Spence, and M. B. Frank. 1976. Application of the lod method to the detection of linkage between a quantitative trait and a qualitative marker: A simulation experiment. *Am. J. Hum. Genet.* 28:167–73.

Lange, K., and D. E. Weeks. 1989. Efficient computation of LOD scores: Genotype elimination, genotype redefinition, and hybrid maximum likelihood algorithms. *Ann. Hum. Genet.* 53:67–83.

Lange, K., D. Weeks, and M. Boehnke. 1988. Programs for Pedigree Analysis: MENDEL, FISHER, and dGENE. *Genet. Epidemiol.* 5:471–72.

Lathrop, G. M., J. Chotai, J. Ott, and J. M. Lalouel. 1987. Tests of gene order from three-locus linkage data. *Ann. Hum. Genet.* 51:235–49.

Lathrop, G. M., A. B. Hooper, J. W. Huntsman, and R. H. Ward. 1983. Evaluating pedigree data: I. The estimation of pedigree error in the presence of marker mistyping. *Am. J. Hum. Genet.* 35:241–62.

Lathrop, G. M., J. M. Lalouel, C. Julier, and J. Ott. 1984. Strategies for multilocus linkage analysis in humans. *Proc. Natl. Acad. Sci. USA* 81:3443–46.

———. 1985. Multilocus linkage analysis in humans: Detection of linkage and estimation of recombination. *Am. J. Hum. Genet.* 37:482–98.

Lathrop, G. M., J. M. Lalouel, and R. L. White. 1986. Calculation of human linkage maps: Likelihood calculations for multilocus linkage analysis. *Genet. Epidemiol.* 3:39–52.

Lathrop, G. M., P. O'Connell, M. Leppert, Y. Nakamura, M. Farrall, L.-C. Tsui, J.-M. Lalouel, and R. White. 1989. Twenty-five loci form a continuous linkage map of markers for human chromosome 7. *Genomics* 5:866–73.

Lathrop, G. M., and J. Ott. 1990. Analysis of complex diseases under oligogenic models and intrafamilial heterogeneity by the LINKAGE programs. *Am. J. Hum. Genet.* 47:A188 (abstr.).

Lawrence, J. B., R. H. Singer, and J. A. McNeil. 1990. Interphase and metaphase resolution of different distances within the human dystrophin gene. *Science* 249:928–32.

Leal, S. M., and J. Ott. 1990. Expected lod scores in linkage analysis of autosomal recessive traits for affected and unaffected offspring. *Am. J. Hum. Genet.* 47:A188 (abstr.).

Lewis, M., D. J. Anstee, G. W. G. Bird, E. Brodheim, J.-P. Cartron, M. Contreras, M. C. Crookston, W. Dahr, G. L. Daniels, C. P. Engelfriet, C. M. Giles, P. D. Issitt, J. Jørgensen, L. Kornstad, A. Lubenko, W. L. Marsh, J. McCreary, B. P. L. Moore, P. Morel, J. J. Moulds, H. Nevanlinna, R. Nordhagen, Y. Okubo, R. E. Rosenfield, P. Rouger, P. Rubinstein, C. Salmon, S. Seidl, P. Sistonen, P. Tippett, R. H. Walker, G. Woodfield, and S. Young. 1990. Blood group terminology 1990. *Vox Sang.* 58:152–69.

Li, C. C. 1987. A genetical model for emergenesis: In memory of Laurence H. Snyder, 1901–86. *Am. J. Hum. Genet.* 41:517–23.

———. 1988. Pseudo-random mating populations. *Genetics* 119:731–37.

Liberman, U., and S. Karlin. 1984. Theoretical models of genetic map functions. *Theor. Popul. Biol.* 25:331–46.

Lichter, P., C. C. Tang, K. Call, G. Hermanson, G. A. Evans, D. Housman, and D. C. Ward. 1990. High-resolution mapping of human chromosome 11 by in situ hybridization with cosmid clones. *Science* 247:64–69.

Lichter, P., and D. C. Ward. 1990. Is non-isotopic in situ hybridization finally coming of age? *Nature* 345:93–95.

Lindenbaum, S. 1979. *Kuru sorcery.* Palo Alto, Calif.: Mayfield.

Linder, D., B. Kaiser McCaw, and F. Hecht. 1975. Parthenogenetic origin of benign ovarian teratomas. *N. Engl. J. Med.* 292:63–66.

Louis, T. A. 1982. Analysis of categorical data: Exact tests and log-linear models. In *Statistics in medical research*, edited by V. Miké and K. E. Stanley, 402–31. New York: John Wiley.

McAlpine, P. J., T. B. Shows, C. Boucheix, L. C. Stranc, T. G. Berent, A. J. Pakstis, and R. C. Douté. 1989. Report of the nomenclature committee and the 1989 catalog of mapped genes. *Cytogenet. Cell Genet.* 51:13–66.

McGuffin, P., and P. Huckle. 1990. Simulation of mendelism revisited: The recessive gene for attending medical school. *Am. J. Hum. Genet.* 46:994–99.

McKusick, V. A. 1990. *Mendelian inheritance of man.* 9th ed. Baltimore: Johns Hopkins University Press.

McKusick, V. A., and F. H. Ruddle. 1977. The status of the gene map of the human chromosomes. *Science* 196:390–405.

McWilliam, P., G. J. Farrar, P. Kenna, D. G. Bradley, M. M. Humphries, E. M. Sharp, D. J. McConnell, M. Lawler, D. Sheils, C. Ryan, K. Stevens, S. P. Daiger, and P. Humphries. 1989. Autosomal dominant retinitis pigmentosa (ADRP): Localization of an ADRP gene to the long arm of chromosome 3. *Genomics* 5:619–22.

Majumder, P. P. 1989. Strategies and sample-size considerations for mapping a two-locus autosomal recessive disorder. *Am. J. Hum. Genet.* 45:412–23.

Mather, K. 1936. Types of linkage data and their value. *Ann. Eugen.* 7:251–64.

———. 1938. Crossing-over. *Biol. Rev. Cambridge Philosophic Soc.* 13:252–92.

Maynard Smith, J. 1989. *Evolutionary genetics.* Oxford: Oxford University Press.

———. 1990. The Y of human relationships. *Nature* 344:591–92.

Meagher, R. B., M. D. McLean, and J. Arnold. 1988. Recombination within a subclass of restriction fragment length polymorphisms may help link classical and molecular genetics. *Genetics* 120:809–18.

Melki, J., S. Abdelhak, P. Sheth, M. F. Bachelot, P. Burlet, A. Marcadet, J. Aicardi, A. Barois, J. P. Carriere, M. Fardeau, D. Fontan, G. Ponsot, T. Billette, C. Angelini, C. Barbosa, G. Ferriere, G. Lanzi, A. Ottolini, M. C. Babron, D. Cohen, A. Hanauer, F. Clerget-Darpoux, M. Lathrop, A. Munnich, and J. Frezal. 1990. Gene for chronic proximal spinal muscular atrophies maps to chromosome 5q. *Nature* 344:767–68.

Mendel, G. 1866. Versuche über Pflanzen-Hybriden. *Verh. Naturforsch. Ver. Brünn* 4:3–47.

Mérette, C., and J. Ott. 1991. Small sample bias in tests of locus order due to unequal marker heterozygosity (in preparation).

Meyers, D. A., P. M. Conneally, F. Hecht, E. W. Lovrien, E. Magenis, A. D. Merritt, C. G. Palmer, M. L. Rivas, and L. Wang. 1975. Linkage group I: Multipoint mapping. *HGM* 2:381–89.

Meyers, D. A., P. M. Conneally, E. W. Lovrien, R. E. Magenis, A. D. Merritt, J. A. Norton, C. G. Palmer, M. L. Rivas, L. Wang, and P. L. Yu. 1976. Linkage group I: The simultaneous estimation of recombination and interference. *HGM* 3:335–39.

Middleton-Price, H. R., A. E. Harding, J. Berciano, J. M. Pastor, S. M. Huson, and S. Malcolm. 1989. Absence of linkage of hereditary motor and sensory neuropathy type I to chromosome 1 markers. *Genomics* 4:192–97.

Miller, D. A., O. J. Miller, V. G. Dev, S. Hashmi, R. Tantravahi, L. Medrano, and H. Green. 1974. Human chromosome 19 carries a poliovirus receptor gene. *Cell* 1:167–73.

Mittmann, O. 1938. Vererbung durch ein Genpaar und Mitwirkung des Restgenotypes im statistischen Nachweis. *Z. Indukt. Abst. Vererb.* 75:191–232.

Mohr, J. 1954. *A study of linkage in man.* Copenhagen: Munksgaard.

———. 1964. Practical possibilities for detection of linkage in man. *Acta Genet.* 14:125–32.

Monaco, A. P., and L. M. Kunkel. 1988. Cloning of the Duchenne/Becker muscular dystrophy locus. *Adv. Hum. Genet.* 17:61–98.

Monk, M. 1990. Variation in epigenetic inheritance. *Trends Genet.* 6:110–14.

Morgan, T. H. 1928. *The theory of genes.* New Haven, Conn.: Yale University Press.

Morton, N. E. 1955. Sequential tests for the detection of linkage. *Am. J. Hum. Genet.* 7:277–318.

———. 1956. The detection and estimation of linkage between the genes for elliptocytosis and the Rh blood type. *Am. J. Hum. Genet.* 8:80–96.

———. 1978. Analysis of crossingover in man. *Cytogenet. Cell Genet.* 22:15–36.

Morton, N. E., and V. Andrews. 1989. MAP, an expert system for multiple pairwise linkage analysis. *Ann. Hum. Genet.* 53:263–69.

Morton, N. E., and A. Collins. 1990. Standard maps of chromosome 10. *Ann. Hum. Genet.* 54:235–51.

Morton, N. E., J. Lindsten, L. Iselius, and S. Yee. 1982. Data and theory for a revised chiasma map of man. *Hum. Genet.* 62:266–70.

Motulsky, A. G., G. R. Fraser, and J. Felsenstein. 1971. Public health and long-term genetic implications of intrauterine diagnosis and selective abortion. *Birth Defects* 7(no. 5):22–32.

Muller, J. 1916. The mechanism of crossing over. *Am. Nat.* 50:193–207.

Murphy, E. A., and G. A. Chase. 1975. *Principles of genetic counseling.* Chicago: Yearbook Medical Publishers (reprinted 1990 by UMI Out-of-Print Books on Demand).

Musarella, M. A., R. G. Weleber, W. H. Murphey, R. S. L. Young, L. Anson-Cartwright, M. Mets, S. P. Kraft, R. Polemeno, M. Litt, and R. G. Worton. 1989. Assignment of the gene for complete X-linked congenital stationary night blindness (CSNB1) to Xp11.3. *Genomics* 5:727–37.

Nakamura, Y., M. Leppert, P. O'Connell, R. Wolff, T. Holm, M. Culver, C. Martin, E. Fujimoto, M. Hoff, E. Kumlin, and R. White. 1987. Variable number of tandem repeat (VNTR) markers for human gene mapping. *Science* 235:1616–22.

Nakashima, H., A. Fujiyama, S. Kagiyama, and T. Imamura. 1990. Genetic polymorphisms of gene conversion within the duplicated human α-globin loci. *Hum. Genet.* 84:568–70.

Neugebauer, M., and M. P. Baur. 1991. A comprehensive pedigree analysis tool: FAP (Family Analysis Package). In *Recent progress in the genetic epidemiology of cancer,* edited by H. T. Lynch and P. Tautu, 145–49. Heidelberg: Springer.

Nordström, S., and W. Thorburn. 1980. Dominantly inherited macular degeneration (Best's disease) in a homozygous father with 11 children. *Clin. Genet.* 18:211–16.

O'Connell, P., G. M. Lathrop, M. Law, M. Leppert, Y. Nakamura, M. Hoff, E. Kumlin, W. Thomas, T. Elsner, L. Ballard, P. Goodman, E. Azen, J. E. Sadler, G. Y. Cai, J.-M. Lalouel, and R. White. 1987. A primary genetic linkage map for human chromosome 12. *Genomics* 1:93–102.

Olson, J. M., and M. Boehnke. 1990. Monte Carlo comparison of preliminary methods for ordering multiple loci. *Am. J. Hum. Genet.* 47:470–82.

Olson, M., L. Hood, C. Cantor, and D. Botstein. 1989. A common language for physical mapping of the human genome. *Science* 245:1434–35.

Ott, J. 1974a. Estimation of the recombination fraction in human pedigrees: Efficient computation of the likelihood for human linkage studies. *Am. J. Hum. Genet.* 26:588–97.

———. 1974b. Computer simulation in human linkage analysis. *Am. J. Hum. Genet.* 26:64A (abstr.).

———. 1976. A computer program for linkage analysis of general human pedigrees. *Am. J. Hum. Genet.* 28:528–29.

———. 1977a. Linkage analysis with misclassification at one locus. *Clin. Genet.* 12:119–24. Erratum in *Clin. Genet.* 12:254 (1977).

———. 1977b. Counting methods (EM algorithm) in human pedigree analysis: Linkage and segregation analysis. *Ann. Hum. Genet.* 40:443–54.

———. 1978. A simple scheme for the analysis of HLA linkages in pedigrees. *Ann. Hum. Genet.* 42:255–57.

———. 1979a. Maximum likelihood estimation by counting methods under polygenic and mixed models in human pedigrees. *Am. J. Hum. Genet.* 31:161–75.

———. 1979b. Detection of rare major genes in lipid levels. *Hum. Genet.* 51:79–91.

———. 1983. Linkage analysis and family classification under heterogeneity. *Ann. Hum. Genet.* 47:311–20.

———. 1986a. Y-linkage and pseudoautosomal linkage. *Am. J. Hum. Genet.* 38:891–97.

———. 1986b. The number of families required to detect or exclude linkage heterogeneity. *Am. J. Hum. Genet.* 39:159–65.

———. 1986c. Linkage probability and its approximate confidence interval. *Genet. Epidemiol. Suppl.* 1:251–57.

———. 1989a. Statistical properties of the haplotype relative risk. *Genet. Epidemiol.* 6:127–30.

———. 1989b. Computer-simulation methods in human linkage analysis. *Proc. Natl. Acad. Sci. USA* 86:4175–78.

———. 1990a. Genetic interpretation of disease clustering. In *Convergent issues in genetics and demography*, edited by J. Adams, D. A. Lam, A. I. Hermalin, and P. E. Smouse, 245–55. New York: Oxford University Press.

———. 1990b. Invited editorial: Cutting a Gordian knot in the linkage analysis of complex human traits. *Am. J. Hum. Genet.* 46:219–21.

———. 1991. Genetic linkage analysis under uncertain disease definition. In *Molecular genetics and biology of alcoholism, Banbury report 33*, edited by C. R. Cloninger and H. Begleiter. Cold Spring Harbor, N.Y.: Cold Spring Harbor Laboratory Press.

Ott, J., S. Bhattacharya, J. D. Chen, M. J. Denton, J. Donald, C. Dubay, G. J. Farrar, G. A. Fishman, D. Frey, A. Gal, P. Humphries, B. Jay, M. Jay, M. Litt, M. Mächler, M. Musarella, M. Neugebauer, R. L. Nussbaum, J. D. Terwilliger, R. G. Weleber, B. Wirth, F. Wong, R. G. Worton, and A. F. Wright. 1990a. Localizing multiple X chromosome-linked retinitis pigmentosa loci using multi-locus homogeneity tests. *Proc. Natl. Acad. Sci. USA* 87:701–4.

Ott, J., J. Caesar, M. Mächler, A. Schinzel, and W. Schmid. 1990b. Presymptomatic exclusion of myotonic dystrophy in a one-generation pedigree of half-sibs. *Hum. Hered.* 40:305–7.

Ott, J., and C. T. Falk. 1982. Epistatic association and linkage analysis in human families. *Hum. Genet.* 62:296–300.

Ott, J., and M. Frater-Schröder. 1981. Absence of linkage between transcobalamin II and ABO. *Hum. Genet.* 59:164–65.

Ott, J., and G. M. Lathrop. 1987a. Goodness-of-fit tests for locus order in three-point mapping. *Genet. Epidemiol.* 4:51–57.

———. 1987b. Estimating the position of a locus on a known map of loci. *Cytogenet. Cell Genet.* 46:674 (abstr.).

Ott, J., D. Linder, B. Kaiser McCaw, E. W. Lovrien, and F. Hecht. 1976. Estimating distances from the centromere by means of benign ovarian teratomas in man. *Ann. Hum. Genet.* 40:191–96.

Ott, J., E. J. B. M. Mensink, A. Thompson, J. D. L. Schot, and R. K. B. Schuurman. 1986. Heterogeneity in the map distance between X-linked agammaglobulinemia and a map of nine RFLP loci. *Hum. Genet.* 74:280–83.

Ott, J., H. G. Schrott, J. L. Goldstein, W. R. Hazzard, F. H. Allen, Jr., C. T. Falk, and A. G. Motulsky. 1974. Linkage study in a large kindred with familial hyper-cholesterolemia. *Am. J. Hum. Genet.* 26:598–603.

Ozelius, L., P. L. Kramer, C. B. Moskowitz, D. J. Kwiatkowski, M. F. Brin, S. B. Bressman, D. E. Schuback, C. T. Falk, N. Risch, D. de Leon, R. E. Burke, J. Haines, J. F. Gusella, S. Fahn, and X. O. Breakefield. 1989. Human gene for torsion dystonia located on chromosome 9q32-q34. *Neuron* 2:1427–34.

Palotie, A., P. Väisanen, J. Ott, L. Ryhänen, K. Elima, M. Vikkula, K. Cheah, E. Vuorio, and L. Peltonen. 1989. Predisposition to familial osteoarthrosis linked to type II collagen gene. *Lancet* 1:924–27.

Paris Conference (1971): Standardization in human cytogenetics. 1972. *Birth Defects* 8(no. 7). Also in *Cytogenet. Cell Genet.* 11:313–62.

Paris Conference (1971), Supplement. 1975. *Birth Defects* 11(no. 9). Also in *Cytogenet. Cell Genet.* 15:201–38.

Pascoe, L. L., and N. E. Morton. 1987. The use of map functions in multipoint mapping. *Am. J. Hum. Genet.* 40:174–83.

Penrose, L. S. 1935. The detection of autosomal linkage in data which consist of pairs of brothers and sisters of unspecified parentage. *Ann. Eugen.* 6:133–38.

Pfanzagl, J. 1966. *Allgemeine Methodenlehre der Statistik II.* Sammlung Göschen Band 747/747a. Berlin: Walter de Gruyter.

Ploughman, L. M., and M. Boehnke. 1989. Estimating the power of a proposed linkage study for a complex genetic trait. *Am. J. Hum. Genet.* 44:543–51.

Prochazka, M., E. H. Leiter, D. V. Serreze, and D. L. Coleman. 1987. Three recessive loci required for insulin-dependent diabetes in nonobese diabetic mice. *Science* 237:286–89.

Rao, C. R. 1973. *Linear statistical inference and its applications.* New York: John Wiley.

———. 1989. *Statistics and truth.* Calcutta: Eka Press.

Rao, D. C., B. J. B. Keats, J. M. Lalouel, N. E. Morton, and S. Yee. 1979. A maximum likelihood map of chromosome 1. *Am. J. Hum. Genet.* 31:680–96.

Rao, D. C., B. J. B. Keats, N. E. Morton, S. Yee, and R. Lew. 1978. Variability of human linkage data. *Am. J. Hum. Genet.* 30:516–29.

Reeders, S. T., M. H. Breuning, M. A. Ryynänen, A. F. Wright, K. E. Davies, A. W. King, M. L. Watson, and D. J. Weatherall. 1987. A study of genetic linkage heterogeneity in adult polycystic kidney disease. *Hum. Genet.* 76:348–51.

Reich, T., J. Rice, R. Cloninger, R. Wette, and J. James. 1979. The use of multiple thresholds and segregation analysis in analyzing the phenotypic heterogeneity of multifactorial traits. *Ann. Hum. Genet.* 42:371–90.

Reik, W. 1989. Genomic imprinting and genetic disorders in man. *Trends Genet.* 5:331–36.

Renwick, J. H. 1969. Progress in mapping human autosomes. Br. Med. Bull. 25:65–73.

Renwick, J. H., and D. R. Bolling. 1967. A program complex for encoding, analyzing and storing human linkage data. *Am. J. Hum. Genet.* 19:360–67.

———. 1971. An analysis procedure illustrated on a triple linkage of use for prenatal diagnosis of myotonic dystrophy. *J. Med. Genet.* 8:399–406.

Renwick, J. H., and J. Schulze. 1961. A computer program for the processing of linkage data from large pedigrees. *Excerpta Med. Int. Congr. Ser.* 32:E145 (abstr.).

———. 1965. Male and female recombination fraction for the nail-patella:ABO linkage in man. *Ann. Hum. Genet.* 28:379–92.

Rice, J. P., J. Endicott, M. A. Knesevich, and N. Rochberg. 1987. The estimation of diagnostic sensitivity using stability data: An application to major depressive disorder. *J. Psychiatr. Res.* 21:337–45.

Risch, N. 1988. A new statistical test for linkage heterogeneity. *Am. J. Hum. Genet.* 42:353–64.

———. 1990. Linkage strategies for genetically complex traits: II. The power of affected relative pairs. *Am. J. Hum. Genet.* 46:229–41.

Risch, N., E. Claus, and L. Giuffra. 1989. Linkage and mode of inheritance in complex traits. In *Multipoint mapping and linkage based upon affected pedigree members: Genetic Analysis Workshop 6,* 183–88. New York: Alan R. Liss.

Risch, N., and L. Giuffra. 1990. Multipoint linkage analysis of genetically complex traits. *Am. J. Hum. Genet.* 47:A197 (abstr.).

Risch, N., and K. Lange. 1979. An alternative model of recombination and interference. *Ann. Hum. Genet.* 43:61–70.

Romeo, G., M. Devoto, G. Costa, L. Roncuzzi, L. Catizone, P. Zuchelli, G. G.

Germino, T. Keith, D. J. Weatherall, and S. T. Reeders. 1988. A second genetic locus for autosomal dominant polycystic kidney disease. *Lancet* 2:8–11.

Rossen, R. D., E. J. Brewer, R. M. Sharp, J. Ott, and J. W. Templeton. 1980. Familial rheumatoid arthritis: Linkage of HLA to disease susceptibility locus in four families where proband presented with juvenile rheumatoid arthritis. *J. Clin. Invest.* 65:629–42.

Rotter, J. I. 1981. The modes of inheritance of insulin-dependent diabetes mellitus. *Am. J. Hum. Genet.* 33:835–51.

Rouyer, F., Simmler, M.-C., Johnsson, C., Vergnaud, G., Cooke, H. J., and J. Weissenbach. 1986. A gradient of sex-linkage in the pseudoautosomal region of the human sex chrommosomes. *Nature* 319:291–95.

Ruano, G., K. K. Kidd, and J. C. Stephens. 1990. Haplotype of multiple polymorphisms resolved by enzymatic amplification of single DNA molecules. *Proc. Natl. Acad. Sci. USA* 87:6296–6300.

Rubinstein, P., M. Walker, C. Carpenter, C. Carrier, J. Krassner, C. Falk, and F. Ginsberg. 1981. Genetics of HLA disease associations: The use of the haplotype relative risk (HRR) and the "haplo-delta" (Dh) estimates in juvenile diabetes from three racial groups. *Hum. Immunol.* 3:384 (abstr.).

Ruddle, R. F., and K. K. Kidd. 1989. The human gene mapping workshops in transition. *Cytogenet. Cell Genet.* 51:1–2.

Ryder, L. P., A. Svejgaard, and J. Dausset. 1981. Genetics of HLA disease association. *Annu. Rev. Genet.* 15:169–87.

Sager, R. 1989. Tumor suppressor genes: The puzzle and the promise. *Science* 246:1406–12.

St George-Hyslop, P. H., J. L. Haines, L. A. Farrer, R. Polinsky, C. Van Broeckhoven, A. Goate, D. R. Crapper McLachlan, H. Orr, A. C. Bruni, S. Sorbi, I. Rainero, J.-F. Foncin, D. Pollen, J.-M. Cantu, R. Tupler, N. Voskresenskaya, R. Mayeux, J. Growdon, V. A. Fried, R. H. Myers, L. Nee, H. Backhovens, J.-J. Martin, M. Rossor, M. J. Owen, M. Mullan, M. E. Percy, H. Karlinsky, S. Rich, L. Heston, M. Montesi, M. Mortilla, N. Nacmias, J. F. Gusella, and J. A. Hardy. 1990. Genetic linkage studies suggest that Alzheimer's disease is not a single homogeneous disorder. *Nature* 347:194–97.

Sandkuyl, L. A., and J. Ott. 1989. Determining informativity of marker typing for genetic counseling in a pedigree. *Hum. Genet.* 82:159–62.

Scheffer, H., G. J. Te Meerman, P. Van der Vlies, R. J. Houwen, and C. H. C. M. Buys. 1989. Multipoint analysis places the tightly linked D13S12 marker distal to the Wilson disease locus (WND). *Cytogenet. Cell Genet.* 51:1075 (abstr.).

Seizinger, B. R., G. A. Rouleau, L. J. Ozelius, A. H. Lane, A. G. Faryniarz, M. V. Chao, S. Huson, B. R. Korf, D. M. Parry, M. A. Pericak-Vance, F. S. Collins, W. J. Hobbs, B. G. Falcone, J. A. Iannazzi, J. C. Roy, P. H. St George-Hyslop, R. E. Tanzi, M. A. Bothwell, M. Upadhyaya, P. Harper, A. E. Goldstein, D. L. Hoover, J. L. Bader, M. A. Spence, J. J. Mulvihill, A. S. Aylsworth, J. M. Vance, G. O. D. Rossenwasser, P. C. Gaskell, A. D. Roses, R. L. Martuza, X. O. Breakefield, and J. F. Gusella. 1987. Genetic linkage of von Recklinghausen neurofibromatosis to the nerve growth factor receptor gene. *Cell* 49:589–94.

Shannon, C. E., and W. Weaver. 1949. *The mathematical theory of communication.* Urbana: University of Illinois Press.

Shapiro, J. A. 1983. *Mobile genetic elements.* New York: Academic Press.

Sherman, S. L., P. A. Jacobs, N. E. Morton, U. Froster-Iskenius, P. N. Howard-Peebles, K. B. Nielsen, M. W. Partington, G. R. Sutherland, G. Turner, and M. Watson. 1985. Further segregation analysis of the fragile X syndrome with special reference to transmitting males. *Hum. Genet.* 69:289–99.

Sherrington, R., J. Brynjolfsson, H. Petursson, M. Potter, K. Dudleston, B. Barraclough, J. Wasmuth, M. Dobbs, and H. Gurling. 1988. Localization of a susceptibility locus for schizophrenia on chromosome 5. *Nature* 336:164–67.

Siddique, T., R. McKinney, W.-Y. Hung, R. J. Bartlett, G. Bruns, T. K. Mohandas, H.-H. Ropers, C. Wilfert, and A. D. Roses. 1988. The poliovirus sensitivity (PVS) gene is on chromosome 19q12→q13.2. *Genomics* 3:156–60.

Simpson, N. E., K. K. Kidd, P. J. Goodfellow, H. McDermid, S. Myers, J. R. Kidd, C. E. Jackson, A. M. V. Duncan, L. A. Farrer, K. Brasch, C. Castiglione, M. Genel, J. Gertner, C. R. Greenberg, J. F. Gusella, J. J. A. Holden, and B. N. White. 1987. Assignment of multiple endocrine neoplasia type 2A to chromosome 10 by linkage. *Nature* 328:528–30.

Sing, C. F., and E. D. Rothman. 1975. A consideration of the chi-square test of Hardy-Weinberg equilibrium in a non-multinomial situation. *Ann. Hum. Genet.* 39:141–45.

Smith, C. A. B. 1953. The detection of linkage in human genetics. *J. R. Statist. Soc.* 15B:153–84.

———. 1957. Counting methods in genetical statistics. *Ann. Hum. Genet.* 21:254–76.

———. 1959. Some comments on the statistical methods used in linkage investigations. *Am. J. Hum. Genet.* 11:289–304.

———. 1961. Homogeneity test for linkage data. *Proc. Sec. Int. Congr. Hum. Genet.* 1:212–13.

———. 1963. Testing for heterogeneity of recombination fraction values in human genetics. *Ann. Hum. Genet.* 27:175–82.

———. 1975. A non-parametric test for linkage with a quantitative character. *Ann. Hum. Genet.* 38:451–60.

———. 1989. Some simple methods for linkage analysis. *Ann. Hum. Genet.* 53:277–83.

Smith, R. J. H., J. D. Holcomb, S. P. Daiger, C. T. Caskey, M. Z. Pelias, B. R. Alford, D. D. Fontenot, and J. F. Hejtmancik. 1989. Exclusion of Usher syndrome gene of much of chromosome 4. *Cytogenet. Cell Genet.* 50:102–6.

Sneel, R. G., L. P. Lazarou, S. Youngman, O. W. J. Quarrell, J. J. Wasmuth, D. J. Shaw, and P. S. Harper. 1989. Linkage disequilibrium in Huntington's disease: An improved localization for the gene. *J. Med. Genet.* 26:673–75.

Snell Dohrenwend, B., and B. P. Dohrenwend. 1981. Life stress and illness: Formulation of the issues. In *Stressful life events and their contexts*, Monographs in Psychosocial Epidemiology 2, edited by B. Snell Dohrenwend and B. P. Dohrenwend. New York: Neale Watson Academic Publications.

Southern, E. M. 1975. Detection of specific sequences among DNA fragments separated by gel electrophoresis. *J. Mol. Biol.* 98:503–17.

Spence, M. A., N. K. Spurr, and L. L. Field. 1989. Report of the committee on the genetic constitution of chromosome 6. *Cytogenet. Cell Genet.* 51:149–65.

Stassen, H. H., C. Scharfetter, G. Winokur, and J. Angst. 1988. Familial syndrome patterns in schizophrenia, schizoaffective disorder, mania, and depression. *Eur. Arch. Psychiatry Neurol. Sci.* 237:115–23.

Stebbins, N. B., and P. M. Conneally. 1982. Linkage of dominantly inherited Charcot-Marie-Tooth neuropathy to the Duffy locus in an Indiana family. *Am. J. Hum. Genet.* 34:195A (abstr.).

Stern, C. 1973. *Principles of human genetics.* San Francisco: Freeman.

Stockert, E., E. A. Boyse, H. Sato, and K. Itakura. 1976. Heredity of the G_{IX} thymocyte antigen associated with murine leukemia virus: Segregation data simulating genetic linkage. *Proc. Natl. Acad. Sci. USA* 73:2077–81.

Sturt, E. 1976. A mapping function for human chromosomes. *Ann. Hum. Genet.* 40:147–63.

Sturtevant, A. H. 1913. The linear arrangement of six sex-linked factors in *Drosophila*, as shown by their mode of association. *J. Exp. Zool.* 14:43–59.

Suarez, B. K. 1978. The affected sib pair IBD distribution for HLA-linked disease susceptibility genes. *Tissue Antigens* 12:87–93.

Suarez, B. K., and P. Van Eerdewegh. 1984. A comparison of three affected-sib-pair scoring methods to detect HLA-linked disease susceptibility genes. *Am. J. Med. Genet.* 18:135–46.

Sutton, J. G., and R. Burgess. 1978. Genetic evidence for four common alleles at the phosphoglucomutase-1 locus (PGM1) detectable by isoelectric focusing. *Vox Sang.* 34:97–103.

Sykes, B., D. Ogilvie, P. Wordsworth, G. Wallis, C. Mathew, P. Beighton, A. Nicholls, F. M. Pope, E. Thompson, P. Tsipouras, R. Schwartz, O. Jensson, A. Arnason, A.-L. Børresen, A. Heiberg, D. Frey, and B. Steinmann. 1990. Consistent linkage of dominantly inherited osteogenesis imperfecta to the type I collagen loci: COL1A1 and COL1A2. *Am. J. Hum. Genet.* 46:293–307.

Terwilliger, J. D., and J. Ott. 1991. A multi-sample bootstrap approach to the estimation of maximized-over-models lod score distributions. *Cytogenet. Cell Genet.* (in press).

Terwilliger, J. D., D. E. Weeks, and J. Ott. 1990. Laboratory errors in the reading of marker alleles cause massive reductions in lod score and lead to gross overestimates of the recombination fraction. *Am. J. Hum. Genet.* 47:A201 (abstr.).

Thompson, E. A. 1984. Information gain in joint linkage analysis. *IMA J. Math. Appl. Med. Biol.* 1:31–49.

———. 1986. *Pedigree analysis in human genetics.* Baltimore: Johns Hopkins University Press.

Trevor-Roper, P. D. 1952. Marriage of two complete albinos with normally pigmented offspring. *Br. J. Ophthalmol.* 36:107–10.

U.S. Congress, Office of Technology Assessment. 1988. *Mapping our genes. Genome projects: How big, how fast?* Baltimore: Johns Hopkins University Press.

Urabe, K., A. Kimura, F. Harada, T. Iwanaga, and T. Sasazuki. 1990. Gene conversion in steroid 21-hydroxylase genes. *Am. J. Hum. Genet.* 46:1178–86.

Väisänen, P., K. Elima, A. Palotie, L. Peltonen, and E. Vuorio. 1988. Polymorphic restriction sites of type II collagen gene: Their location and frequencies in the Finnish population. *Hum. Hered.* 38:65–71.

Vance, J. M., G. A. Nicholson, L. H. Yamaoka, J. Stajich, C. S. Stewart, M. C. Speer, W. Y. Hung, A. D. Roses, D. Barker, and M. A. Pericak-Vance. 1989. Linkage of Charcot-Marie-Tooth neuropathy type 1a to chromosome 17. *Exp. Neurol.* 104:186–89.

Vieland, V., D. A. Greenberg, S. E. Hodge, and J. Ott. 1991. Linkage analysis of two-locus diseases under single-locus and two-locus analysis models. *Cytogenet. Cell Genet.* (in press).

Vilkki, J., J. Ott, M.-L. Savontaus, P. Aula, and E. K. Nikoskelainen. 1991. Optic atrophy in Leber hereditary optic neuroretinopathy is probably determined by an X-chromosomal gene closely linked to DXS7. *Am. J. Hum. Genet.* 48:486–91.

Vilkki J., M.-L. Savontaus, and E. K. Nikoskelainen. 1989. Genetic heterogeneity in Leber hereditary optic neuroretinopathy revealed by mitochondrial DNA polymorphism. *Am. J. Hum. Genet.* 45:206–11.

Vogel, F., and A. G. Motulsky. 1986. *Human genetics.* New York: Springer.

Voss, R., E. Ben-Simon, A. Avital, S. Godfrey, J. Zlotogora, J. Dagan, Y. Tikochinski, and J. Hillel. 1989. Isodisomy of chromosome 7 in a patient with cystic fibrosis: Could uniparental disomy be common in humans? *Am. J. Hum. Genet.* 45:373–80.

Wald, A. 1947. *Sequential analysis.* New York: John Wiley.

Wallace, D. C. 1989. Report of the committee on human mitochondrial DNA. *Cytogenet. Cell Genet.* 51:612–21.

Wallace, D. C., G. Singh, M. T. Lott, J. A. Hodge, T. G. Schurr, A. M. S. Lezza, L. J. Elsas II, and E. K. Nikoskelainen. 1988. Mitochondrial DNA mutation associated with Leber's hereditary optic neuropathy. *Science* 242:1427–30.

Warren, A. C., S. A. Slaugenhaupt, J. G. Lewis, A. Chakravaarti, and S. E. Antonorakis. 1989. A genetic linkage map of 17 markers on human chromosome 21. *Genomics* 4:579–91.

Watson, J. D. 1990. The human genome project: Past, present, and future. *Science* 248:44–49.

Watson, J. D., N. H. Hopkins, J. W. Roberts, J. Argetsinger Steitz, and A. M. Weiner. 1987a. *Molecular biology of the gene.* 4th ed. Vol. 1, *General principles.* Menlo Park, Calif.: Benjamin/Cummings.

———. 1987b. *Molecular biology of the gene.* 4th ed. Vol. 2, *Specialized aspects.* Menlo Park, Calif.: Benjamin/Cummings.

Weber, J. L., and P. E. May. 1989. Abundant class of human DNA polymorphisms which can be typed using the polymerase chain reaction. *Am. J. Hum. Genet.* 44:388–96.

Weeks, D. E. 1988. New mathematical methods for human gene mapping. Ph.D. diss., University of California, Los Angeles.

———. 1991. Human linkage analysis: Strategies for locus ordering. In *Advanced techniques in chromosome research*, edited by K. W. Adolph, 297–330. New York: Marcel Dekker.

Weeks, D. E., and K. Lange. 1987. Preliminary ranking procedures for multilocus ordering. *Genomics* 1:236–42.

———. 1988. The affected-pedigree-member method of linkage analysis. *Am. J. Hum. Genet.* 42:315–26.

———. 1990. Linkage methods for identifying genetic risk factors. In *Genetic variation and nutrition*, edited by A. P. Simopoulos and B. Childs, 35–48. Basel: Karger.

Weeks, D. E., T. Lehner, and J. Ott. 1991. Preliminary ranking procedures for multilocus ordering based on radiation hybrid data. *Cytogenet. Cell Genet.* (in press).

Weeks, D. E., T. Lehner, E. Squires-Wheeler, C. Kaufmann, and J. Ott. 1990. Measuring the inflation of the lod score due to its maximization over model parameter values in human linkage analysis. *Genet. Epidemiol.* 7:237–43.

Weeks, D. E., and J. Ott. 1989. Risk calculations under heterogeneity. *Am. J. Hum. Genet.* 45:819–21.

Weeks, D. E., J. Ott, and G. M. Lathrop. 1990. SLINK: A general simulation program for linkage analysis. *Am. J. Hum. Genet.* 47:A204 (abstr.).

Weinberg, W. 1912. Zur Vererbung der Anlage der Bluterkrankheit mit methodologischen Ergänzungen meiner Geschwistermethode. *Arch. Rass. Ges. Biol.* 6: 694–709.

Weir, B. S. 1989. Locating the cystic fibrosis gene on the basis of linkage disequilibrium with markers? In *Multipoint mapping and linkage based upon affected pedigree members: Genetic analysis workshop 6*, edited by R. C. Elston, M. A. Spence, S. E. Hodge, and J. W. MacCluer, 81–86. New York: Alan R. Liss.

———. 1990. *Genetic data analysis*. Sunderland, Mass.: Sinauer Associates.

Weissmann, C. 1989. Sheep disease in human clothing. *Nature* 338:298–99.

White, R., and J.-M. Lalouel. 1987. Investigation of genetic linkage in human families. In *Advances in human genetics*, edited by H. Harris and K. Hirschhorn, 121–228. New York: Plenum.

White, R. L., J.-M. Lalouel, Y. Nakamura, H. Donis-Keller, P. Green, D. W. Bowden, C. G. P. Mathew, D. F. Easton, E. B. Robson, N. E. Morton, J. F. Gusella, J. L. Haines, A. E. Retief, K. K. Kidd, J. C. Murray, G. M. Lathrop, and H. M. Cann. 1990. The CEPH consortium primary linkage map of human chromosome 10. *Genomics* 6:393–412.

White, R., M. Leppert, D. T. Bishop, D. Barker, J. Berkowitz, C. Brown, P. Callahan, T. Holm, and L. Jerominski. 1985. Construction of linkage maps with DNA markers for human chromosomes. *Nature* 313:101–5.

Wright, E. C., D. E. Goldgar, P. R. Fain, D. F. Barker, and M. H. Skolnick. 1990. A genetic map of human chromosome 17p. *Genomics* 7:103–9.

Wright, J. E., Jr., K. Johnson, A. Hollister, and B. May. 1983. Meiotic models to explain classical linkage, pseudolinkage, and chromosome pairing in tetraploid derivative salmonid genomes. In *Isozymes: Current topics in biological and medical research*. Vol. 10, *Genetics and evolution*, edited by M. C. Rattazzi, J. G. Scandalios, and G. S. Whitt, 239–60. New York: Alan R. Liss.

Xie, X., and J. Ott. 1990. Determining the effect of a change in affection status on the lod score. *Am. J. Hum. Genet.* 47:A205 (abstr.).

Yamamoto, F., H. Clausen, T. White, J. Marken, and S. Hakomori. 1990. Molecular genetic basis of the histo-blood group ABO system. *Nature* 345:229–33.

Ying, K.-L., and E. J. Ives. 1968. Asymmetry of chromosome number 1 pair in three generations of a phenotypically normal family. *Can. J. Genet. Cytol.* 10: 575–89.

Zhao, L. P., E. Thompson, and R. Prentice. 1990. Joint estimation of recombination fractions and interference coefficients in multilocus linkage analysis. *Am. J. Hum. Genet.* 47:255–65.

Zoghbi, H. Y., L. A. Sandkuyl, J. Ott, S. P. Daiger, M. Pollack, W. E. O'Brien, and A. L. Beaudet. 1989. Assignment of autosomal dominant spinocerebellar ataxia (SCA1) centromeric to the HLA region on the short arm of chromosome 6 using multilocus linkage analysis. *Am. J. Hum. Genet.* 44:255–63.

Zonta, L. A., S. D. Jayakar, M. Bosisio, A. Galante, and V. Pennetti. 1987. Genetic analysis of human obesity in an Italian sample. *Hum. Hered.* 37:129–39.

Volumes 1–8 of the international workshops on human gene mapping (HGM) were published by the March of Dimes Birth Defects Foundation in its Birth Defects: Original Article Series (BD:OAS). The reference to an article in the fifth workshop, for example, would normally read as follows: *Human Gene Mapping 5 (1979): Fifth International Workshop on Human Gene Mapping*. Birth Defects: Original Article Series 15, no. 11 (1979); also in *Cytogenet. Cell Genet.* 25 (1979). Starting with volume 9, the proceedings of the HGM workshops have been published by Karger AG in *Cytogenetics and Cell Genetics*.

Workshop Number	Volume in BD:OAS	Volume and Year in *Cytogenet. Cell Genet.*
HGM 1	10, no. 3	13 (1974)
HGM 2	11, no. 3	14 (1975)
HGM 3	12, no. 7	16 (1976)
HGM 4	14, no. 4	22 (1978)
HGM 5	15, no. 11	25 (1979)
HGM 6	18, no. 2	32 (1982)
HGM 7	20, no. 2	37 (1984)
HGM 8	21, no. 4	40 (1985)
HGM 9	—	46 (1987)
HGM 10	—	51 (1989)

Index

Jurg Ott received a Ph.D. in zoology from the University of Zurich in 1967 and an M.S. in biomathematics from the University of Washington in 1972. He is a professor in the Department of Genetics and Development and the Department of Psychiatry at Columbia University, and a research scientist at the New York State Psychiatric Institute. He serves on various editorial boards, is editor-in-chief of *Human Heredity,* and is a member of HUGO. He wrote the first generally available computer program on linkage analysis (LIPED).

Designed by Glen Burris
Set in Times Roman by G&S Typesetters, Inc.
Printed on 60 lb. Glatfelter Hi-Brite and bound in Holliston Aqualite cloth by
The Maple Press Company